the year i met my brain

I wish to acknowledge the Bunurong people of Kulin Nation, the traditional owners of the land on which this book was written, and whose sovereignty was never ceded. I also wish to acknowledge all traditional owners of Country throughout Australia, and the important contributions Aboriginal and Torres Strait Islander people have made and continue to make in Australian society. They are the land's first storytellers, and I pay my respect to Elders past and present.

the year i met my brain

A travel companion for adults who have just found out they have ADHD

matilda boseley

Illustrations by Evie Hilliar

LIFE

*To my amazing partner, Anthony, for loving me,
supporting me, and always remembering to
take the bins out on bin day.*

contents

Why I use the word neurodiversity

While writing this book I put a lot of thought into whether to use the terms 'neurodiversity', 'neurodivergent' and 'neurotypical', as they're a topic of heated debate among autistic and ADHD communities (as well as many others, I'm sure).

If you haven't come across these words before, 'neurodiversity' is a way of talking about groups of people within our society whose brains have developed or function differently from the majority. These people are described as 'neurodivergent', while those with more, I guess, factory-standard brains are 'neurotypical'.

There's no absolute consensus on who 'counts' as neurodivergent, but the term generally encompasses those with autism spectrum disorder (ASD); attention-deficit/hyperactivity disorder (ADHD); dyslexia and its lesser-known cousin conditions, dyscalculia, dysgraphia and dyspraxia (which create difficulties with maths, writing and coordination respectively). Some also broaden this out further to include those with an array of other neurological disorders, mental health conditions and acquired brain injuries.

The term was coined by Australian sociologist Judy Singer in the 1990s. Notice I said sociologist, not psychologist. That's because 'neurodiversity' isn't a medical term, nor is it intended to be. Instead, it's a cultural and political one born out of the autistic self-advocacy movement.

It's a way of moving away from the idea that there are 'healthy' or 'normal' brains on one side of the line and 'diseased' ones on the other. It leaves room to acknowledge the neutral and positive parts of having the minds that people with neurological differences do. And, most importantly, it allows us to widen the conversation and discuss how society can create a world that accommodates the way our brains work, rather than solely focusing on how to 'cure' or 'fix' us.

But the term isn't universally accepted. Some people with these conditions feel that the concept of 'neurodiversity' is a form of toxic positivity that's ultimately dangerous to disabled communities. Now, I do understand where they're coming from, because, yes, in the hands of some, the seemingly harmless sentiment that these conditions 'aren't just disabilities, they're superpowers' can quickly turn into 'and therefore it's unnecessary, perhaps even evil, to diagnose and treat them', and 'these medications are being used to turn our kids into robots', and 'stop complaining and asking for accommodations, you've been given a gift'. In fact, some large online ADHD communities have denounced and even banned the use of 'neurodiversity' and related terms for this very reason.

But, honestly, I think this is a massive overgeneralisation and pretty behind the times. That extreme 'disabilities don't exist' mindset was not how I was introduced to these words, and I have never seen them used this way among younger generations. Language is constantly evolving, so while in the past 'neurodiversity' may have been more aligned with these (entirely incorrect) views, this is not what they mean to the vast majority of people now. For me, the term has always been about acknowledging that neurodevelopmental disorders are disabilities, but that's not *all* they are. For many people, conditions like ADHD and autism are part of their identity, they're a way of travelling through the world, and they represent so much more than just a list of impairments in a diagnostic handbook.

I've always seen 'neurodivergent' as a neutral or even an empowering term, so ultimately that's why I decided to use it in this book.

However, I acknowledge that there's a more nuanced discussion to be had about the neurodiversity movement and how, if we're not careful, moving away from a purely medical view of neurological disabilities could potentially endanger those with a higher level of support needs. So, just know that I'm not ignoring this issue, and I'll be diving into it more in later chapters.

Introduction

If you'd asked me at twenty-two to describe ADHD, I would have told you about the noisy kids in my class back in primary school. They would jump around during reading time and interrupt the teachers constantly. They would ask questions that had just been explained, and if there was a fight in the playground, chances are they were involved. I actually have no idea if these kids even had ADHD, but that's what our parents told us, and the impression stuck. The kids I always thought of as the ADHDers were young, loud, disruptive, hyperactive and, most importantly, they were boys.

It had never occurred to me to imagine ADHD as a young woman crying in the bath because she's forgotten her doctor's appointment for the second time in a week, utterly exhausted by the simple act of trying to keep her world in order.

She's just finished university, moved out of home and started her first full-time job. Sure, she's bright, and she's always been a high achiever, but now that the scaffolding of formal education and the daily support provided by living with her parents has fallen away, everything has become so much harder.

She's bought an expensive weekly planner, but she's never written in it. The vegetables in her fridge keep rotting before she remembers to use them. She can't find the energy to unstack the dishwasher, she hasn't replied to her boss's last urgent email, and when she looks around at her peers it feels like everyone can deal with 'life' so much better than she does.

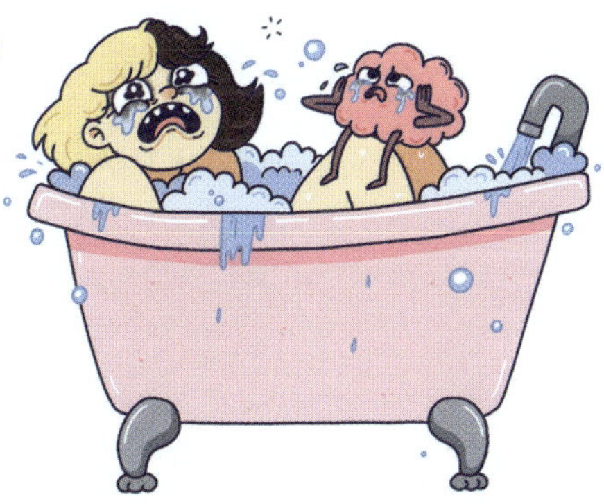

That's what ADHD looked like for me, but it's taken twenty-four years of ignorance and one tumultuous year of self-doubt, grief, relief, excitement and mess to get to a place where I can admit that.

The issue is, ADHD is way more complicated and diverse than we give it credit for. So what is it? Well, the short answer is that it's a condition characterised by a persistent pattern of **inattention** and/or **hyperactivity** and/or **impulsivity** that interferes with your functioning and negatively affects daily life. The long answer is, well, the rest of this book.

I was diagnosed a couple of days before my twenty-fourth birthday. It had been months of doctor's visits, referrals and waiting to book a psychiatrist appointment, but somehow when I got one I still managed to forget to take the afternoon off at the *Guardian*, where I work as a journalist. I was reporting from home, so I took my laptop into my bedroom when my allotted time came around, prayed no major news would break while I was gone, closed the doors in case my housemates decided to start yelling at the PlayStation, and settled in.

The global COVID-19 pandemic dictated that the consultation would take place over video chat, and when the psychiatrist's face appeared he seemed blithely uninterested and busy. After a hurried hello he asked me to tell him the story of my life – I assume to get a sense of how ADHD-y it was – so I went down the laundry list, which I will paraphrase for you thus . . .

'Well, I was born in Melbourne. My family is very nice and middle-class, and by all accounts I should be well adjusted. But I was bullied a lot as a child and I had trouble making friends with the other girls.

'I was usually near the top of my class, but I was told off a lot for interrupting, or getting distracted, or forgetting to check my work, or not colouring neatly within the lines.' (This isn't some profound metaphor for the education system's unwillingness to accept difference, by the way. As a kid I just could never find the patience required to sit and colour properly.)

'And, oh, I was terrible at spelling. I'm not sure if that's important.

'When I got to high school I was really bad at remembering to write things in my diary, or keep all my work together. Sometimes notes or worksheets, or honestly whole textbooks, would get buried in a drawer and I would completely forget they were there. And actually, this still happens with all sorts of things, like – there's probably a dozen shirts at the bottom of my wardrobe right now that I have no clue I even own. "Out of sight, out of mind" is a very literal phrase for me.

'I did well in high school, except I found it super hard to get started with homework. And I know that isn't that weird, but once I did get started, sometimes I'd almost go into a trance and then work for hours and hours without even realising.

'Anxiety has also been a huge factor in my life,' I told him, hoping his utterly blank expression meant he was still listening. 'I'd constantly have these little breakdowns. Things would build up and get too much and I'd be snappy and rude to my family and then cry for hours, especially in my final year of school.

'Some things definitely came easily to me, but other times it felt as if I had to try so much harder to keep up with others. And I think, looking back, I used to really rely on my parents to help me to look after myself. It's embarrassing to admit, but I was seventeen and I still sometimes needed my mum to remind me to take a shower or ask me before I left the house if I'd put on deodorant, and that's obviously not a good feeling at all.

'And there was also just lots of "girl" stuff that other girls seemed better at than me, or just came naturally to them. My phone screen was always smashed, I was constantly biting my nails and ripping off hangnails. I could never leave a spot on my face un-squeezed and, oh my god, having a regular night-time skincare routine was just impossible.

'Oh, and also when I'm doing . . . you know, sex, sometimes I get so caught up in my thoughts and thinking about all the things that I have to do and all the people I've let down, and even just like all the cracks in the paint on my walls, that I'll legitimately forget that I'm actually doing it.

'And my partner is really good at sex, so that's not the issue.'

In retrospect, I probably didn't need to clarify that last point.

'Anyway, now I'm a journalist, and I think I'm pretty good at it, but I often leave writing my articles till the last hour or two of the day, and my boss called to tell me that I need to start proofreading my work before filing it. But I do proofread, it's just that often I get this overwhelming feeling of just needing it to be done, so I'll end up skimming and hitting send too soon and regretting it.

'Then I went on TikTok and it kept giving me more and more videos about adult ADHD, and I realised that I was relating to almost all of them, so I thought maybe I should talk to someone professional about that. Anyway, that's my life, I think.'

When I was done, the psychiatrist went 'hmmm' and then opened up a checklist of thirty or so diagnostic statements. It's hard to remember the exact details, but after every sentence he told me to answer on a scale between 'strongly disagree' and 'strongly agree', and, wow, the 'strongly agrees' were coming thick and fast.

'I often feel fidgety or restless.'

'Strongly agree.'

'I often have problems remembering obligations or appointments that I've made.'

'Strongly agree.'

'In conversation, I'll often start replying before the person I'm talking to . . .'

'Strongly agree.'

At the end he tallied my score, we chatted some more, and forty-five minutes later he looked down the eye of his laptop camera and said, 'Well, it seems clear to me that you have ADHD and you've had it since you were a child.'

I started to sob uncontrollably. 'I'm sorry! Sorry about this,' I said between heaves.

'I know it can be very overwhelming and difficult to hear,' he replied.

'No,' I said, my breaths sounding like hiccups between the waves of tears. 'I think I just spent my whole life wondering why everyone was just better at being a person than me, and why [*sniff*] I was just failing [*sniff*], and it's just such a relief to know there was actually a reason, you know. Like, I'm not just *bad*,' I gasp out, dissolving into a snotty mess.

He paused, looking unblinkingly down the webcam at me. 'Okay . . . Anyway . . .'

I learnt two important things that day:

1. **There's something notably different about the way my brain works, and this has had far-reaching, profound implications for nearly every aspect of my life.**
2. **Despite dedicating their life to mental health, it seems most psychiatrists aren't big fans of all that touchy-feely shit.**

At the end of the session he wrote me a prescription for 5-milligram short-acting dexamfetamine tablets, spoke vaguely about my brain 'not having enough **dopamine**', told me to read up on the disorder, and gave me the number of an 'ADHD coach'. And that was the end of the video call.

I have a bad habit of thinking about my life in terms of a movie or TV series, organising events into scenes, turning people into character archetypes and viewing traumatic moments as 'climaxes' (most likely as a way of intellectualising and distancing myself from my emotions, combined with the effects of watching way too much *Gossip Girl* at an impressionable age). That moment, staring at the 'call ended' screen on my laptop, felt like an end-of-season cliffhanger. The twist had been revealed, I was at the start of a whole new section of my life, and I mistakenly assumed that a couple of months spent watching educational ADHD TikTok videos and securing a clinical **diagnosis** meant that I was prepared for the season ahead.

I didn't know about the three different **presentations** of ADHD. I didn't know what **executive dysfunction** was, or that the condition could affect my social skills and emotional regulation, too. I'd only vaguely heard of '**time blindness**' through social media, and assumed '**object permanence**' and '**rejection sensitivity dysphoria**' were official, clinical terms. I didn't know having the brain I do put me at higher risk of addiction, death by suicide and car accidents,[1] nor did I have any clue about just how much hard, painful emotional work was ahead of me to undo the damage that the **undiagnosed** decades had done to my **self-esteem**.

I had a prescription, but I didn't know there were so many things I could and should be doing on top of taking medication to reduce my **symptoms**, or how many tricks, hacks and behavioural systems I could put in place to complement the way my brain works and make life more liveable. It felt like after years lost at sea I'd been handed a map, and yet the faint lines and lack of detail never brought me within sight of land.

I spent the next year stumbling through my new identity. I knew some people worked intensively with their psychiatrist after being diagnosed, but even if I could have afforded that sort of treatment, it certainly wasn't presented to me as an option. The few appointments I had with that doctor over the next year were about ten minutes long. He'd ask me if the medication was working, I'd say 'Kinda but maybe not that much', he'd up my dosage a little and we'd say goodbye.

I really did try to take his advice about reading up on the disorder, but, honestly, it's extremely hard as an individual armed only with an internet connection and no medical degree to know which information to trust. If you google 'adult ADHD', you might learn the basics and some useful tips on how to keep your room tidy, but you could just as easily come away believing that ADHD is all a giant conspiracy orchestrated by 'big pharma' to get our young ones hooked on speed.

When I looked for resources, I was flooded with articles teaching parents how to help their ADHD kids. There were structures and schedules and tips, but even if you ignore the fact that all the articles are centred on how to get your seven-year-old to sit still in class, the tactics they provided relied on there being a non-ADHD adult to keep everything going. Turns out it's really hard to adopt healthy habits to help treat your neurological condition when the very neurological condition you're trying to treat makes it really hard to adopt healthy habits. And if you want information that's not aimed at parents, it's probably buried in the densest academic articles on earth. Again, having ADHD makes the chances of getting through something like that pretty darn slim, and I may or may not have been reduced to tears multiple times reading them while researching for this book.

I assumed the first year following my diagnosis would be a revelation, filled with reawakening, discovery and self-understanding. Yet here I was, a year in, and my understanding of ADHD didn't extend much beyond thinking of myself as 'clinically forgetful'. And while, sure, my new medication helped me focus at work, my day-to-day life was still kind of a mess.

But, of course, ADHD is so much more than 'clinical forgetfulness' and a pill you pop to get some emails done. So, when the first anniversary of my diagnosis rolled around, I came to a conclusion: 'If I'm ever going to get my act together out there, I'm going to have to actually understand what's going on up here.'

I'd said 'hi' to my brain a few times, but now it was time for me to actually meet it. Perhaps then I might finally figure out how we could work together to get our life in order.

But as soon as I began this journey, I realised how difficult it was. I'm a journalist who has been trained in how to do research, understand academic jargon and get in touch with experts in the field. These are advantages and resources that the vast majority of people don't have access to, and yet I was still struggling. Getting the information you need to live successfully as an adult with ADHD shouldn't be this hard. But then I remembered that, as a journalist, I'm trained in how to do research, understand academic jargon and get in touch with experts in the field. This was a problem I could actually help solve.

I'm not a psychiatrist, nor am I in possession of any medical degree or PhD. I've taken to quietly diagnosing fictional characters with ADHD (Lorelai Gilmore) or **autism** (Rory Gilmore), but as far as I can tell these assessments would not stand up in a court of law. However, what I do have is an acute awareness of what information – if it were easily accessible, reliably sourced and explained in plain English – would have made my life a hell of a lot easier if I'd received it immediately after my diagnosis. So that's what I've set out to create – the book I wish someone had handed me the second that call with my psychiatrist ended, complete with interviews, pictures, diagrams, fun facts, anecdotes and everything that makes sense to my little ADHD brain.

In the first half of the book/year, we'll learn about why our brains work the way they do, how it's impacted our lives and self-esteem so far, and why so many of us were missed in childhood and are now suddenly finding out about ADHD well into our adulthood. We'll also dispel some of the pervasive myths, half-truths and misunderstandings that surround the disorder. In part two, the second half of the year, we'll learn how to actually live with the brains we have, including how to maintain relationships across the ADHD divide and why ADHD medications are nowhere near as scary as the 6 pm news might have you believe. We'll also think about the dangers and delights of the condition, whether it's a disorder or an identity, and what needs to happen next to make the world a more ADHD-friendly place.

When it comes to the science, I'll be relaying what the data shows and backing up my assertions with reliable, usually large-scale, academic studies or the perspectives of some of the world's most renowned experts in ADHD. But this book is more than the cold, hard biological facts. It's an exploration of what actually happens after you suddenly get the answers to the core mystery that's been subconsciously plaguing your entire life. The plot twist has been revealed, the season finale cliffhanger has played . . . Now what?

Even if your story doesn't exactly mirror mine, there's still a lot here for you. Perhaps you were one of those loud, hyperactive kids in the Grade 2 classroom. You were diagnosed back in the day, but as the years stretched on and your school desk turned into a work one, everyone stopped talking about ADHD. They all assume you've grown out of it, that you're just doing fine now. And, sure, you're not jumping off the walls any more, but things are still so bloody hard. In fact, the main thing adulthood has changed is not your condition but the way people no longer give you the benefit of the doubt because of it. So, yes, technically you met your brain back in childhood, but perhaps you feel well overdue for a reintroduction.

Perhaps you only suspect you might have ADHD and want to learn more about the disorder before you commit to an expensive diagnostic consultation. Or, maybe you're **neurotypical** and reading this in the hope of better understanding what's going on in the busy brain of your ADHD partner, friend or child.

Whatever brings you here, together we're embarking on a voyage to figure out what's going on in the stormy seas that are ADHD brains.

So, on to the first order of business: it's time to learn what ADHD actually is.

part one

learning

DIARY ENTRY

Whirlpool afternoons

It's a regular Wednesday afternoon. I've finished work on time for once and have just one simple task to complete – jump on a Zoom call at 6 pm with an important person in the publishing world who it is vital I impress. Usually, when the stakes are this high, I can trust my anxiety to win the battle with my ADHD. But just in case, I set an alarm on my phone. An unlabelled alarm. My first mistake.

With forty minutes to spare, I inexplicably decide to clean the windowsills in my home office, and because I've never done a chore in my life without some additional form of entertainment, I pop my earphones in and start playing an episode of *The Real Housewives of Salt Lake City* on my phone.

I grab a sponge to wipe down the windowsill and immediately trip over a coat I've left on the floor. My arm shoots forward, sending my partner Anthony's beautiful zebra-shaped indoor plant pot hurtling to the ground. (Luckily there's no plant in it.) The pot smashes as it hits the carpet, breaking into just enough pieces to make fixing it difficult but still feasible. A dare from the universe if ever I've seen one.

'I have superglue in the laundry,' I think to myself as I gather up the black-and-white pieces and place them on the living-room table. And there I sit for the next twenty minutes, glue in one hand, zebra parts in the other, as housewives fling cutting insults back and forth on the phone screen in front of me.

It's at this point that my fingers get robustly stuck together. Naturally, I pour a tiny bit of my cheapest vodka (the closest thing I have to rubbing alcohol) into a bowl and soak my fused thumb and ring finger. It doesn't work, and I end up pulling them apart, wincing in pain, hoping I've only sacrificed the top layer of skin.

As I resume my task, it becomes clear that the ceramic surrounding one of the zebra's wooden legs is smashed beyond repair. I need something to fill in the gap. A little alarm goes off on my phone, but, on the cusp of a brilliant idea, I quickly silence it. Last year, I briefly decided to get into making polymer clay earrings, which led to making regular clay jewellery, which led to an interest in making miniature sculptures, which led me to purchase 500 grams of oven-drying terracotta clay, and I swear to god it's still in my art box somewhere.

As the end credits of that episode of *Real Housewives* play, I rush to my room. Huzzah! It's there! I rip open the resealable tab to reveal a very dry and unusable block of clay. 'Well, that's fixable,' I think. 'I've just got to dunk it in some water.'

I don't have a big enough bowl, so I bust out the gigantic Oktoberfest beer stein I bought the week before on impulse from Aldi. I fill the flagon with water and begin ripping off little pieces of clay and dropping them in. After a few minutes of massaging and the accidental spreading of terracotta slurry across the kitchen bench and my clothes, I'm confident it's usable.

I mould the clay securely around the leg of the zebra, then begin pouring the sludgy water into a plastic container – for storage, I guess – when suddenly I hear 'Next time on *The Real Housewives of Salt Lake City*' and my heart drops. That's the second time I've heard this. This is the end of the second 45-minute episode. Then my mind races back. Oh god, that was my phone alarm. Oh god, the meeting!

I rush to my computer to see an email sent at 6.09 pm: 'Hey Matilda, just sitting here on Zoom. Are you still able to make it?' That was thirty-eight minutes ago. I desperately write back, apologising and blaming the recent change to daylight savings time, leaving my mobile number and telling them to call any time.

As I press send, I begin to cry. Before I can consciously register what I'm doing, I call my mum, desperate for her to tell me everything will be okay.

Because here's the thing about my ADHD – sometimes I feel as if it turns me into someone I'm not. I don't want to seem selfish, I don't want to be careless with other people's time. I don't want to be caught in this whirlpool of unaccomplished chores, unanswered emails and disappointed family, friends and co-workers, but sometimes it feels like I'll never be able to row fast enough to break out.

And when I can't break out, I break down. Between my sobs, my mum suggests I run myself a bath, 'and set a timer too', given the flooding incident in the apartment the week before.

I sit in the bath, knees up against my chest, washing the clay from between my fingers, crying harder than I've cried in a long time, terrified I might have permanently burnt a vital professional bridge. But just then, the eddy of self-loathing is disrupted by the ringing of my phone.

It's them! I'm so ecstatically relieved that I pick up, forgetting that I'm sitting entirely naked in the bath. Thank god it's only a voice call. As I apologise again and thank them for making the time, I ever so slowly pull my body from the water, desperately trying not to splash.

I'm so excited, I barely care that I've forgotten to bring a towel into the bathroom and, as my housemates are now home, I have no choice but to conduct this ninety-minute professional conversation while curled up naked on the bathmat.

I laugh about it in retrospect, but you know what? Right now, sitting in my room next to my earring stand is a plastic box half full of water and some now extraordinarily over-hydrated terracotta clay. But, hey, I can't throw it away. I might need it someday.

1

Why is everyone suddenly talking about ADHD?

At first I was pretty embarrassed by the way I found out I have ADHD. Because the truth is, it wasn't my parents, my teachers or my psychologist who first clocked that there might be something different going on in my brain. No, it was the 'dancing app', TikTok.

I'd been a casual viewer on the app throughout 2019, but when the COVID pandemic struck and the world shut down, I was utterly consumed, watching people make frothy coffees and do elaborate craft projects for hours each day.

I can't exactly remember when I saw the first ADHD video, but it was titled something like 'Five little-known signs of ADHD in women', and I found it mildly interesting. When the video ended, I played it again and counted on my fingers all the things I related to, then hit the little heart-shaped 'Like' button at the side of the screen, saving the video in case I wanted to rewatch it later.

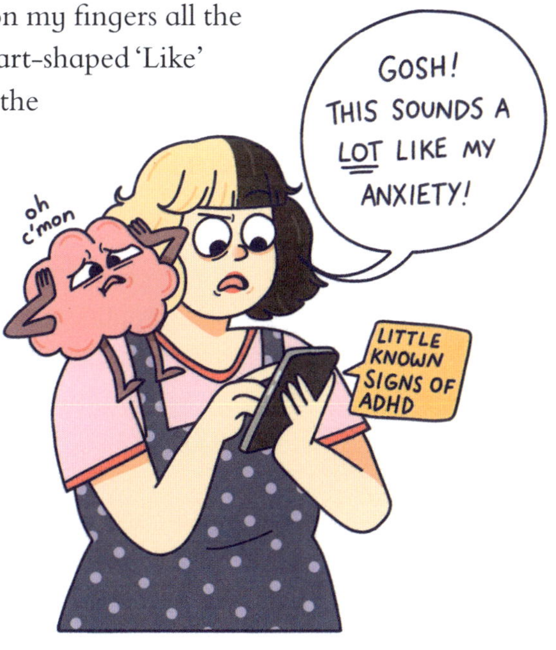
GOSH! THIS SOUNDS A LOT LIKE MY ANXIETY!
oh c'mon
LITTLE KNOWN SIGNS OF ADHD

But this simple act must have alerted the AI overlords that I had at least a passing interest in the topic, so they shot a couple more ADHD videos my way. And just as predicted, I watched them, liked them and maybe even visited the creators' pages to check out some more. This is gold for a company such as ByteDance, which owns the app – it had found a topic that kept me on its app and therefore kept me consuming its ads. So, like the dystopian megamind it is, the algorithm kept showing me more and more of these videos, desperate to extract every possible advertising cent my eyeballs could buy.

But as a **side effect**, my feed was suddenly filled with not just content about ADHD, but content made by women with ADHD, for women with ADHD. It was the first time in my life that I'd ever really considered that women could even have the condition, and, wow, a lot of the things they were talking about really did sound a lot like my anxiety.

After a few weeks, it began to dawn on me. I wasn't only interested in these videos because it was cool to fall down a new internet rabbit hole. I was transfixed because the women on my phone were talking about me. It was as if they were reaching into my brain, pulling out everything that had ever made me feel weird and different but could never formulate into words, and listing them off in sixty seconds or less.

I know it's corny to say, but watching these videos made me realise how lonely a little part of me had felt for all these years. Without even knowing it, I'd been keeping this secret shame tucked away, too scared to even admit there was something I was hiding. And here these people were, sharing it with hundreds of thousands, if not millions who all felt the same.

So I talked to my GP, who told me to talk to my psychologist, who, although surprised by my hypothesis, agreed there was probably something to it. She sent me back to my GP, who gave me a referral to a psychiatrist – and five months and $700 later I had my answer. TikTok was right.

Through some accidental quirk of late-stage capitalism, ByteDance had built a computer program that knew my brain better than I did. And I'm certainly not alone in this. Psychiatrists

I've spoken to from all around the world have told me about the uptick of people, adult women in particular, talking to them about the videos they'd seen on TikTok and wondering if they might have ADHD.

An app that deals entirely in short, funny videos, delivering repeated bursts of immediate gratification, with an algorithm that has a knack of exposing **undiagnosed** people to educational content about ADHD, would be a game-changer in and of itself. But combine this with a global pandemic that utterly obliterates the concept of 'normal' for billions – toppling many people's carefully built towers of routine, coping mechanisms and workarounds? Well, you've just created exactly the kind of environment that would trigger ADHDers who were missed in childhood to recognise that they need help and then seek a **diagnosis**.

It's a big call, but I believe we'll look back on the early years of the 2020s as one of the most pivotal moments in the history of ADHD, and one that fundamentally restructured the way our society thinks about **neurodivergence** in general.

However, as with any cultural turning point, this new, more adult chapter in the ADHD story has brought with it heavy criticism and a touch of moral panic, with copious articles and think pieces written about how 'everyone has ADHD these days' and 'it's even more overdiagnosed than before' and how people are 'turning to medications rather than putting in the hard yards to get their lives together'.

All three of these statements are extremely incorrect. But given they do dominate so much of the conversation and can cause those of us navigating our newfound identities significant anxiety, it might be wise to start our journey by clarifying exactly how common ADHD is, and why underdiagnosis, not overdiagnosis, is the far more pressing concern.[1]

You may have noticed that so far, I've only used the term ADHD, not ADD, and there's a reason for that. Many people, even plenty of doctors and experts, use the two terms as if they describe similar but slightly different conditions – one with **hyperactivity** and one without. But this is a common misconception. ADD is actually just the old name for ADHD before it was updated in 1987. But by then, people had kind of gotten used to the term and it stuck around. Nowadays, it's mostly used colloquially to describe what's officially known as the inattentive **presentation** of ADHD.

Now, I don't think attention-deficit/hyperactivity disorder is a particularly accurate or useful name for the condition either, but when we're only presented with bad options, we may as well pick the one that's in the most up-to-date textbooks.

How many of us have ADHD?

It's actually quite hard to tell how common ADHD really is, because obviously the number of people diagnosed isn't the same as the number of people who actually have it. The best method for estimating its worldwide **prevalence** is to take a random group of people and, through the use of clinical interviews, screen them all for ADHD. Some of the most robust data we have – where hundreds of studies and hundreds of thousands of data points are all combined and compared in what's known as a **meta-analysis** – suggests that between 5.9 per cent[2] and 7.2 per cent of children and teens[3] have ADHD, and 2.8 per cent of adults.[4,5] (But that adult figure is likely a bit on the low side, given the studies used an older, less grown-up-friendly version of the ADHD **diagnostic criteria**.)

But how many of these people actually know they have it? Unfortunately, most countries only track the number of people who are prescribed ADHD medications rather than the number of actual diagnoses, so it's hard to get a good sense of the real-world detection rate. But the picture we can paint suggests an aggressive pattern of underdiagnosis.

For example, if we apply those (likely conservative) global prevalence figures to the latest Australian census data,[6] we would expect there to be between 892,000 and 967,000-ish ADHDers down under. However, according to the most recent data, just 334,000 people accessed any kind of ADHD medication through the country's pharmaceutical benefits scheme (the PBS) in 2020.[7] Barely a third of us. Now, this number has likely gone up in the years since, and of course plenty of people choose not to medicate – so, let's be generous and say the number of diagnosed ADHDers is double that: around 668,000. That's still somewhere between 25 and 40 per cent of Australians with ADHD falling through the cracks.

Adding to that, a 2018 study suggested that, globally, just 0.39 per cent of people aged nineteen or over are medicated,[8] or just one in every seven people we suspect have ADHD, and stats can dip even lower in some countries. For example, in South Korea it's just 0.04 per cent of the total population.[9] In fact, one of the only countries where ADHD treatment rates even come close to outstripping global prevalence estimates is the US, and even then only in some states.

So, is overdiagnosis an issue at all? Well, kind of . . . just not a systematic, global one, and it's very much the exception, not the rule.

The US-sized elephant in the room

I'm not going to sit here and tell you that no person has ever been misdiagnosed with ADHD. This is a condition that has a huge amount of **symptom** overlap with a bunch of other disorders – so its diagnosis can be pretty tricky. Anxiety, depression, PTSD, **autism** and many mood and personality disorders can cause issues with attention or **impulsivity**. I mean, even an underlying sleep disorder might produce symptoms that share a shocking resemblance. To make matters even more confusing, pretty much all of the conditions I just listed can also be **comorbid** (aka commonly co-occur) with ADHD. This is why it's so important to seek a proper professional **diagnosis**. ADHD is a tangled knot that needs an expert's hand to unravel. Generally, this process involves multiple in-depth clinical interviews, symptom-screening questionnaires and even gathering corroborative evidence such as school reports or statements from family members to ascertain that symptoms were present in childhood and occur across multiple areas of life. It's when the diagnostic processes for ADHD don't meet these standards that we potentially start to see inflated diagnosis rates.

In Stephen Hinshaw and Richard Scheffler's book *The ADHD Explosion* – which looks at the current ADHD landscape in the US – they noted that in some areas, doctors were diagnosing ADHD with as little as a fifteen-minute appointment, which is likely nowhere near enough time to rule out the array of possible other causes. They also discussed how, for several decades starting in the 1990s, the US education system began introducing laws (including a policy you might have heard of called 'No Child Left Behind') that incentivised schools to improve their graduation rates or performances on standardised tests, and sanctioned those schools that fell behind – even potentially shutting them down if students persistently underperformed. This is important because an official diagnosis of ADHD and several other conditions often allowed a child extra accommodations, such as additional time on tests. For a time, some districts even allowed schools to exclude a kid's results from that school's score averages altogether.[10]

The states that have had these systems in place the longest tend to be the ones with the highest rates of ADHD. This might help explain why there are such huge variations in diagnosis rates across the country. From 6 per cent of children in California and Nevada (still a little under the global prevalence estimate) to a whopping 16 per cent in Mississippi and Louisiana, according to a 2019 survey from the country's Centers for Disease Control and Prevention (CDC).[11] (It's worth noting that in many areas it is primarily boys driving these numbers up, while a sizeable portion of girls go undetected.)

The US education system has undergone some serious policy shifts in recent years, so I reached out to Stephen Hinshaw to see if he thought education policy was still *the* driving factor in the US's diagnosis rates.

'It certainly used to be – but the abolition of the policy that "special ed" kids (including those with ADHD) get deleted from the school district's test scores, a decade ago, has probably "depressed" that tendency,' he tells me. 'My guess is that the highly medicalised views in the US, along with piss-poor diagnostic practices, are the main reasons now.' Hinshaw isn't a man to mince words.

In this and so many other ways the US is an outlier when it comes to ADHD, yet extremely US-specific statistics and concerns unfortunately still seem to dominate the conversation. And this disproportionate focus (and, dare I say it, moral panic) surrounding overdiagnosis is a huge problem because it overshadows the much larger and genuinely life-threatening issues of under-recognition, underdiagnosis and undertreatment that the vast majority of the world faces.

The trendy diagnosis

I was the first person in my immediate circle to be diagnosed with ADHD, but I certainly wasn't the last. Since then, every couple of months another one of my close friends or extended family or co-workers will mention that they've just received their diagnosis. And while this is extraordinarily brilliant news for them, I have to admit that a tiny part of me started to worry there was something in the water leaching all the **dopamine** from our brains, or maybe the critics were right: ADHD was just a 'trendy diagnosis' and we were all simply overreacting to not being able to sit through a TV show without being on our phones any more.

But neither of those options is correct. Population-wide prevalence has been remarkably steady for decades.[12] So, really, it's not so much that there are more people with ADHD nowadays but simply that more people know they have it. It's just a pretty darn common disorder. I mean, about 2 per cent of children have red hair, which means – even by conservative estimates – a kid is three times more likely to be an ADHDer than to be a ginger.

The rise in diagnosis over the past decade, and even the somewhat sharper increase in adult referrals during the COVID era, aren't some sign of the end of days or proof that ADHD isn't real. Instead, this is a much-needed and long-overdue course correction based on decades of underdiagnosis and undertreatment. It's good news! Sure, it might feel weird that you know ten different people with ADHD, but it affects nearly 3 per cent of the adult population. I'm sure you know more than 300 people, so that's just basic maths.

The overdiagnosis question isn't the only controversy that surrounds ADHD. There are plenty of misunderstandings, conspiracy theories and downright misinformation out there, and for a while I considered including a section debunking all of them. But I feel the same way about these ideas as I do about climate change denial. There's a vast, broad, comprehensive body of data and research proving time and time again that this is a legitimate, genetic and widespread condition. Spending our precious time trying to combat every naysayer would be giving them more airtime than they deserve. There are already plenty of resources and books tearing these theories to shreds. I just want to get on with learning to live with my ADHD rather than justifying its very existence.

The age of ADHD

Giving the exact rate of persistence of ADHD into adulthood is complicated by the fact that many of the largest studies have relied on older criteria from the *Diagnostic and Statistical Manual of Mental Disorders*, fourth edition (DSM-IV), which is significantly more geared towards children. However, a growing number of smaller, more recent studies (using the **DSM-5** definition) are starting to suggest that fully diagnosable ADHD may well persist in a substantial majority of people, and even that the entire idea of 'growing out of' ADHD might be a flawed concept to begin with.[13, 14, 15] One group of ADHD researchers realised that most of the 'recovery' data we have only really indicates whether formerly ADHD kids still have the disorder at one single point in their adult life – the day they get assessed. When the researchers reassessed their subjects eight times across a sixteen-year period, they found that most of them actually drifted in and out of the 'diagnosable' range throughout their life.

This was a relatively small study that only looked at those with **ADHD-C** (combined), so I wouldn't take it as gospel, but it found that only 9 per cent of those who had entered **remission** stayed there for the rest of the study (i.e. recovered), and only 10 per cent met the full diagnostic criteria the entire time.[16] While genetics may well play a part in deciding how persistent someone's ADHD will be, the researchers posited that someone's life circumstances likely also play a significant role. Maybe in moments of dramatic change, high stress and low sleep, their subjects' symptoms got worse or the way their brain functioned became a lot more inconvenient and *bam!* they are impaired enough to meet the full clinical criteria. At other times, when things were calm, their health was good, their routine solid and support abundant, their symptoms quietened down, their slightly different brain function wasn't really an inconvenience and they slipped back below the diagnosable threshold. Anyhow, my point is that it's seeming more and more likely that lifelong ADHD, and therefore adult ADHD, may well be the norm, not the exception.

So, now that we've established how common ADHD is, it's probably time to get down to brass tacks. What does this condition that affects such a huge portion of the world's population actually, well, do?

DIARY ENTRY

Swan poo

Because of my job as a reporter and my insatiable need for every person on the planet to think I'm funny, I've developed a bit of a following online. Nothing life-changing, but still enough that I was known by at least a portion of the experts I reached out to for this book. This has, however, created the situation where several times when I've mentioned over the course of these conversations that I myself have ADHD, they've replied, 'Oh, I thought so. Yeah, that doesn't surprise me at all.'

One such person was A/Prof Katherine Johnson from the University of Melbourne, who has been incredibly helpful throughout the writing of this book. Before I even had the chance to ask what had given my ADHD away, she said, 'Yeah, I've wondered about you since I read the story about the bike.'

And suddenly everything made sense.

At the start of 2021, a few days before my ADHD assessment, I managed to spectacularly ruin my New Year's resolution, and decided to deal with the profound embarrassment and shame in a very normal and healthy way – by writing an article about it for the international news platform I work for.

I figured that the two most common New Year's resolutions are to spend less money and to lose weight, and as someone who had just moved out of home and had a problematic preoccupation with trying to get their university clothes to fit again, I decided to combine both by riding my bike to and from work every day.

So, the first day I could, I helmeted up and hit the road, confident that I'd left myself more than enough time to arrive at work punctually.

I had not.

Google Maps is very good at estimating driving time, but it has an unrealistic idea of my cycling fitness, and in my productivity euphoria,

I forgot about the 39-degree-Celsius heatwave forecast for the city that day. By the time I wheeled my extremely heavy but aesthetically pleasing bike into the lift at work, I was fifteen minutes late, my dress was drenched in sweat and my face was as red as an apple.

But I made the best of it, did my day's work and, after submitting my story – which, in a moment of ominous foreshadowing, was all about being safe near waterways over the coming long weekend – I wheeled my bike out and headed home.

To avoid Melbourne's peak-hour traffic I cut across to Albert Park – the big park with a lake at the centre that the Formula One cars zoom round once a year. But the evening cool change had brought a colossal number of joggers to the water, and the normal bike path was filled.

'No problem,' I incorrectly thought to myself. 'I'll just ride on the footpath right next to the lake.'

As I zoomed along, I looked out at a magnificent family of swans gliding through the wobbly reflection of the city, with five fluffy grey cygnets trailing behind, and I thought to myself, 'How lucky I am that I get to do this every day.'

This was my last thought before I heard a loud *thunk* as something caught in my wheel. I veered wildly off course and, as I overcorrected, looked up to see myself headed directly towards the water half a metre below.

Full disclosure: the previous year, when I was only a few weeks into my job, I'd spilt a full cup of tea into my work laptop keyboard, causing it to, well, explode, filling my room with the scent of burnt plastic and requiring a new computer to be couriered urgently from Sydney. It was horrifically mortifying and so, as I splashed into the water, I was determined not to let it happen again.

After surfacing like the Loch Ness monster from the murky depths,

I pulled my bike out of the swan-poo sediment, ripped the laptop from my drenched backpack and computer case, and tried to climb out. But the slimy concrete lake wall gave me no purchase.

A muscled jogger ran up and asked if I was okay, but instead of responding like a sane person, I screeched at him, 'TAKE MY LAPTOP!' A little shocked, and probably concerned about my mental health, he did. Next, he tried to grab my arms and hoist me out, but it was no good: the walls were too high and I guess I was too heavy. This meant I had no choice but to stand there for five whole minutes, looking up at him and making awkward small talk while we tried to flag down another strong man.

When one eventually came along, they grabbed an arm each and pulled my soaking body, crucifixion style, up onto land, my floral dress now stinking of pond scum and swan faeces. After repeatedly asking if I was sure I was okay, they gave me one last concerned look as I thanked them profusely, hopped back on my bike and rode away, leaving a snail-like trail of drips in my wake.

Luckily my laptop survived, but the next morning as I headed out to work, humbled and still vaguely stinking, I realised that I'd never recovered my building pass from the water. It was now impossible for me to ride my bike to the office, as I couldn't get in. My New Year's resolution didn't even make it one round trip.

'Oh, yeah,' I chuckled to Dr Johnson on the phone, 'I guess in retrospect that is a pretty ADHD-ish thing to do.'

'No, you don't understand,' Johnson laughed. 'There's a German children's book called *Der Struwwelpeter* where each page is a little poem about a kid getting into some predicament. But it was written by the psychologist Dr Heinrich Hoffmann, and so rather than just being a kids' story, every child actually represents a different mental condition.'

'Oh,' I said, my eyes widening.

'And the child with ADHD, he falls straight in a lake.'

'Oh my god,' I say.

'And guess why,' Dr Johnson enthused.

'Why?'

'Because he was so distracted looking at some birds, he walked right off the ledge.'

Sometimes I really wonder how I wasn't diagnosed with ADHD earlier. Because, sure, I might not be a textbook case, but I'm certainly a picture-book one.

2

What's wrong with me?

ADHD is full of contradictions and paradoxes, and one of the most unfortunate, counterintuitive examples of this is that, despite it being one of the most common **neurodevelopmental** disorders in the world, our culture's general understanding of ADHD is pretty bloody awful.

We're here to correct this, so let's start with the basics. How does one actually become an ADHDer?

Who's to blame?

We still don't know precisely what causes someone to get a case of the fidgety brain, but those in the neuroscientific field are fairly sure it's a combination and/or accumulation of genetic and environmental factors. Or, put more simply, certain genes make it possible for you to have ADHD, and being exposed to specific conditions while in the womb, or in very early childhood, can increase your chance of developing the disorder.

A decent body of evidence suggests there's a **correlation** between an increased risk of developing ADHD and factors such as low birth weight,[1] being born prematurely,[2] and even things such as exposure to lead[3] during gestation or at a young age.

It's unlikely that any single environmental factor will straight-up cause a baby to have ADHD. Instead, each factor just bumps up the chances little by little. And, of course, we can't chalk up all ADHD cases to external factors alone, because it's well known that the jittery genes tend to run in the family.

A note on the word 'correlation'. When used in academia it's a way of saying that there's enough evidence to show that two things are related in some way or often occur together, but not that one necessarily causes the other. For example, there's a correlation between 'having *Family Guy* as your favourite TV show' and 'being a terrible person to talk to at parties', but we don't know if one caused the other or if they both stem from a third unknown factor.

So, while there's some evidence for environmental conditions contributing to the likelihood of developing ADHD, this hasn't been proven definitively. For example, a number of large-scale studies have linked mothers smoking while pregnant to increased cases of ADHD in their children. But given that ADHD is largely **hereditary** and also increases the chances of developing nicotine dependence to begin with, it's possible that mothers who have ADHD themselves just happen to be more likely to smoke while pregnant.[4] Thus 'correlation', not 'causation', is the more accurate term.

Because we've only cottoned on to the idea that adults can have the condition relatively recently, the sample sizes of family-based ADHD studies tend to be small. But the data we have suggests that around 50 per cent of families with an ADHD child will have at least one ADHD parent.[5,6] A number of other studies suggest that 40 to 57 per cent of children with ADHD parents will receive a **diagnosis** themselves.[7] Also, if your older sibling has been diagnosed with ADHD, your odds of being diagnosed are thirteen times higher.[8] It's worth bearing in mind, though, that the underdiagnosis of the disorder likely warps such statistics a little.

My basic point is that if you've been diagnosed, it might be worth having a look around at your immediate family and seeing which of them has the most unfinished craft projects lying around the house.

While researching, I've been playing a fun game with my family called 'Who's to blame?' where I slowly and sneakily ask them about their childhood to see if they could potentially fulfil the official **diagnostic criteria** for ADHD. The results of this extremely unscientific study are still pending, but there are a few of them whose legs are suspiciously jiggly during family dinners.

No 'one' ADHD

It would be nice if I could simply tell you, in one short sentence, the exact genetic quirks that are responsible for ADHD – if there was a single gene that I could point to and say, 'That's the culprit, get him, boys!' But when I asked the University of Melbourne's Professor David Coghill, one of Australia's (and the world's) foremost experts on ADHD, he told me that there were likely hundreds, if not thousands of culprits. 'It's not just one gene or two genes. It's many, many, many genes, each having a very small effect.'

The data we have suggests that around 50 per cent of families with an ADHD child will have at least one ADHD parent.

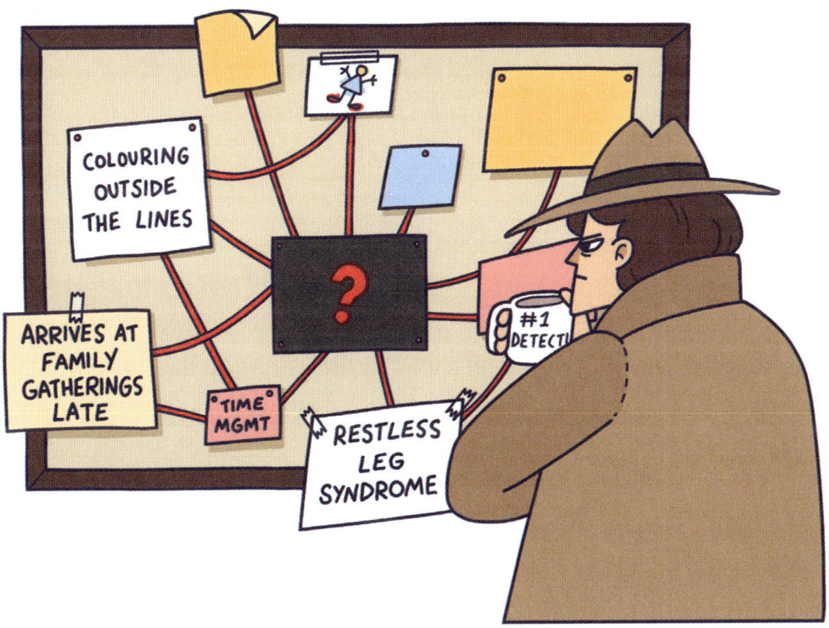

These all eventually add up to create ADHD, but the truly mind-boggling thing is that these genetic variations can occur and combine in millions of different ways. 'There is no "one" ADHD,' Professor Coghill tells me. 'ADHD comes in lots of different flavours and lots of different colours. And the balance of ADHD [symptoms] in each person can be quite different.'

Personally, I like thinking about ADHD this way: not as a single monolithic thing, but perhaps as something closer to a spectrum, or a lucky dip of related **symptoms**. I remember in the early days, getting so stressed if I read something about an ADHD trait I'd never experienced, wondering if that meant my diagnosis was wrong. But no, it's all different strokes for different folks in the world of **neurodivergence**.

But the medical community loves categorisation. Diagnosis is merely a shorthand way for medical professionals to communicate what's going on with a patient. So, simply saying 'I guess the vibe of their ADHD is more energetic, but they also like to doodle on their leg in meetings and they cry a bit too often' isn't that helpful. So, in the end the medical professionals seem to have reached a compromise, with three overarching terms that describe the variations of the disorder.

The flavours of ADHD

As described by the *Diagnostic and Statistical Manual of Mental Disorders*, fifth edition (**DSM-5**), the three **presentations** of ADHD are:

1. **primarily hyperactive/impulsive (ADHD-H)**
2. **primarily inattentive (ADHD-I)**
3. **combined (ADHD-C).**

I'm a combined presentation gal myself and, let me tell you, it's double the dysfunctional fun.

The *Diagnostic and Statistical Manual of Mental Disorders*, fifth edition, is basically a giant tome that lists the characteristics and diagnostic criteria for every mental disorder. It's by no means perfect, but it's the most widely accepted manual in the field of psychiatry across the world, so it's the one on which I'll be basing my official description of ADHD.

The World Health Organization (WHO) has its own version of the DSM called the International Classification of Diseases (ICD), but this didn't officially recognise 'ADHD' until very recently. Instead, it listed something called 'hyperkinetic disorder' (HKD), which had more conservative and restrictive criteria, potentially including less than half of the people who would meet the DSM definition of ADHD. For example, there was a while there when you couldn't be diagnosed with HKD if you also had anxiety and depression, despite these two conditions potentially occurring in half of all people with ADHD. There was also a much greater focus on **hyperactivity**, which isn't that helpful for girls and adults. This was updated in the ICD-11, which includes a condition called 'ADHD' with a very similar definition to the DSM-5. A preview of these changes came out in 2018 but only officially came into effect in 2022, and because it's so recent, barely any studies reference it, which is why you won't see me talking about it too much.

So let's take a look at what each of these flavours of ADHD entails.

The class clown: ADHD's predominantly hyperactive/impulsive presentation

When people think about that stereotypical, ants-in-his-pants, can't shut up to save his life, energetic little boy – chances are they're thinking about the hyperactive/impulsive presentation of ADHD (**ADHD-H**). One of the official symptoms in the DSM-5 is that people with this presentation are constantly 'on the go' or 'acting as if driven by a motor', but the symptoms aren't all about literally jumping off tables; they can be more subtle, too. Maybe they can't stop fidgeting, or they can talk the leg off a table. The impulsive aspect of the disorder could mean they struggle at not interrupting or at waiting their turn.

THE CLASS CLOWN

ADHD-H (HYPERACTIVE/IMPULSIVE)

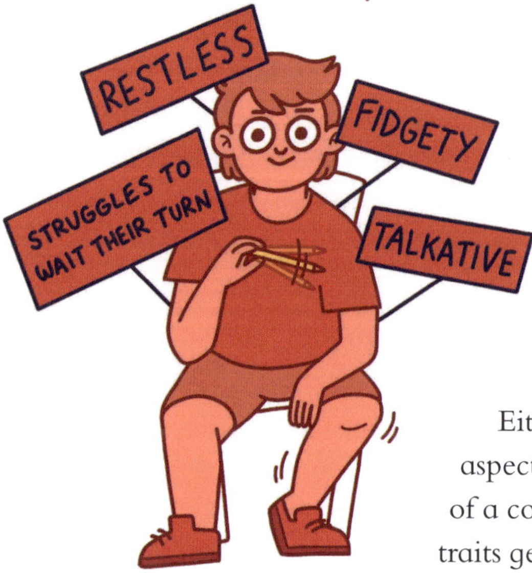

The reason you might automatically associate these traits with children is that ADHD's style of hyperactivity tends to become much more internalised with age. This could be due to something about the genetics or biology of the condition, or maybe just because society has a lot less patience for adults jumping up and down in the middle of a meeting or repeatedly talking over their boss. So, we have to mask it in order to survive. Either way, in adulthood the hyperactive aspect of the condition tends to present as more of a constant inner **restlessness**.[9] The impulsive traits generally tend to stick around longer, though, and these are the ones that tend to continue causing issues.

Notionally, those with the primarily hyperactive/impulsive symptoms don't really struggle with **inattention** to any great degree. So, while they may be bouncing off the walls in class, actually holding their attention on a topic for a sustained period of time wouldn't be that much harder for them than for their **neurotypical** peers, provided they can stay seated. However, this ADHD presentation – where someone has only hyperactive symptoms and no significant issues with attention – is the least common.

It's pretty difficult to estimate how common each ADHD presentation actually is, for all the same reasons it's hard to estimate the overall **prevalence** of the disorder. But it seems ADHD-H is most common in preschool-aged children, where it potentially makes up more than half of all cases. But this shrinks to around a quarter by primary school and even less by the time high school rolls around.[10] Usually this isn't because the kids were 'cured' of ADHD altogether, but simply that their condition has shifted to either the combined or inattentive presentation. This has led some to question whether ADHD-H – at least as it's described by the current diagnostic criteria – is actually a valid presentation in adults,[11] or even in those older than six.[12]

The space cadet: ADHD's predominantly inattentive presentation

Probably the most misunderstood and overlooked version of ADHD is the primarily inattentive presentation (**ADHD-I**). Someone presenting this way will have a much harder time staying focused and might be prone to making careless mistakes in their work. Unless they find a task super engaging, it might be difficult or even impossible for them to keep their attention homed in on it, and distractions are a constant challenge. They might zone out when people are talking to them, forget the instructions they were just told, and find that they're constantly losing or misplacing important things.

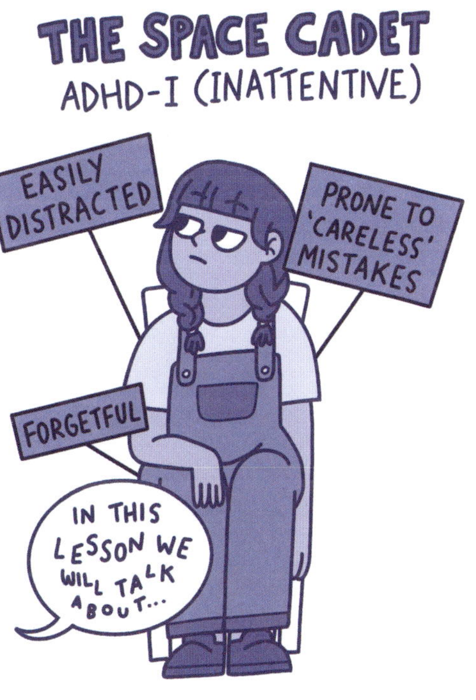

That's not to say that they can never focus – in fact, quite the opposite. ADHD brains of all varieties have the capacity for extreme prolonged attention if the topic or the activity is interesting to them – a phenomenon colloquially known as '**hyperfocus**'. They might be able to play a video game for hours and hours without a break, or read a book series they love for days on end. And although they can easily stay up till 3 am googling all the history and lore of Frank Herbert's

Dune universe, they may still be unable to get their tax return done even if it's nine months overdue and, oh my god, Matilda, it would literally take, like, fifteen minutes tops to finish. That's part of the reason why the name 'attention-deficit/hyperactivity disorder' is kind of bad at actually describing the condition.

It's not that we have a deficit in attention; we have a deficit in control over it.

Jumping back to the classroom, those with primarily inattentive ADHD probably aren't going to be the kids tripping over chairs and interrupting. They're more likely to be sitting there quietly, gazing off into the middle distance or focusing on the way the bird hops from branch to branch in the tree outside the window. Because these kids aren't necessarily all that prone to disrupting class time, their disorder is much more likely to go unnoticed and thus **undiagnosed**. But despite their symptoms being more internalised, they can still be exceedingly destructive and impairing.

While the prevalence of ADHD-H might decrease with age, ADHD-I increases, and by adulthood makes up about 47 per cent of all cases.[13] (At least based on the DSM-IV criteria.)

The hurricane: ADHD's combined presentation

Now we come to the grand finale, and my own presentation – combined hyperactive/impulsive and inattentive (**ADHD-C**). Plenty of people with ADHD-I (inattentive) are still going to have a touch of hyperactivity and **impulsivity**, and those with ADHD-H (hyperactive/impulsive) will have shades of inattention too, but ADHD-C is the diagnosis you get when you tick lots of boxes from both columns. Basically, it's the 'all of the above' flavour, so focus is difficult, impulsivity is strong and the brain is always on the go. It's a lot.

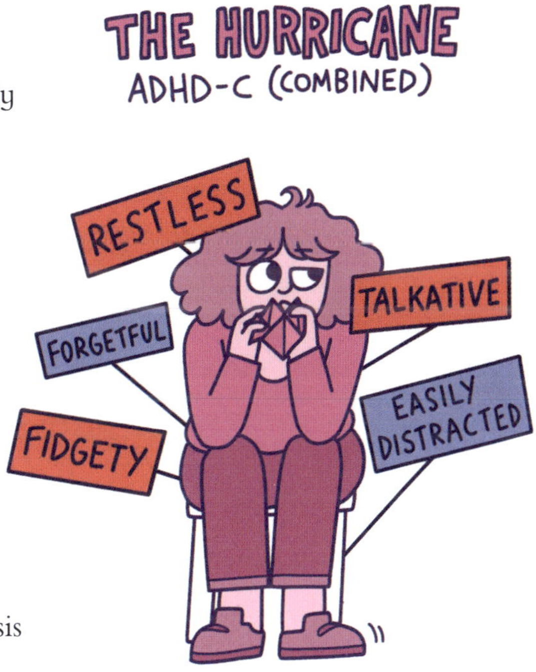

Generally speaking, inattentive ADHD symptoms tend to be more closely associated with academic **impairment**, trouble with employment and low **self-esteem**, while hyperactive/impulsive symptoms are more directly linked with peer rejection, risky driving and accidentally injuring oneself.[14] So, you can imagine having both is a real hoot and a half.

There's a bit of mixed information about whether ADHD-I or ADHD-C is the most common presentation. One meta-analysis study suggested that the predominantly inattentive presentation may actually be the most prevalent, but that those with a combined presentation are more likely to be referred for clinical services, so it tends to get the most attention.[15] (At least this is the case with children; reliable presentation-specific adult data is much harder to come by).

You might also have heard these presentations described as 'subtypes', but that name changed in 2013 (when the DSM-5 came out), after it became clear that an individual's experience of ADHD isn't set in stone. People can, and often do, change presentations over the course of their life.

It's not that we have a deficit in attention; we have a deficit in control over it.

When I started properly educating myself about the symptoms of this condition it was almost as if I could feel the earth jolt and start shifting under my feet. Suddenly, so many strange events from my childhood were starting to make sense. Moments where I was struggling, seemingly for no reason, had potential explanations. I could tell I was on the edge of a complete perspective shift.

But I'd still only learnt the end results of the way my mind worked. To really begin the process of recontextualising my life up to this point, I'd need to know why my brain did what it did. Oh, and why on earth everyone kept talking about **dopamine** all the time.

Planning to be spontaneous

The really annoying thing about my personal experience of ADHD is that I didn't get the fun, thrill-seeking version of impulsivity. I'm not a daredevil who free-solos giant mountains or paddles my kayak down white-water rapids. I'm not booking spur-of-the-moment trips around the world. I'm not impulsively dancing in the rain. My version of impulsivity is just interrupting people a lot, making dumb jokes in work meetings, accidentally electrocuting myself by trying to get the dimensions of a switched-on light socket using a metal tape measure, and struggling to kick a mild nicotine addiction. I know that risk-taking behaviour is a serious safety issue for a lot of people with ADHD, but I can't help but feel a tiny bit jealous of my neurodivergent peers who manage to be spontaneous as well as socially awkward.

When reading up on all the ways ADHD impulsivity can manifest, I racked my brain for some wild story to tell, but the truth is, I've only ever done one truly, traditionally impulsive thing in my whole life.

It's about five years ago and I'm in Nepal, on a three-week study tour with university students from all around Australia. The country is beautiful and breathtaking, but the coursework we all need to complete is really starting to drag. My antidote to this dullness is to get close to one of the boys from another state.

In fact, extremely close. Like spending eleven days straight hanging out close. Like hiking up to the top of the nearby hill and lying on the grass with the tops of our heads touching, staring out at the Himalayas as a meteor shower sends shooting stars trailing across the sky and talking about who in the group we'd make out with if we had the chance – close. Like him pausing for a second and saying 'No one', and then pausing for a second more and saying, 'Well, actually it's you' – close. But then immediately following that sentence up with, 'The thing is, I have a girlfriend.' Which really feels like information he could have shared at the bottom of the hill, to be honest.

I spend the last days of my trip stewing in my own guilt, embarrassment and longing, and by all metrics listening to far too much Elton John. That is until my mate from uni, Simon, who has been politely pretending not to see the melodramatic tears that periodically roll down my face, says, 'Okay, but we have to go paragliding.'

The thing is, I've been specifically told over and over that paragliding is not covered by my travel insurance, and was also made to pinky-promise my parents that I wouldn't do it because, as they reminded me repeatedly, if I got injured and needed a ventilator or something, it would cost hundreds of thousands of dollars to get me back to Australia. So I tell Simon no and resign myself to a day of solitude, masala tea and 'Rocket Man' on repeat.

Usually I'm utterly terrified to break rules, but not engaging in emotional affairs with guys who are already in a relationship is kind of a rule, and that ship seems to have left the harbour. Plus, the perverse pleasure I was taking in fully giving myself over to misery isn't getting me anywhere. And then all of a sudden, before I realise what I'm doing, I'm running onto the road (well, the hotel driveway) as the minibus filled with my daredevil buddies is pulling away and yelling, 'Let me in!' They open the doors, I hand a wad of rupees to the confused tour operator, and I sit down, 100 per cent confident in my spur-of-the-moment decision.

By the time we get to the top of the mountain I'm thoroughly questioning what the fuck I'm doing. I haven't even looked up the safety record of the paragliding company, for god's sake. I see Simon get strapped onto a muscly Nepalese man with a giant parachute trailing behind him and, just as I see the fear dawn in my friend's eyes, the pair start running together straight off the edge of the plateau, lift into the air, and he is gone!

I meet my tandem guide, an adrenaline-junkie American dude who moved here for the 'sick air currents'. He jokes that it's his first day on the job. I smile politely without looking away from the cliff as he assures me he's kidding. I strap in. We run. I feel my feet exit the ground, and my heart exit my butt, and we're up, sailing around in majestic circles. And even though the day is exceedingly foggy and I can barely see the lake below, I'm awed by the grandeur and feel tears of delight rolling down my face. I release all the built-up anger and longing in a squeal of delight and terror, and imagine the credits starting to roll, superimposed on the clouds ahead of us.

The moment is totally shattered when we land and Simon says, 'So, like, what should we do for the rest of the day?'

But that's my one truly 'fun' impulsive moment – the one time my ADHD actually helped me be the spontaneous person I always wished I was.

Except, now that I see it all written down, I realise it wasn't actually that spontaneous, was it? Doing something specifically so you can have a powerful ending scene in the made-up movie of your life? And, feeling so guilty about the fact that you just risked bankrupting your family that you ring your parents on the drive home to apologise doesn't really scream 'daredevil'.

So, yeah, when it comes to impulsivity, I got the boring end of the stick. Or, more specifically, the overly dramatic, failed-theatre-kid end. And perhaps that's even worse.

3

What's going on inside my brain?

If there was any doubt in your mind as to whether ADHD was actually a real, physical condition, know that there's a growing body of evidence to suggest that you can literally see the structural differences in scans of ADHD and **neurotypical** brains.[1] It's not a hard line in the sand – there's a gradient of differences – but it's still significant enough that people are investigating whether we could use MRI scans to diagnose ADHD in the future.

This probably won't mean much unless you are a neuroscientist, but in case you're interested, those consistent differences in brain structure are a slightly smaller amygdala, nucleus accumbens, caudate nucleus, hippocampus and putamen, and a reduction in the intracranial volume. A number of other studies have been looking into differences in grey matter volume, too. Thrilling stuff indeed!

Where's the dopamine gone?

But what's happening in ADHD brains to make them so different? Before I dived head-first (or brain-first) into the wild world of **neurotransmitters**, this whole **dopamine** thing never made much sense to me. Pop culture and my high school's mandated drug-awareness lectures had taught me that dopamine is the 'pleasure chemical' and you get a rush of it when you fall in love or eat a piece of cake or smoke the devil's lettuce or have sex. Then, after my **diagnosis**, it was drilled into me that dopamine is something ADHD brains don't have enough of.

But if I have less of the pleasure chemical in my brain, shouldn't that just make me depressed instead of making me spend $150 on embroidery needles, Aida cloth and bamboo tension hoops at 3 am because I saw *one video* about cross-stitch? And what on earth does this have to do with attention, or **hyperfocus**, or not being able to stop myself interrupting people when they're talking?

As it turns out, it didn't make sense to me because pretty much everything I assumed about dopamine and the chemical side of ADHD was wrong. Firstly, dopamine isn't the only brain chemical implicated in ADHD. Its friend **noradrenaline** (aka norepinephrine, which is like adrenaline for the brain and helps with alertness) probably also plays an important role.

Secondly, we're not actually 100 per cent sure what the relationship between ADHD and dopamine even is. We know there's a link, because the most common type of ADHD medication – stimulants – generally work by increasing the levels of dopamine in certain areas of the brain, which decreases the **symptoms** of the disorder. But it's not quite as simple as saying ADHD brains 'don't have enough of it', although this is often used as a shorthand way of talking about the neurology of ADHD.

I had assumed that every time you did something good, your body would pump some of this sweet, sweet feel-good dopamine into your skull, then your brain would bathe in it for a little while, soaking up the pleasurable feeling. And if you just naturally didn't get enough, then your brain would be constantly darting your attention around, trying to find something else stimulating so it could get another hit.

But that's not how ADHD, or brains, work at all.

You might know that your brain is made up of tens of billions of cells called **neurons**, which are very nearly – but not quite – touching the neurons next to them. In extremely simplistic terms, these cells talk to each other by shooting a few molecules of certain chemicals, known as neurotransmitters, across that little gap to their next-door neighbours. When the molecules land in the next neuron's specially shaped receptors, that gives the cell the green light to squirt out some neurotransmitters to the next neuron down the line, and so on and so forth, millions of times in a big chain reaction, until eventually the message makes it to its destination and that bit of the brain does what it's meant to do.

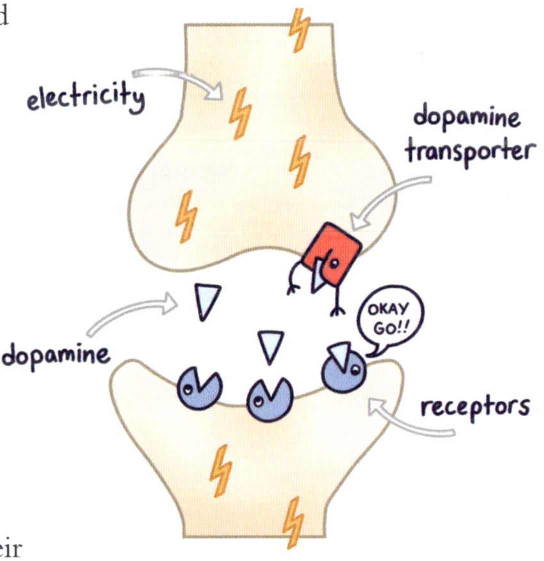

Different neural pathways and sections of the brain use different chemicals to achieve this, but the ones we care about use dopamine primarily as their molecule of choice. The most widely held theory about what causes ADHD is that a number of these **dopaminergic** (i.e. dopamine-regulated) pathways aren't functioning quite as you'd expect. Perhaps ADHD brain cells don't have enough dopamine to begin with, or the bit of the neuron that the dopamine is meant to land in (the receptor) is shaped weirdly, or the first cell's dopamine transporters suck the molecules back up too fast, or there's some other problem entirely that the extra dopamine and noradrenaline in ADHD medication simply helps compensate for. Who bloody knows! The academic world has been arguing about this for years, but the end result is that the messaging systems in certain parts of the ADHD brain are a bit shonky and don't work as consistently or reliably as we'd like.

The ~~pleasure~~ *motivation* chemical

The third common misconception about dopamine is that it's the 'pleasure chemical'. It actually has numerous roles in the brain and body (including, oddly enough, controlling lactation). But when it comes to ADHD, it's probably best known as the chemical that regulates the **mesolimbic pathway** (don't worry – this is one of the last science terms I'll make you learn), which connects all the areas that make up the brain's reward system. In this way, dopamine is actually more related to motivation than pleasure.

This is no doubt an egregious oversimplification, but one theory of dopamine is that when we do something that helps us survive as a species – such as eating juicy berries or having sex with that handsome, strong hunter in our stone-age community – those mesolimbic neurons start shooting off dopamine to each other, activating that reward system and basically bookmarking the experience with a little note that says, 'Hey, this was good and made you feel good.' Then, the next time we think about those berries or glistening prehistoric abs, our brain revs up those dopaminergic reward system neurons in anticipation, reminding us how good it was last time and motivating us to do it again. This is important, because what if it's horrifically cold and rainy and your loincloth is chafing? It would be a real pain in the arse to go out and pick those berries. Staying by the warm fire feels nice in the moment, but getting enough food to survive would feel good in the long run. Dopamine helps bridge that gap to get us out and gathering again. Or, you know, slipping into that hunky, hunky hominid's shelter.

Nowadays we might not be battling against the wilderness for survival, but we might need to battle against filling out an extremely long and boring job application in order to experience the pleasure of a better-paying position – and it's those little bursts from our mesolimbic pathway that keep us focused, motivated and typing away. Or at least that's what happens in neurotypical brains.[2]

Regardless of the exact cause, the end result is that in ADHD brains the reward system doesn't function as effectively as it should. We don't get to experience that same level of anticipation and motivation while ploughing through uninteresting tasks, so it makes sense that we might constantly be scouring our surroundings for stimulating distractions, or impulsively jumping into a new activity when there's nothing reminding us of the pleasure that updating our résumé will eventually bring.[3]

Regardless of the exact cause, the end result is that in ADHD brains the reward system doesn't function as effectively as it should.

Obviously, this struggle with motivation doesn't map out the entirety of the ADHD labyrinth. But the reward system isn't the only part of your brain that dopamine controls. And with that, it's probably time I introduce you to the mesolimbic pathway's next-door neighbour, the **prefrontal cortex** – home of the brain's executive functions.

Executive dysfunction: let's meet Ethel

If you've recently been diagnosed with ADHD, chances are you've heard the term **executive dysfunction**. It's the most widely accepted theory about what's going on cognitively inside most ADHD minds, and, at least for me, learning about it was what made everything click. But, as Professor Coghill was quick to point out, not everyone with ADHD has trouble with this stuff, so if you don't relate to what I'm about to say, it doesn't necessarily mean you don't have ADHD. A million different flavours, remember.

Executive functions are all the higher-order self-regulation skills our brains use to organise themselves and make it easy for us to get complicated things done. Controlling inhibitions, sustaining attention, problem-solving, switching between tasks or ways of thinking, and moving numbers around in our head to figure out how much this new Lego Botanicals bonsai tree set is going to cost now that it's 35 per cent off; these are all executive functions. The prefrontal cortex also needs just the right level of dopamine in order to function, but rather than acting as the motivation chemical, in this section of the brain dopamine is more the **working-memory** chemical, the resisting-impulse chemical and the cognitive-flexibility chemical. The theory is that because there is something going awry in this area of the brain, too, a large number of ADHD symptoms can ultimately be traced back to these executive functions *not functioning* the way they should.

When learning about executive functioning, it helped me to picture my mind as a little office, where each department is in charge of a different brain function, and my thoughts are the paperwork telling them all what to do. At the front of the office sits the executive-function lady, and it's her job to fill out all those forms and send them to the correct departments for action. I like to think her name is Ethel, and she wears thick, rectangular glasses, blue eyeshadow and huge clip-on earrings. She's got a massive job to do, so she likes to keep a tub of nutritious dopamine biscuits on her desk to give her energy, and a cup of bitter noradrenaline coffee by her side to keep her alert.

It's not that ADHD offices have dodgy paperwork or crappy departments. It's just that our Ethels are super overwhelmed, underpaid and, to be honest, pretty bloody tired. But really, it's hard to blame her for being a bit under the weather, because her work is relentless.

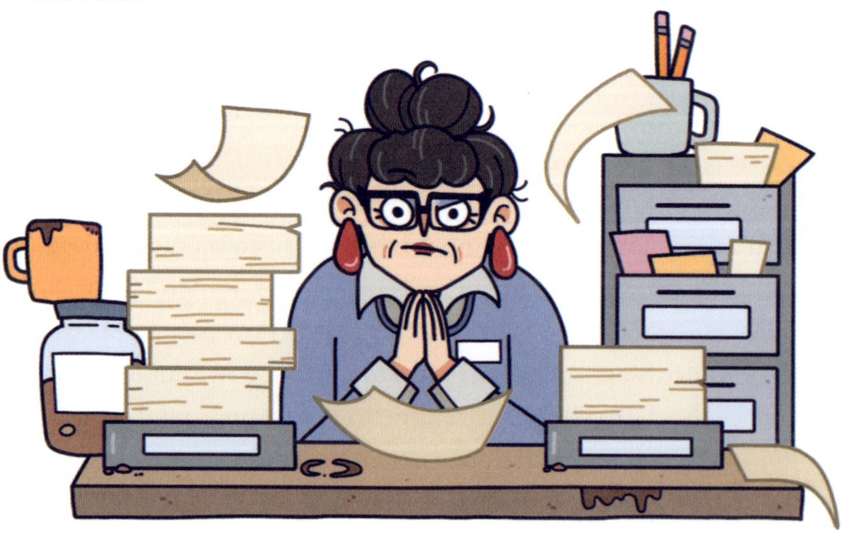

Let's say you want to wash the dishes. This is what her next few minutes are going to look like: first, you'll have to actually notice that the dishes need to be done – that's some paperwork for her to fill out. Then, when you get into the kitchen and see the kettle, you'll need to ignore the impulse to make a cup of tea. So Ethel needs to catch that 'tea' memo as it goes into her inbox and throw it in the shredder. She also needs to get rid of that emotional memo urging you to get upset and start crying when you see how big the pile of dishes is, and the one that appears when it occurs to you that the peace lily growing on the kitchen windowsill might need a little water.

Next up, you need to plan out all the mini-tasks involved in washing the dishes. You need to find the plug. You need to get the dirty cups from your bedside. You need to put the right amount of soap in the sink. You need to get some rubber gloves. Each of those is a form, and Ethel then has to take all this paperwork over to the working-memory desk, rearrange it into the most efficient order, run over to the long-term memory cabinet, pull up the report from when you scalded your hand with hot water last time and staple that to the bundle so you don't do it again, chuck all that in a folder and send it to the right department.

Plus, while this has been happening, nineteen more distracting impulse memos have hit Ethel's inbox and at this point she's using her feet to urgently throw them in the shredder and keep you on task.

Then Ethel needs to help you problem-solve when you realise the detergent bottle is empty. That's paperwork. She needs to make sure you're keeping track of all the time this is taking. That's paperwork. She needs to pull up the report reminding you not to use a scouring brush on the non-stick frying pan that your grandma gave you as a house-warming present. That's paperwork too.

By the time the plates are in the drying rack, your Ethel has likely filled out, filed, shredded and altered upwards of a thousand forms, and then, without a second's rest, she has to sweep absolutely everything off her desk, change your mindset and move on to the next thing.

All Ethels miss memos and bugger up reports occasionally, but in an ADHD brain – where her dopamine biscuit tin is often empty and her noradrenaline coffee cup keeps running dry – the right paperwork getting to the right department can become really hit or miss.

The pile: classic executive dysfunction

Every so often since I've learned about executive dysfunction, a memory will pop up in my brain and I'll suddenly see it in a whole new light.

I was eighteen and sitting on my bed, the fitted sheet coming off at the bottom back corner. There were textbooks, used teacups and who knows what covering every square centimetre of available desk space, and the giant pile of clothes loomed over me, threatening to topple at any second.

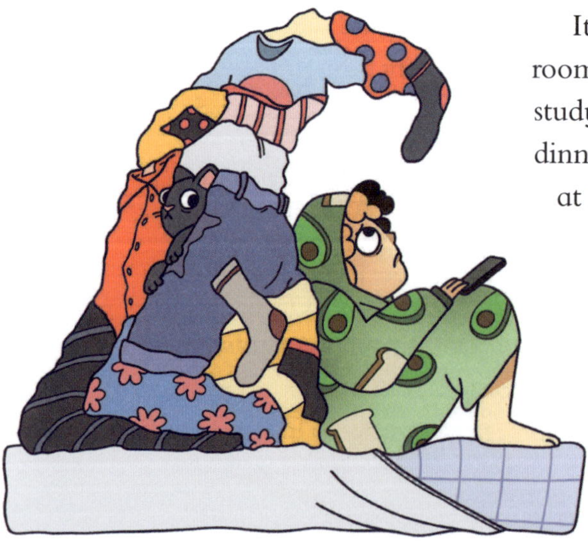

It didn't even take that long for my room to get like this, just a week of intense studying and my friend Olivia's birthday dinner on Friday requiring me to try on at least eight outfits that, obviously, I tossed on my bed rather than hang back up. When Olivia's mum dropped me back home at 12.30 am, I simply pushed the clothes to the floor, and then I put them back on the bed when I woke. Thus the pile grew.

I remember staring at my phone, desperately angry at myself for being so goddamn lazy and not just standing up and starting to tidy. I hated my room when it was like this. I wanted a clean space so badly, and realistically it would only take me forty-five minutes to get it there. Yet there I was, an hour and a half into scrolling through Instagram. That's laziness . . . right?

Even then, I knew that word didn't quite feel right. It wasn't that I couldn't be bothered to clean. Honestly, I'd have loved nothing more. I simply couldn't force myself to hit the lock button on my phone and get started. But lazy was the only word I had, so it's how I labelled myself, and little labels like that, repeated thousands of times across childhood and adolescence, can take their toll.

I know now that moments such as this were examples of acute executive dysfunction. My Ethel just didn't have it in her to clear her whole working-memory desk of all the easy, entertaining social media paperwork and start filling out the huge pile of tidying forms.

Don't underestimate how much you're asking when you tell your ADHD brain to turn away from a high-dopamine, low-effort activity to something laborious and dull. That's even tough for neurotypical people.

It was just as I was starting to descend into the rabbit hole of anxiety that my mum popped her head into the room.

'Come on,' she said, and I bristled, waiting to be told off. 'Let's chuck on a podcast and get this done.'

So that's what we did. And the cleaning wasn't even that hard. In no time, my Ethel was sitting up straighter and powering through her paperwork. In this instance, she just needed help getting started.

Ironically, re-examining and recontextualising memories like this based on new information requires the use of one of the core executive functions, cognitive flexibility – so my Ethel is at work right now.

Playing life on 'Expert' mode

The mesolimbic pathway (connecting the brain's reward system) and the prefrontal cortex (Ethel's workstation) certainly aren't the only things affected by ADHD.

I could fill this book with the different theories about how a hundred different brain pathways, grey matter mass and neurotransmitters all combine and correlate to create ADHD (and in fact, many people have written whole books about this). So while the theories I've touched on here don't explain everything, I hope they've helped you start to make sense of why some things that come so easily to neurotypical people are so much harder for us.

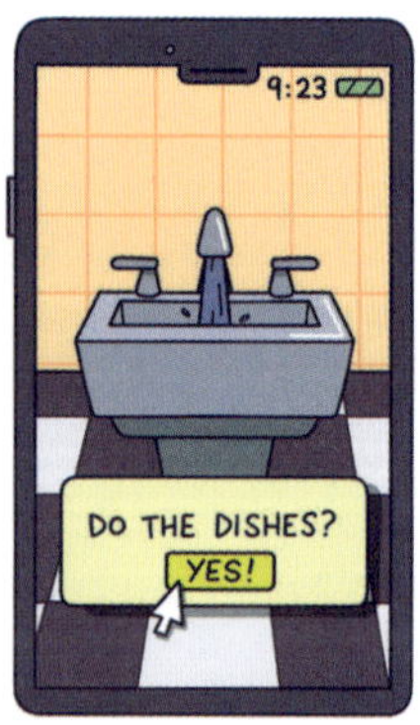
9:23
DO THE DISHES?
YES!

For me, ADHD sometimes feels like everyone is playing the same video game, *Organising Everyday Life*, but someone secretly switched me to the 'Expert' difficulty setting without telling me. I went along for so many years accepting that I was worse at playing than everyone else, but turns out, for us dopamine- and noradrenaline-challenged people, the game is just harder.

It's not your fault things are difficult, and it's not really Ethel's fault either. There's a small chance it might be partly the fault of the lead mine that was up the road from your mother's house while she was pregnant with you, but most of the time ADHD is just a fact of nature. It's an extra challenge that a big chunk of the world's population has to deal with. And, as complicated as my feelings about my condition may be, it does come with a sense of pride, knowing that my achievements represent that little bit extra because the challenges genuinely were bigger.

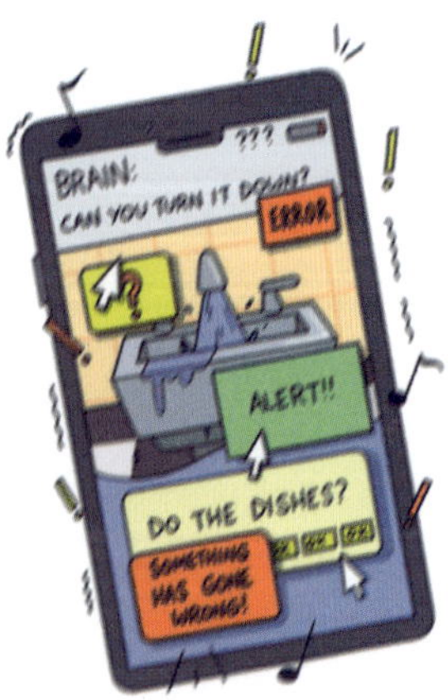
???
BRAIN:
CAN YOU TURN IT DOWN?
ERROR
ALERT!!
DO THE DISHES?
SOMETHING HAS GONE WRONG!

But learning about ADHD did make me wonder what other aspects of my life it had been affecting that had never even occurred to me – and what impact all these years of trying to live up to the standards of a neurotypical world has had.

The warning signs

I'm curled up on the couch one morning with a bowl of leftover pasta, reading an article about ADHD (as usual, written with parents of ADHD kids in mind), when a particular passage catches my eye. It said one warning sign worth looking out for is if your child is constantly popping out of bed to ask for another glass of water, one last hug, or to sleep in the big bed with you. And, *thunk*, just like that, another missing puzzle piece from the jigsaw of my childhood clicks into place. Why did no one warn me an adult ADHD diagnosis would come with so many earth-shattering, mind-altering existential moments of terrifying clarity in the most mundane of situations? I was only looking for something to read while I ate breakfast. I'm not even wearing socks yet.

See, when I was a little kid, bedtime was my worst enemy. I would spend all afternoon dreading it. I would beg my parents to let me stay up just a bit later. I would try to force my sleep-oriented older sister, Perrin, to stay up and talk to me. I would toss and turn, filled with a pure, visceral boredom that felt close to physical pain, which my four-year-old self had no capacity to articulate or understand.

I would get up at least three or four times every night, asking for some milk or complaining of a made-up tummy ache or pretending I'd had a bad dream, despite having been in bed for barely fifteen minutes. I remember standing flat against the wall outside the lounge room, listening to President Bartlet and C.J. argue about the upcoming election in *The West Wing*, trying to piece together what was going on from the sliver of TV screen I could see when I dared to crane my neck around the corner. I would always get found out, and told, 'Come on, Mattie, time to get back to bed.' Resigned, I'd go and then lie there, willing myself not to get up again, knowing Mum and Dad's patience would be wearing thin, but I just couldn't force my little body to stay put.

'I've never met a child who resists going to sleep as much as you do,' my mum told me once, no doubt on her fourth round of taking me back to my room for the night. But it turns out there are lots of kids who did the same thing as me, it's just no one had ever told my parents that this was a symptom of ADHD, or that ADHD was something that little girls like me could even have.

In class I always found it easier to listen when I could doodle and draw, so the teachers who allowed us to do that were always my favourites. I used to get so excited when they would let us have stress balls or squishy toys in class, because it gave me something to do with my hands besides shredding the corners of whatever worksheet I had in front of me. Now that I think about it, the squishy-toy thing was definitely an accommodation the teachers were making for the known ADHD kids. Did no one notice that it was also working suspiciously well for me?

One time in primary school, when a group of us were making a paper-mosaic shark, I got so stubborn and caught up in it being realistically coloured that literally every member of my group asked to move to the turtle team. However, I, totally transfixed on gluing down the little squares, didn't even notice it had happened till I was totally alone at the table. Sometimes I look back on that and laugh, and then other times I wonder why the teacher was so willing to accept that I was just a bossy pain in the arse. Why didn't they start asking more questions?

A few years later, during the worst bout of being bullied, I was taken out of class by a nice lady, who in retrospect was most definitely a counsellor, to talk about some of the harassment that was going on. I remember telling her that it was difficult to concentrate in class, but I guess when you've been called in to talk to a primary schooler about trauma, you'd expect the kid to be having trouble concentrating.

Towards the end of primary school, my teacher called my mum to ask if things were going wrong with my friendships again because I seemed to be acting up a bit in class, interrupting with jokes at inappropriate moments, and that this sort of behaviour was often the result of a kid's growing insecurity and anxiety. But the funny thing was, this period was the first time in a long time that I wasn't struggling socially. In fact, it was the most comfortable and relaxed I'd felt in years. Of course, there's something else that can lead a kid to display poor impulse control and a decreased ability to interpret social cues . . .

But ultimately, no one's thoughts went to ADHD. Maybe because I was still doing well in class academically. Maybe because a history of being bullied seemed like a more obvious explanation. Maybe because I was just talking too much rather than running around like the hyperactive boys the teachers saw every day. But also, maybe, because when most people look at a girl, the idea of ADHD never even crosses their minds.

4

What does ADHD mean for a grown-up?

I promise I don't hate children.

Overall they're fine. In fact, most of them are pretty neat. But as a recently diagnosed ADHD adult, one specific thing constantly rubs me the wrong way. I'll go to look up something about my condition, find a reputable health information website, get four paragraphs into an article and then read 'which is a great way to help your child sit still in the classroom'. It makes me want to throw my laptop out of a window. (But, like, a ground floor one, maybe onto some grass. I really can't afford the cost of repairs right now.)

The issue is, despite the recent uptick in adults being diagnosed with ADHD, we're contending with centuries of research where the condition was assumed only to affect children – overwhelmingly, little hyperactive (and usually white) boys.

I'm not joking when I say 'centuries', by the way. The first description in medical literature of an ADHD-like disorder affecting children was by the German physician Melchior Adam Weikard in 1775. The first hint that the disorder might continue into adulthood, however, wasn't published until 1956.[1] It took humankind's greatest scientific minds 180 years to figure out that distracted kids sometimes become distracted adults, and it took decades more for this to be widely recognised and understood. (To be honest, we're still working on it.)

Part of the problem is that until 1980, the DSM required someone to be hyperactive in order to be diagnosed with ADHD[2] – and, as we now know, **hyperactivity** is the element of the disorder that's most likely to fade as we age. Basically, it was harder to see that adults were struggling, so for hundreds of years we just assumed they weren't. But now that we've got our shit together (slightly), we know that many, perhaps even the majority, of ADHD kids will carry **symptoms** into their adult life.

The problem is, this condition looks drastically different in childhood and adulthood, and all these child-focused resources probably aren't going to be particularly helpful. So, why don't we chat about the nitty-gritty of the legal-voting-age version of ADHD.

No more bouncing off the walls

Probably the biggest sticking point for me when I was trying to reconcile the idea that I might have ADHD was my belief that hyperactivity only manifested as running around and being filled with boundless energy. As a 23-year-old, I didn't have any problems staying seated at work or lying down on the couch to watch TV. I didn't feel like I was bursting at the seams with energy – in fact, I was bloody tired all the time.

Even the updated, more adult-friendly **DSM-5** lists plenty of symptoms that only really make sense if you're thinking about a seven-year-old. 'Often leaves the seat in situations when remaining seated is expected.' Sorry, I have to pay rent, I'm not about to stand up and walk out in the middle of a meeting. 'Often unable to play or engage in leisure activities quietly.' My friend, I'm **burnt-out**. The only leisure activities I have are watching TikToks, getting expensive food delivered to my apartment and having sex; and I have to be quiet doing that one because I have roommates. See above: rent is expensive.

Even once I was diagnosed, I didn't properly recognise my own hyperactivity symptoms for many months. I can't remember if my psychiatrist told me about my **ADHD-C** (combined)

presentation status during that first appointment, but if he did, it didn't stick, and when I started to learn about the different presentations, I just assumed I was inattentive. So, when I double-checked with my psychiatrist a few appointments later, I was genuinely shocked to learn I was wrong.

The thing is, when hyperactivity does persist into adulthood, it often moves inwards. The physical manifestations may be confined to jiggling a leg or tippity-tapping one's fingers[3] – which, much to the annoyance of my family and friends, I'm perpetually guilty of.

However, the years have barely dulled my voracious love of talking (deep apologies to anyone who has ever had to listen to my rants post 1.5 glasses of wine), and although my body might be collapsed on the couch, my mind is still relentlessly on the go.

I find it really hard to just sit down after a long day at work and unwind. I'm racked with guilt about not doing some household chores, or the week's shopping, or extra interviews for work. I'm constantly planning my next move. It's just that now, as an adult, I'm often too tired to actually make the move.

One realisation this year has brought is that I've actually been **self-medicating** with alcohol for a while in order to control my hyperactivity – using a glass of red or a whisky on the rocks to bring me down to a more relaxed place after a day of intense work. It's not an addiction, but it's something I need to be conscious of, because **substance abuse** is shockingly common for ADHDers,[4] and it's theorised that conscious or unconscious self-medication might be a major reason for that.[5] This is why it's so important for us to understand the symptoms of adult ADHD – they come with adult consequences. Learning about grown-up hyperactivity allowed me to connect the dots, identify the start of an unhealthy habit and monitor it with the care it deserves.

Bigger impulses with bigger costs

As we saw in Chapter 2, despite being grouped with hyperactivity in the DSM-5 presentations, the impulsive component of ADHD tends to stick around longer than its jittery cousin. Many of us will spend our whole lives leaning to the impulsive side of the spectrum, and if we're not cognisant of how it's affecting our decision-making, that can spell trouble.

Many of the most serious potential outcomes of adult ADHD are linked to **impulsivity**, including unplanned pregnancies, higher imprisonment rates, car accidents, accidental injuries and a reduced life span in general – but we'll get into that more in Chapter 15. For now, I want to focus on the more subtle ways impulsivity expresses itself in day-to-day life. This can be as simple as a tendency towards impatience, acting before thinking or struggling with impulse buying (as the tiny projector that does nothing but shine a single pixelated image of the moon onto the wall that arrived in the mail for me today can attest).

It's exceedingly hard for me not to interrupt people when what they're saying sparks a new idea in my head. I've never been that great at 'healthy eating' because the moment I'm a little emotionally raw I can't stop myself reaching for comfort food. And never in my life have I noticed a little bump on my face without immediately running to a mirror to squeeze it.

Many of us are natural **novelty seekers**, which can lead to amazing creative ventures but may also see us rejecting healthy structure and stability in favour of excitement and adventure, no matter the emotional cost. This might lead some to jump from job to job and relationship to relationship. Or it could mean constantly seeking out thrilling, stimulating experiences,[6] like jumping out of a plane or seeing how many f-bombs you can drop in front of your grandpa before he tells you off.

Lack of life glue

When we think about ADHD **inattention** in childhood, the most common example is constantly drifting off when a teacher is talking to the class – probably because when you're a kid that's one of the only scenarios where your ability to focus on something boring is really put to the test. But as an adult, 'attention' is so much broader.

Adults with ADHD might find it tough to keep a planner up to date, they might forget meetings, they might find themselves sitting at their desk for hours unable to get work done. Things that other people find easy might be insurmountably difficult, such as keeping their house tidy, or calling their dad back, or remembering to put in an expense claim at work for a taxi ride.

If a co-worker is talking too loudly it might be impossible to drown the sound out, or the flickering fluorescents might ruin their chances of getting an important task done that day. They might get takeaway every night because they never remember to buy the ingredients to make a proper dinner, only for their credit card to be declined because they haven't kept track of their spending and now have nothing in their account until next Tuesday. And oh my god, where is their phone? This is the third time today!

Learning about grown-up hyperactivity allowed me to connect the dots, identify the start of an unhealthy habit and monitor it with the care it deserves.

As you grow up, and especially once the omnipresent sense of structure many people get from living with parents or guardians falls away, attention becomes a fundamental part of keeping your life in order. So it's no surprise that my first year after moving out of home was total chaos. (It's still pretty chaotic now, but at least I know what's causing it.)

Those are the most straightforward ways that ADHD expresses itself in adult life, but there's plenty of weirder, less obvious stuff too.

Beyond the DSM-5

When talking about the experience of ADHD, I sometimes find it makes the most sense to think of the symptoms existing in several rings. (In my mind, they are the multiple walled rings of the Earth Nation kingdom of Ba Sing Se from *Avatar: The Last Airbender* – the Ba Sing S-ADHD, if you will – but feel free to substitute your preferred circular visual aid.)

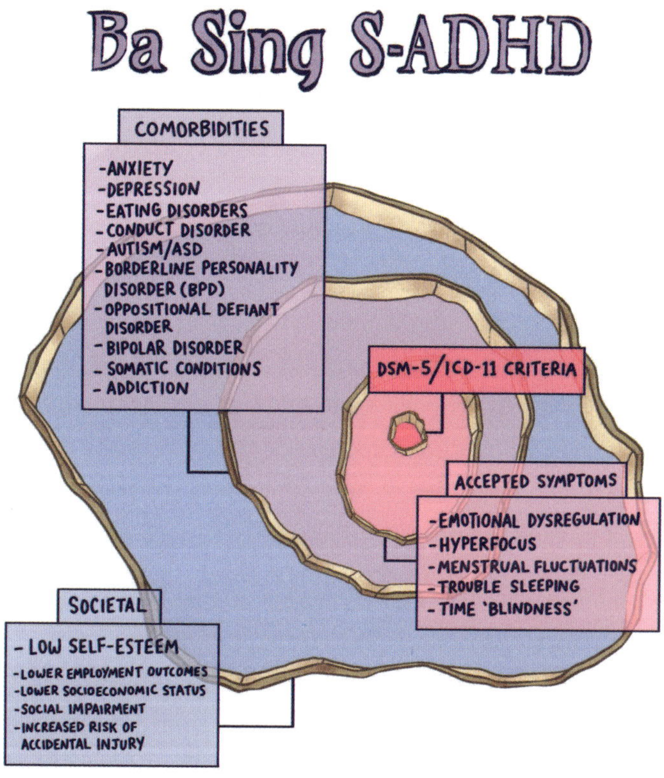

Right in the middle are the written-in-stone clinical symptoms listed in the DSM-5 or ICD-11. These are the ones for which there are piles of data and evidence and widespread **consensus**, and they're the main traits a physician looks for when making a **diagnosis**. But as you're probably starting to gather, the DSM and ICD might be the medical world's diagnostic bibles but, just like the actual Bible, they have a couple of pretty significant issues and omissions. That's why it's important that we venture a little further afield.

So now I welcome you to the second ring – where we find a group of symptoms that aren't officially part of the **diagnostic criteria** but go hand in hand with ADHD for a huge number of people, and still have a decent whack of psychological studies to back up their existence.

Emotional dysregulation

One of the most overlooked characteristics of ADHD is the way it changes how one experiences emotions. Around 70 per cent of ADHD adults experience higher levels of '**emotional dysregulation**', which basically means more rapid and drastic emotional shifts,[7] with frequent highs and lows.[8] It also seems the more severe our ADHD symptoms are, the more intensely we tend to feel negative emotions specifically.[9]

If, until now, most of your exposure to ADHD information has come from social media (no judgement, been there), you might be expecting me to discuss '**rejection-sensitive dysphoria**' right about now. While RSD and other popular internet terms such as '**object permanence**' and '**ADHD paralysis**' can be incredibly useful for communicating the ADHD experience, and are legitimate points of discussion, they have a bit of a complicated relationship with hard-and-fast scientific data. Don't worry, we'll cover them, but just a little later when we chat about ADHD internet culture in Chapter 8.

As part of my attempt to get to know my brain better during this year, I've had many, many conversations with my parents about what I was like as a child, and one thing that came up again and again was just how deeply little me felt every emotion.

'When you were happy you were so, so happy, and you used to make us all happy,' my mum told me. 'But I guess . . . I guess I also wished that things could just be a little closer to the middle for you, too. Because when things went wrong, you'd feel that sadness so deeply as well.' She paused for a moment. 'But then again, I've never met someone who is able to turn a bad day around as well as you. I've also never met someone who benefits so much from just going for a walk.'

And it's true, even to this day I can be in the throes of absolute devastation, and a twenty-minute walk with Mum, Dad or my partner, Anthony, can bring me right back to that 'middle'. Mum generously attributes this to strength of character, and, look, maybe she's right, but I tend to think I just get distracted and forget what I'm upset about. Say what you want about ADHD, but that short attention span can come in handy sometimes.

A number of large studies have concluded that emotional dysregulation is a core element of ADHD for many people[10, 11, 12, 13] and contributes significantly to their level of day-to-day **impairment**.[14] Some experts have even called for ADHD-related emotional volatility symptoms to be included in the next edition of the DSM, which, if it happens, could be a game-changer for ensuring that people with more internally rather than externally disruptive symptoms (particularly girls and women) don't fall through the diagnostic cracks.

Time blindness

Your run-of-the-mill poor time management is a pretty fundamental inattentive symptom of ADHD.[15] This is one of the reasons why physical fitness is important for us, because we regularly have to sprint the last 200 metres to catch our train. But our issues with time get way weirder and more cerebral than this.

Now, the passage of time is a bit wonky for everyone, right? Your first week at a new job feels ten times longer than your fiftieth week. An hour spent playing *The Legend of Zelda: Breath of the Wild* passes much faster than an hour trapped in bumper-to-bumper traffic.

Often in online ADHD communities, we hear people say that a common symptom of ADHD is '**time blindness**'. But this is more of a nickname than an official diagnostic term. See, it's not that we have some totally alien or unique perception of time, it's just that the way we perceive its passing is a bit wonkier than usual.

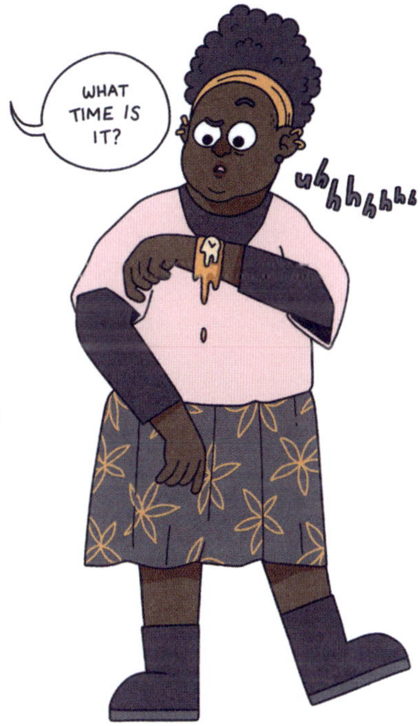

It's been theorised that ADHDers, particularly those with severe hyperactive/impulsive symptoms, tend to experience time very much in the here and now. Dr Russell Barkley (a highly respected ADHD expert and probably the world's best known) has described it as a 'near-sightedness to the future'. He even goes so far as positing that, at its core, ADHD *is* 'time blindness' and its ramifications.[16] This is by no means the clinical consensus – I'm not sure I even totally agree with it myself. But I'm including it because recognising how profoundly ADHD actually impacts my ability to judge, estimate or even really conceptualise time has been an extremely important step in my quest to understand how my brain works.

As usual, we tend to see more of a research focus on kids in this area, with a growing but still significant body of evidence suggesting that ADHD children and teenagers are, on average, considerably worse at estimating how much time has passed than their **neurotypical** peers. Specifically, they tend to overestimate, leading experts to theorise that their 'internal clock' runs slightly faster than the normal person's, meaning they potentially perceive time as moving more slowly.[17] Although far from conclusive, some small studies suggest this applies to ADHD adults as well,[18, 19] but the symptoms do tend to decline with age.

Time blindness part two: delay discounting edition

ADHD impulsivity also plays a big role in our time-related struggles. The ability to choose a larger, more delayed and distant reward over a smaller but immediate pleasure is something that's kind of important for an adult. It's how you do things like 'saving up for a house', 'getting good grades at university' or 'not participating in that third round of king's cup because you don't want to be desperately hungover at your aunt's birthday brunch tomorrow'.

The perceived value of a reward, and therefore your motivation to work towards it, is based, in part, on how far into the future it is. Basically, the further away it is, the less valuable it feels. This effect is called '**delay discounting**' and it's something all humans experience.

Unfortunately, ADHD amplifies these delay discounting tendencies,[20, 21] meaning that if you were to graph out how much we value a reward, its decline as it gets further into the future would be way sharper. For example, if a neurotypical person was asked to choose a packet of chips now or a free five-course gourmet feast in a year's time, chances are they'd choose the feast. An ADHDer might instead think about how much they want those delicious sweet chilli and sour cream chips in their tummy and grab the packet. (This is not a clinically tested example, by the way. And I'm deeply sorry if I've now made you crave sweet chilli and sour cream chips.)

This ADHD tendency towards delay discounting also means the consequences for our actions can feel way less important if we won't face them for some time. This helps contextualise why deadlines and procrastination can be so torturous for people with ADHD, because that pressure of 'Holy shit, I'm about to ruin my life if I don't start writing this essay right now' might not kick in until much closer to D-day than for someone with a neurotypical brain. For many of us, leaving things till the last minute isn't just an occasional hurdle to overcome, it's a way of life.

Delay discounting can also make it really hard to do things like eat healthily or quit smoking, where you're being asked to deprive yourself of dozens of short bursts of pleasure every day and the only motivating factor is the distant, nebulous reward of 'still being alive and healthy when you're seventy'.

Trouble sleeping

Issues with sleep have been associated with ADHD for a really long time, and although it's not part of that core symptom ring, there's a strong argument that it should be. In fact, 'moves about excessively during sleep' was actually on the DSM-III diagnostic criteria list back in the 1980s.[22]

While there's fairly robust research on ADHD sleep issues in children, hard-and-fast data on adults is significantly harder to come by. (Noticing a theme here?) Unfortunately for us sleep-deprived dopamine goblins, the little research we do have estimates that up to 85 per cent of ADHD adults report excessive sleepiness during the day and a poorer quality of sleep in general, including having more trouble drifting off and waking more often during the night.[23] (This is why some in the research world refer to ADHD as a '24-hour disorder'.[24])

Our sleep issues seem to be caused by a combination of factors. Some are pretty straightforward: it's hard to get to sleep if you can't quieten down the 800 million thoughts currently rushing through your head, and struggling with **impulse control** can make it difficult to simply switch off a great TV show or put down an amazing book just because 10 pm rolls around.

Then there's the complicating factor of stimulants – the most common form of ADHD medication. As paradoxical as it sounds, stimulant medications actually help some people with ADHD get to sleep. But for me and many others, they create yet another barrier between us and the sweet escape of unconsciousness, and forgetting to take them until later in the day can mean hours of tossing and turning that night. (We'll get much more into ADHD medications in Chapter 14.)

ADHD also regularly occurs alongside more official sleep disorders and syndromes, such as insomnia disorder, sleep-disordered breathing,[25] restless leg syndrome[26] and narcolepsy. But possibly most interestingly, at least one **meta-analysis** has concluded there is consistent evidence that ADHD is associated with a delayed **circadian rhythm**.[27]

You know that innate instinct of 'when the sun is up, wake up, when the sun is down, get sleepy and go to sleep'? That is your circadian rhythm, and one of the main chemicals that helps control circadian rhythm is **melatonin**. Again, there's more data for children[28] than adults, but one study has shown that night-time melatonin production kicks in nearly an hour and a half later for people with ADHD,[29] meaning that we might not even begin feeling drowsy until well after our intended bedtime. This isn't too much of a drama for people who can just get up later, but if you have any 'am' commitments, for example, a job that requires you to be there at 7 or 9 am, it may mean you're consistently getting significantly less sleep than you'd like.

There appears to be a **correlation** between how severe someone's ADHD symptoms are and how much they struggle with reduced sleep,[30] delayed sleep onset[31] and sleeping disorders in general.[32] But the question is, do the symptoms worsen the sleep issues, do the sleep issues worsen the symptoms, or is there something biological happening in our brains that causes them both? We don't know yet, and it may well be a mix of all three.[33] But it does mean that, for ADHDers, getting a good night's sleep needs to be a priority. If only it weren't so bloody difficult. (Don't worry – we'll talk about some tactics to help with this in Chapter 10.)

Did you know sleep, inattention and impulsivity are all so closely linked that sleep deprivation can even cause ADHD-like symptoms in neurotypical folk?[34] This is part of why ADHD diagnosis can be so complicated, and why a physician may want to rule out the possibility that your issues are entirely sleep-related before prescribing you stimulant medication.

Shark week

I used to joke that when my life started falling apart, I knew my period was coming. It turns out I was probably onto something, because a small but growing body of research suggests that ADHD symptoms and the menstruation cycle are pretty closely linked . . . in the most annoying way possible.

The thing about oestrogen is that, while it's mostly found in the ovaries, it's also produced in the brain, and is known to affect cognitive ability and the functioning of **dopamine**.[35] Thus, menstrual cycles have been found to impact levels of attention, impulsivity, memory, mood regulation and **executive functioning** in general.[36] Which is especially important to factor in when you've got a brain that struggles with these things to begin with.

When oestrogen is high and progesterone is low – such as just before ovulation – it seems cognitive abilities are improved, mood is heightened and ADHD symptoms are diminished. But when oestrogen is low and progesterone is high – such as in the week leading up to one's period – everything, well, kind of goes to crap. Not only do ADHD symptoms become more impairing, but anxiety and depression (conditions that often occur alongside ADHD) may worsen too.[37]

There's also speculation that increased oestrogen and progesterone might negatively impact the efficacy of ADHD medications, particularly as someone goes through 'female' puberty.[38] This has led some researchers to suggest that physicians adjust ADHD medication dosages in line with a patient's menstrual cycle[39] – but this is hardly a widespread practice just yet, and you should never independently adjust your medication regime without consulting a doctor. Nevertheless, if you menstruate, it's probably worth tracking your period and remembering to go easy on yourself as the crimson wave approaches.

Hyperfocus

While the psychological world hasn't spent too much time so far researching the intense bursts of **hyperfocus** experienced by many ADHDers, they're still a widely discussed aspect of the disorder. At least one moderately sized study has shown a clear correlation between adult ADHD and a higher intensity and frequency of hyperfocus across multiple settings.[40]

In my experience, hyperfocus sometimes takes the form of a burst of energy that allows me to get all my work done, clean my entire home top to bottom, and briefly live out my productivity dreams. But it more often means becoming unreasonably obsessed with some random TV show, or convincing myself I'm going to become the kind of person who sews all their own clothes, including designing the patterns (turns out, not as easy as it seems) and purchasing a tiny $50 sewing machine that breaks the first time I try stitching through sherpa fleece and then lies abandoned under my couch for the next year. These bouts of **hyper-fixation** are exceedingly fun, but they don't help all that much with putting away the dishes.

Addiction

As I alluded to earlier, one of the most damaging and dangerous parts of adult ADHD is the way it makes us vulnerable to substance abuse and addiction.

Like, did you know, as an ADHDer you're about three times as likely as your neurotypical pals to become dependent on nicotine?[41] I didn't, and golly gosh I wish I had, because I probably wouldn't have been as blasé about purchasing a disposable vape 'just so I have something to do when I want to step outside a loud party to talk with people'. I knew a number of people who kept one in the back of a drawer somewhere that they'd pull out for a night out, put back when they got home and not think about again for weeks. I assumed I'd be able to do the same, and even though an occasional puff still wasn't particularly healthy, in my mind it didn't seem like a real risk to my wellbeing. But my little stimulation-starved mind couldn't just casually dip in and out of nicotine use. I couldn't simply 'not think about' that vape when I was at home. The temptation of an easy dopamine hit proved too great and, little by little, puff by puff, I gave myself a habit that's taken more than a year, dozens of attempts and a ridiculous amount of mental energy to shake . . . mostly.

ADHDers don't have the luxury of simply not thinking too much about our consumption habits. We're more than twice as likely as a non-ADHD person to develop an alcohol problem, and the risk of us developing any other kind of drug addiction is somewhere between two and three times as high.[42]

Addiction is heavily associated with the brain's reward system, with addictive drugs producing powerful surges of dopamine. So it's not that much of a stretch to assume that this would be particularly hard to resist when you have a hard time with impulse control to begin with and your brain's **dopaminergic** pathways are desperate for a boost.

We also know **self-esteem** plays a big part in substance abuse, something many ADHDers already struggle with. And of course there's that element of self-medication I mentioned earlier, be it using depressants such as alcohol or weed to relax, or using stimulants like caffeine or cocaine because they increase the levels of **noradrenaline** and dopamine in the brain and (potentially) assist with focus.

ADHD's comorbid crew

ADHD very rarely travels alone. It has a whole host of friends who like to tag along. These are known as common **comorbidities**, which just means other disorders that for some reason often occur in the same person at the same time.

These are correlated with ADHD, but the exact nature of their relationship isn't always clear. Is ADHD causing the other disorders? Did the other disorders cause ADHD? Is there something similar in the genetic basis of both disorders? Do they share environmental triggers? Who knows! Not scientists, that's for sure.

Anxiety is one of the most common comorbidities, affecting 44.7 per cent of adults with ADHD compared with 4.9 per cent of those without. Depression rates are also right up there, found in around 42 per cent of us versus 4.7 per cent of non-ADHDers.[43] So it's fairly common for people to take some form of anti-anxiety or antidepressant drug alongside their ADHD medication.

ADHDers are also 3.8 times more likely to experience an eating disorder than non-ADHDers, and 5.7 times more likely to have bulimia nervosa specifically.[44] We really don't know enough yet to say why this is the case – some originally thought it was a consequence of the increased level of anxiety disorders in the ADHD population, but the correlation remains even once you control for that. Some leading researchers have suggested that higher levels of impulsivity and inattention may make someone more likely to show bulimic symptoms, while another theory is that ADHD brains may struggle more with some areas of self-awareness, which can thus distort body image.[45] There's also just the issue of how bloody tough having ADHD can be on your self-esteem, which of course puts people more at risk as well.

Other common comorbidities include: obsessive compulsive disorder, where persistent fears and intrusive thoughts lead to compulsive behaviours; borderline personality disorder, which severely impacts the ability to regulate emotions; and bipolar disorder, which causes episodes of depressive lows and manic highs.

While you obviously can have both ADHD and bipolar disorder, it's worth noting that the oscillations between episodes of mania and depression seen in bipolar – which fall at the extreme ends of the emotional spectrum and often last several days – are quite different from the emotional dysregulation common in ADHD, where moods can shift multiple times a day and usually stay within what you could call the 'normal' range of emotions.[46]

People with ADHD are also more likely to struggle with behavioural conditions such as oppositional defiant disorder and conduct disorder. While the former is overwhelmingly found in children, the latter can persist well into adulthood, and is basically an excessive difficulty with following rules, and persistently behaving in a socially unacceptable way, such as showing aggression towards people and animals, destroying property, stealing, lying and breaking laws. These conditions don't appear in many mainstream media conversations about ADHD, but according to the DSM-5 are really quite common, with conduct disorder affecting about a quarter of children and teens with ADHD-C (combined).[47]

AuDHD

About 12.4 per cent of young people with ADHD are also diagnosed with **autism spectrum disorder** (ASD),[48] and a truly whopping 40–70 per cent of people diagnosed with ASD have ADHD.[49] There's even a nickname now for having both conditions – AuDHD – and this sizeable subgroup has begun carving out its own identity and community in online neurodivergent spaces.

This large overlap is particularly interesting given that until 2013, ASD and ADHD were considered mutually exclusive conditions, meaning your doctor had to pick one or the other to diagnose you with, you couldn't have both. This stipulation was removed in the DSM-5, which has likely contributed significantly to the subsequent rise in the diagnosis for both conditions.

ADHDers have a one in eight chance of also having ASD, so if you have a spare fifteen minutes it probably wouldn't hurt to take the RAADS-R autism test, which you can find online. It's a self-administered questionnaire aimed at identifying those with overlooked or subclinical autism traits, and while it absolutely can't diagnose you (nor can any other online test), it can help clarify if it's worth chatting to your doctor about ASD. For reference, my score was fifty-seven, which means I might show some traits but I'm likely not autistic.

One reason they used to be considered mutually exclusive is that high levels of inattention and hyperactivity/impulsivity are also present in most autistic children. But what we are coming to understand is that the conditions (both in childhood and adulthood) actually have a bunch of similar traits, including executive-function difficulties, social impairments, impulse control, sleep disturbances, hyperfixations and difficulty shifting focus, and even some physical similarities, such as variations in grey matter in certain regions of the brain.[50] Plus, there seems to be some genetic link, too, because having a close family member with one disorder increases your chance of having the other.[51]

However, while certain traits may appear identical from the outside, we know now that they are often caused by very different things. The exact characteristics of both conditions vary greatly from person to person, but to use one example, those with ASD may have a harder time in social situations because it's trickier for them to understand facial expressions and social cues, while someone with ADHD may well internalise all the cues, but their hyperactivity and impulsivity may mean they find it way harder to follow them.

There's clearly some connection between the two disorders, but its exact nature is still a topic of research and debate. A common sentiment in neurodivergent circles is that ADHD is just the 'little brother' to ASD, but this isn't really the case. While it's true that some researchers have begun to question if ADHD and ASD exist on a continuum[52] – or are perhaps different manifestations of a shared condition – this is by no means the general consensus. At the moment it seems they are probably more like cousins than siblings – but given we are only a couple of years into even recognising that the pair can coexist, it's not surprising that we don't have that many firm answers yet.

Friends from all around the body

Moving on from the brain, let's talk about the comorbidities that affect the rest of your body (these are called 'somatic' conditions). Although this is not an exhaustive list, it seems that there is a strong link to asthma, obesity (due both to lifestyle and genetic factors) and of course the sleep disorders I mentioned earlier. There's also a less robust connection with migraines, coeliac disease and circulatory system conditions.[53]

Oh, and we're more likely to contract a sexually transmitted infection, too[54] (possibly because poor impulse control and consistent condom usage don't exactly go hand in hand).

•

Look, adult ADHD is complex, confusing and sometimes seemingly contradictory, but we're learning more about it every day. And as more and more people discover their long-hidden neurodivergent identities, it will only become easier to learn from one another.

This sharing of experiences and building of community is vital, because there's one important question that empirical, science-based, hard-and-fast academic studies have a really hard time answering: What effect does growing up in a world that isn't built for you – constantly feeling different and lazy and hopeless but never understanding why – have on your self-worth?

DIARY ENTRY

Once again, it's 3.30 am

Oh my god it's 3.30 am and I can't get to sleep.

I've been lying in bed for four hours now. It's got to the point where I'm trying to convince myself that I've actually been asleep this whole time and was just dreaming about being awake. All I can do is go over and over the maths in my head, calculating the quickly decreasing number of hours of sleep I'd get if I drifted off this second.

The worst bit is that I specifically went to bed early so I could wake up at the crack of dawn tomorrow (god, actually it's *today*) and get in a full day of book work. But now all I can think about is how tired I'm going to be. How many extra hours I'm going to have to sleep in. How late I'm going to have to work and how late I'm going to get to sleep tomorrow.

Obviously that means that I'm going to waste my entire month. I won't finish this book. I'll be embarrassed publicly. I'll be fired from my job. I'll end up miserable and bitter and unloveable, and that will mean Anthony will leave me. So then I'll have to move out of our apartment, I'll waste all my life savings and I'll probably end up dead in a gutter somewhere.

That, or I'll just be really tired tomorrow, and both of those options are pretty bad.

At 12 am I thought maybe I was too cold, so I put on a hoodie. At 12.30 I thought maybe I was thirsty, so I drank some water. At 1 am I thought maybe I was bored, so I tried listening to a podcast. By 1.14 I figured maybe the podcast was too stimulating, so I switched to an audiobook I'd already listened to but, god damn it, now I'm too bored again to get to sleep.

I just can't turn off the anxiety and noise in my brain. Is this because I took my meds too late? Is this because my meds have worn off too fast?

I want to just say screw it and get up at 8 am anyway and force myself into borderline jet lag to stop this pattern where my bedtime creeps later and later. But chances are, instead of a good day's work, I'd just end up with a full-blown anxiety attack and, let's face it, probably then be too exhausted to actually go to sleep.

How on earth am I meant to have good sleep hygiene when I'm on leave from work and there are no devastating consequences for not getting to sleep on time? How am I meant to get to bed when I know I can just sleep in?

How frustrating is that? I even need a deadline to get to sleep.

This passage better end up in the bloody book, otherwise I will have truly just screwed up a whole day of productivity for nothing.

Let. Me. Sleep.

FUCK.

5

Am I okay?

If I could go back in time to that 23-year-old version of myself – the one crying as she hung up from the psychiatrist Zoom call where she found out she had ADHD – and tell her one thing, this is what it would be.

The true harm that ADHD causes isn't that you forget doctor's appointments, or interrupt people, or struggle to keep the house clean. The most impairing, difficult and life-altering thing about ADHD isn't what it does to your brain at all – it's what it does to your **self-esteem**. That erosion of one's fundamental sense of self is what I've come to think of as the largest feature of that outermost ring of the ADHD **symptom** map. It's the one that is the least directly related to genetics and **neurotransmitters**, but is the source of many of our hardest and most omnipresent struggles.

The most impairing, difficult and life-altering thing about ADHD isn't what it does to your brain at all – it's what it does to your self-esteem.

For that reason, the most important thing you personally can do to 'get better' is recognise the trauma that comes from living with ADHD in a society that isn't built for people like us, and learn to forgive yourself for all the things you'll come to realise were out of your control.

I hope by this point I've managed to impress upon you how most of the symptoms of ADHD are just normal human struggles amped up a few (potentially quite a few) notches. But without a proper understanding of your brain, it's extremely easy to assume that you're simply a bit 'worse' than other people.

We call ourselves 'failures' because our brains are filled with all these passions and ideas and ambitions, but for some reason we can't make our actions match our abilities. We tell ourselves we're 'clumsy' and 'stupid' and 'forgetful' and 'lazy' because another Wednesday has come and gone without us taking the bins out. And we tell ourselves we're 'thoughtless', 'hopeless', 'unreliable' and 'selfish', because why in god's name can't we just remember to text our grandad 'Happy birthday'?

We've learnt to talk to ourselves this way because we were taught to.

20,000 criticisms

One figure that gets thrown around a lot is that ADHD children will experience 20,000 more criticisms than a **neurotypical** kid by the time they are ten. People, including me, tend to assume this is based on some massive academic study where kids carried around a counter and clicked it each time a teacher scolded them for not paying attention, or something like that. But the earliest reference to this number that I can find appears to be in an opinion piece in the May 2010 issue of *Clinical Psychiatry News*, where Dr Michael S. Jellinek created a rough estimate based on the idea that it's not unlikely for an ADHD child to receive three criticisms an hour from a teacher, six hours a day, 180 days a year.[1]

Despite the number perhaps not being as scientific as I'd originally believed, the general idea behind it does have merit. Even if we weren't ultra-disruptive in class, chances are we were still told off far more than our neurotypical peers – for forgetting things, for interrupting, for all those 'careless errors' that we were 'too old to be making'. During this formative period, when we were just learning how to view ourselves and figuring out how the world views us, we spent much of our time bouncing from one mistake to another – perhaps able to understand what we were doing wrong, but at a total loss as to how to stop ourselves doing it again. Sure, little cuts like that heal. But when they're inflicted thousands of times, they are bound to leave a scar.

However, this goes so much deeper than purposeful, conscious criticisms adults might level at 'naughty' kids. Because, the thing is, as you grow, ADHD has a way of teaching you to shrink.

Neurotypical lessons, neurodivergent learnings

For me, it started with the practical stuff, like Mum telling me to 'Stop showing off' when guests would come over. It's not unreasonable to want to host a dinner party that's not utterly dominated by a rambunctious five-year-old demanding you watch her dance routine for the fourth time. I don't blame them for wanting a little more peace and quiet at the table.

But most of the time I wasn't 'showing off' out of some desire for constant attention, I was just excited and had no idea that I was even being loud. And, as an accidental result, I didn't take away a lesson about humility and letting others be heard – I simply internalised the idea that the ultra-excitable, boisterous version of myself was somehow wrong and bad.

As I grew up and was expected to clean up after myself at home, I got into trouble time and time again for not closing the soda water lid properly and letting it go flat, for not putting the seaweed crackers back into the commemorative Arnott's Anzac tin, and allowing them to go stale, for leaving my wet towels on the floor in my room in an ever-growing pile.

'You've just got to switch your brain on, bubby,' Mum and Dad would say. 'The house only works if everyone does their bit.'

'I just wish when you start something, you'd finish it properly.'

'You have to start thinking about other people a bit more.'

I wasn't doing it on purpose, but of course they couldn't have known that. I didn't even know why it was all so hard. I knew what I was doing was lazy and selfish and thoughtless, but it never occurred to me that being lazy or selfish or thoughtless were things people *chose* to do. I assumed they were unchangeable traits that you were born with and it was just tough luck that this meant some people – like me – were inherently bad.

I was lucky – my parents were loving and kind and usually patient – but that's not necessarily the norm. Research is limited, but it seems that parents are more likely to criticise their ADHD kids[2] and less likely to show them warmth, which can become especially problematic when you consider that at least one study has shown that high levels of parental criticism may even lead to ADHD symptoms worsening over time.[3] No wonder so many of us struggle to see the good in ourselves when we're told over and over again that we're the problem.

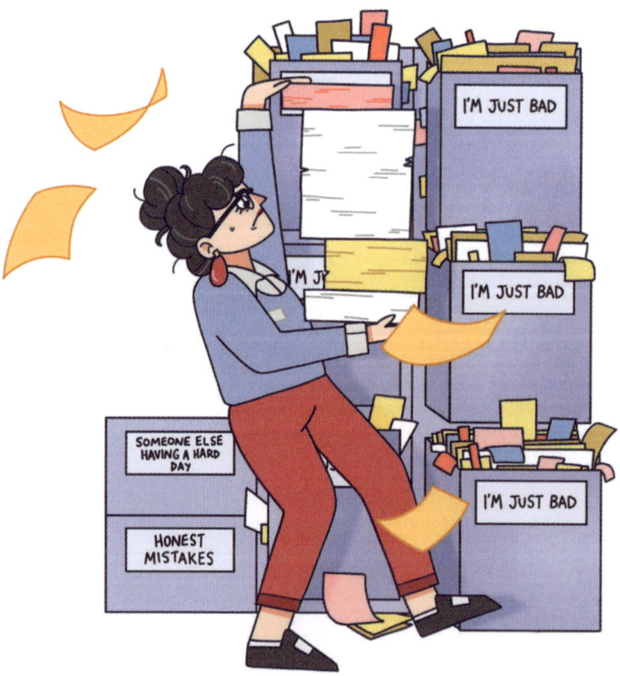

In my first years of school, I was told off a lot for calling out my answers and ideas, with the teacher pulling me aside and telling me that just because I was smart didn't mean it was okay for me to take learning experiences away from other kids. But I wasn't calling out because I wanted to prove I was better than my classmates, or didn't care about them, it was simply that my little brain was brimming with thoughts I wanted to share. Waiting there with my hand in the air, desperately trying to catch my teacher's eye, was so excruciating it was nearly impossible.

Some of my teachers were amazing – they assumed the best of me and found ways to work with my brain, even if they didn't realise it was ADHD causing the classroom issues. But others weren't. So rather than learning about the importance of taking turns and being part of a community, I learnt that voicing my ideas and putting myself in the conversation made me selfish and unfair.

Undercover dumb-dumb

Desperate to be the good kid I believed myself to be but seemed woefully unable to show, I started focusing on the thing I really could be 'good' at: schoolwork. Because even if the teachers sometimes got annoyed at me, they still seemed to like me if I could prove I was smart. Being bright was my way of finding approval, so I clung to it like I clung to my favourite stuffed toy.

Because of this, I probably had a somewhat atypical ADHD experience when it came to academic results. Sure, my school reports had comments here and there about how I needed to focus more and chatter less, but unlike many ADHDers, my youth wasn't marked by the dreaded phrase 'has potential if they only applied themselves'.

For many kids with ADHD, the classroom is one of the most brutal battlegrounds for their self-esteem, and it's through discussions with my close friends who've also recently been diagnosed that I've begun to understand how hard the feeling of early academic struggle can be to shake.

Take Olivia. (I've changed her name, as not all workplaces are as accepting of **neurodivergence** as mine.) We went through all of high school and university together, and despite the fact that she's one of the smartest people I know, throughout those years she would make offhand comments about how she was 'stupid' and 'secretly dumb deep down'. In fact, she said this very thing to me a couple of months back when she was struggling to get started on a big assignment. The issue with this statement? It was an assignment for the final year of her law degree at one of the top law schools in the world.

See, whereas my ADHD eroded my sense of belonging and social acceptance, hers made her mistake struggling to *focus* for struggling to *think*.

'I just couldn't do maths. You saw me trying. It didn't work in my brain at all. And I never got it because I was good at humanities and writing,' she tells me over the phone.

'Looking back, I think *because* some things did come easily to me, I really struggled to actually sit down and force myself to make it click. I just so desperately wanted to do anything else, and I would get so stressed, so it always felt impossible for me to get over that wall.

'I used to be the best-behaved kid in every class and then it would get to maths and I'd constantly fake a tummy ache or a headache and force Mum or Dad to come to get me, or I'd say I needed to go to the bathroom all the time. I just couldn't make myself be there, and I assumed that was because I was too lazy.

'It felt like I had this secret, that I was actually a really dumb person, and I could never let people find out . . . I think that manifested into "Okay, I'll just try to do really well at other subjects and go to law school" and then I can at least say, "Well, I'm a lawyer."'

'But it didn't work, though?' I ask. 'You went to law school and you still felt like that?'

'Oh, 100 per cent,' she laughs. 'In my first year of law, I really was thinking, "Oh my god, I fucking did it," and then second year hit and so did this massive wave of **burnout** and my grades took a drop and that feeling crept up again, where it was just like, "Everyone knows you're stupid, they found out, you haven't proved them wrong."'

But, while a Juris Doctor degree didn't end up being the cure-all Olivia assumed it would be, an ADHD **diagnosis** has managed to take the edge off. 'Previously I would get one bit of negative feedback in a uni assignment or whatever and I'd just crumble,' she said. 'But now, knowing and understanding a bit more, I'm getting to the point where I can get a bad result and can still say to myself, "Well, I'm going all right, you know. Look at me, I live with my partner who I love, I have my cat, my career is going well. It will be fine."'

The social problem

Although schoolwork was never that traumatic for me, school itself was still an excruciatingly difficult experience. Because, like many ADHD kids, I quickly learnt that the playground wasn't the place of respite and joy that it is for others.

School-aged ADHDers are less likely to be liked by their neurotypical peers[4] and more likely to be bullied.[5,6] In fact, many of us have a harder time socialising in general. I mentioned it briefly before, but ADHD has quite a profound impact on a person's interpersonal abilities,[7] especially for those of us with **ADHD-C** (combined).

We know our emotions can be big and hard to control. When we're excited it can be tough for us not to interrupt or talk over people, and having an inattentive, wandering mind can make it difficult to listen to others. As children, we have more trouble with things like sharing and taking turns. It's easy for social cues to get lost in the busyness of our brains, which makes it harder to identify when a social problem has arisen or figure out how to solve it.[8] That kind of stuff is exceedingly difficult for any kid, let alone one whose **prefrontal cortex** is already running on empty.

Not only are ADHD kids often bullied and ostracised, but we – especially the boys – are often written off as troublemakers and pains in the arse. This is where diagnosis can be something of a double-edged sword. While those of us who went through our school years undetected didn't have the relative protection of a clinical explanation that might make teachers more understanding, a number of people who were diagnosed as kids have told me how the label of 'ADHD', in some adults' hands, saw them pigeonholed into being an 'unfixable hooligan' who wasn't worth the effort of trying to help.

I had a lot of trouble with friendships as a kid – I would float from one group to the next, often being told I was too bossy or too annoying to play with. I would find a group of kids I got along with, but arguments were common, and each time I found an incredibly close best friend, the friendship would utterly implode after a couple of years. In fact, looking back, most of my defining heartbreaks and break-ups have been platonic rather than romantic.

I was bullied, too – being thrown off the flying fox, girls trying to trip me down the stairs, a girl hacking into my Yahoo account and sending emails to the other kids, pretending to be me, asking if they thought she was 'a bitch'. (In retrospect, I have to give props to this one. An amazing level of forethought for a ten-year-old.)

Several times throughout my teen years, I had friends tell me I was loud, bossy and self-obsessed. Mostly because I'd interrupt conversations, would always relate other people's stories back to my own similar experiences and would occasionally find myself cracking a joke that crossed the line, seemingly unable to stop talking despite my brain screaming at my mouth to shut up. I'm sure, from my friends' perspective, their comments were justified, but for me, having just come out of several years of intense bullying in primary school, they were absolutely devastating.

I'm not going to pretend I was a total saint – I mean, I was a teenager, and one with a particularly ravenous hunger for attention to boot, so I probably wasn't considering other people's feelings nearly enough. I'm extremely regretful and still hold a little ball of red-hot self-hatred over this – but part of my journey this year has been trying to unpack what was the intentional rudeness of adolescent self-obsession and what was a by-product of the neurological **impairments** I was unknowingly grappling with.

Because, truth be told, a lot of the time I wasn't interrupting because I didn't care what others had to say, but because I'd already worked out the end of their sentence and if I waited rather than blurting out my reply, my thoughts might disappear back into the buzz of noise in my head. Often it was talk now or lose the ability to follow the conversation altogether. And I wasn't relating everything back to my own experiences because I only wanted to talk about myself; it's just that's how I thought you showed someone that you understood and could empathise with what they were going through. I never noticed that it wasn't something everyone did.

So, once again, instead of learning how to be a better friend, the lesson I internalised was that the version of myself I was when I wasn't actively trying to **mask** and fit in was unlikeable and egotistical, and that it was my job to shrink that person down and keep her hidden.

Now, a lot of the time I did like myself. I was proud of my achievements, I was proud of my intelligence, I was proud of being a caring and compassionate friend. And I even loved that I was funny and extroverted. But somewhere deep down, hanging in my semi-conscious awareness, I was convinced that I was merely a bad person who was just desperately trying to be good.

For some, this struggle to process social cues and react appropriately manifests as a perpetual, lingering anxiety – knowing something has gone wrong, and it was probably their fault, but having no clue how to stop it from happening again. At least that's how it felt for Loki: my sister's partner, a close friend and another recently uncovered ADHDer.

'Being hypervigilant and I guess almost paranoid about everything all the time helped me prevent mistakes that I didn't know I was making,' he tells me as we sit on my grandparents' couch.

'For a bit there I thought I might just be really self-centred. I think the idea of being rude is the scariest. You don't want to be rude. You don't want people to think your parents haven't raised you well. I guess all the consequences of not paying attention can add up to be quite heavy.

'Once I moved schools in Grade 5 and was suddenly in this whole other social group and, well, economic class. That was when I leant into being, I guess, the disruptive kid, and the class clown. Because it just seemed easier than trying to fit in. And I do look back at that now and regret it. I think I was pretty unreliable as a friend back then, too.'

'Dude, you were *eleven*. How can an eleven-year-old be unreliable?' I say in a hypocritically annoyed tone.

'Well, I guess with—' he starts, but I interrupt him (our conversations involve a lot of interrupting).

'You were totally overloaded and surrounded by rich kids and stressed out. How did you choose to lean into anything? I mean—'

'Well,' he cuts me off, then pauses. Loki is a conscientious, responsible man, and taking responsibility for his past actions has been an important part of how he's structured his sense of morality. But with late-diagnosed ADHD, accountability isn't always the answer. Sometimes things are just hard, and we fall a little short. Sometimes kids act out. It feels so unfair to me to hear this 29-year-old man talking badly about this little 11-year-old boy. And I realise at that moment that perhaps I've been doing some harsh moral accounting myself – constantly counting the sins of young Matilda in an attempt to shield my present self from failure and guilt.

But there's no time for that kind of self-reflection right now. I'm pretending to be wise and all-knowing – so I stare Loki down.

'Well,' he says again. 'Well, I guess that's just what I decided I'd done when I looked back a few years later.

'I guess it might not have been a super conscious decision.'

I'm not sure he totally believes what he is saying quite yet, but I'll still chalk it up as a win. We'll both get there one day.

The results

Obviously, everyone's experiences with self-esteem will be different, and I'm acutely aware that during my struggles with unidentified ADHD I was in an extremely privileged position. I had relatively low support needs. I was intelligent in a way that allowed me to do well in school despite my attention issues. I had attentive and loving parents who were actively trying to raise a kid with high self-esteem. I grew up middle-class in a wealthy city in a wealthy country. Because I was white and close enough to being conventionally pretty, I was able to play into the 'quirky but loveable weird girl' stereotype and pass off many of my symptoms as socially acceptable *eccentricities*. (I guess I have Zooey Deschanel and Lisa Kudrow to thank for that.) I was extraordinarily lucky . . . and yet my self-esteem was still ripped to absolute shreds by the time I reached adulthood.

Studies have repeatedly shown that ADHD kids and adults end up with significantly lower self-esteem than their neurotypical peers,[9] a problem that's only exacerbated by lack of treatment.[10]

And it's easy to see how this contributes to other negative ADHD outcomes, such as the likelihood of **comorbid** anxiety and depression, higher rates of **substance abuse**, eating disorders and, in the most extreme cases, suicidal ideation and actions.

At least one study has shown that ADHD adults tend to have lower **self-efficacy** as well[11] – meaning we may believe we're less capable of fixing the problems that emerge in our lives, and generally perceive ourselves to be less in control. When you consider the trouble our long-suffering prefrontal cortex has keeping everything in order, it's true that in some ways, we genuinely are in less control of our lives.

If you have ADHD, you've probably spent years trying and failing to get your shit together, being told over and over that you just need to be more determined, more organised, more careful, and yet things don't seem to change. For many of us, pulling ourselves up by our bootstraps through sheer willpower simply isn't possible. That's not because we're bad people. It's just bad advice.

ADHDers can still live a productive, fulfilling life. It just involves changing your world to suit you rather than yourself to suit your world. That's why therapy, introspection and learning to treat yourself with compassion are such integral parts of the treatment process, especially for those diagnosed in late adolescence or adulthood. ADHD is funny that way – it's a disorder where the two most effective medications are strictly regulated stimulant drugs and a profound capacity for self-forgiveness.

Healing from this trauma is possible, though. And I'm not just saying that because of course that's what you're meant to say. I'm saying it because I think I'm starting to feel it happening. I've worked hard to learn about my brain and why I faced the struggles I did. Yes, it's been difficult and painful, but also totally worth it. My anxiety has dropped, my self-worth has gone up, and I'm in the process of rewriting my history so it's filled with more kindness and understanding.

I'm not exaggerating when I say that learning I had ADHD was the most positive, wonderful, hopeful thing that has ever happened to me.

I'm not exaggerating when I say that learning I had ADHD was the most positive, wonderful, hopeful thing that has ever happened to me.

It's still a work in progress, but this change was only possible because I accidentally happened across the right information, recognised ADHD symptoms in myself and managed to get diagnosed.

No single study should be taken as gospel, but it's worth noting that at least one academic paper has concluded that when you compare adults who show symptoms of ADHD, those with an official diagnosis have better-functioning social and family lives than those without. They're more productive at work, they rate their health-related quality of life higher, and, would you look at that, they have significantly better self-esteem.[12]

Now, don't get me wrong: even ADHDers who were diagnosed before they were out of a highchair still face significant, life-altering struggles. But I can't help wondering how much of the damage to my self-esteem could have been avoided if the adults in my life had been given the resources and education that would have allowed them to recognise the warning signs.

DIARY ENTRY

The bad wife

I don't think we talk enough about how isolating having ADHD can be for adult women. ADHD is never easy, but I can't help but feel that the entrenched gender roles that permeate every aspect of our society seem so much more forgiving when it comes to the typical ADHD experience for a cisgender, straight man – diagnosed or not.

Imagine a nineteen-year-old guy. He's struggling with ADHD but has no idea he has it. He's finished school, moved out of home, and naturally ends up living in a shared house with a few of his mates. The apartment is a mess, there's dust filling every corner, the only food in the fridge is leftover pizza and the dishes are stacked shoulder-high in the sink.

All of those are manifestations of ADHD, but it's also typical for young men. There's barely any shame attached to it. The fact that our guy is living on takeaway and there's no toilet paper in the bathroom are just goofy aspects of the socially accepted young bachelor lifestyle.

This doesn't mean he's okay or coping, but everyone still gives him the benefit of the doubt and assumes he'll grow out of it.

And the thing is, he does. By the time he's in his mid-twenties and people start getting a little less forgiving, chances are he's found himself a serious girlfriend, and probably a neurotypical one to boot.

He proposes to her, or they at least move in together, and suddenly he isn't a bachelor. And no matter how much feminist theory either of them has read, it's still totally normal and accepted that she's the one who'll keep track of what needs to get done in the home.

She does the shopping because it's easier than explaining everything they need to him. She makes most of the meals because she has more cooking experience. She wants the house to stay nice, but even if they divide the chores equally, she still tells him what to clean and when. She's organising the dinner parties and buying his mum a birthday gift. And when they do eventually have kids, she's the one ensuring that all excursion slips get signed and handed in.

Yes, work is still much tougher for him than for his neurotypical colleagues, but luckily he now has the time and mental energy to ensure he stays afloat.

It's not on purpose, it's not even his fault. But because women are still ultimately expected to be running the household, no one will bat an eyelid when she's left in charge of the logistics of his life, unconsciously carrying so much of his executive-functioning burden. Not even her. Not even him.

But for girls with ADHD, things are different.

Sure, when the young ADHD woman moves out of home, there's a bit of leeway for her messy shared house and her empty fridge, but people do think to themselves, 'She really should be eating healthier and wasting less money on food delivery' and 'Gosh, no wonder her boss isn't taking her seriously; she left all her clothes crumpled up in a pile on the floor.'

By the time she's twenty-two, people are already wondering if she'll ever get her shit together, but unlike for her male counterpart, there isn't really a finish line in sight. Because when she gets into her mid-twenties, finds a nice neurotypical boy and they decide to settle down, all those taxing, executively demanding tasks don't suddenly fade away. They double.

Her partner is well-meaning, but he never learnt to cook properly or competently execute a weekly shopping trip. He never got judgemental comments about his messy shared house from relatives, so it doesn't occur to him to clean things up without prompting.

When the two of them were growing up, it was always their mums who dealt with the school stuff like buying uniforms and signing forms, so without ever consciously thinking about it, when they have kids they both assume she'll be in charge of that too.

Ultimately, societal norms dictate that she's the person running the day-to-day functioning of the house. And she's failing at it.

She never manages to get everything she needs at the supermarket or finish the cleaning. Cooking dinner nearly brings her to tears, and she constantly forgets that little Andy doesn't like tomatoes. The kids' lunchboxes are filled with packaged snacks because that's just easier, but, oh my god, now the school has sent home a letter saying it's trying to reduce waste.

On top of this, she's trying desperately to keep her head above water at work but she's already exhausted by the time 9 am rolls around, let alone 5 pm.

People with ADHD are often incompetent homemakers. But that's only a crime for one side of the gender binary. The traditional female role is about self-control and organisation and caring for others constantly, while still finding time to care for yourself when no one is watching. That's difficult for all women, but having ADHD as a girlfriend, wife or mother is a shameful transgression of womanhood that carries its own personal brand of trauma.

I'm lucky. I'm queer, but as a woman in a relationship with a man, I hit the jackpot when I found my partner, Anthony, who's managed to shed the constraints of toxic masculinity better than anyone I've ever met. He's caring and precise, and willing not only to divide those high-executive-functioning tasks down the middle, but to take on so much of my load too. He's never made me feel less worthy because I can't fulfil the homemaker role the way society expects, and his generosity has allowed me to flourish. I'm so grateful for him.

But also, that's the problem, right? The fact that I'm so grateful. If he were the woman and I were the man, it would probably never even occur to me to be grateful for the role he plays in our home. That would have been the norm.

ADHD men and women both struggle, but ADHD men – at least the straight ones – are almost guaranteed to find some respite in a relationship. ADHD women – at least the straight ones – have to win the relationship jackpot just to keep the difficulty level of their lives the same as it would be if she were on her own.

6

Where did all the girls go?

The other day I was playing around with an AI image-generator bot that uses information from all around the internet to create a picture of whatever prompt you type in. I'd seen a few videos of people inputting the names of different disorders and getting awesome artistic results, so I put in 'ADHD' just to see what might come up – expecting something like an abstract pattern or a hurricane of objects showing how fast everything moves in the ADHD brain.

But instead, what I got was a seven-ish-year-old white boy sitting at a desk, staring at a worksheet, one arm flailing around in the air, the other pulling at his hair in frustration. And that's the issue, right? Scour all the internet, base your information on our cumulative collective understanding of ADHD, and a hyperactive little white boy is what you get.

It's widely accepted that women with ADHD are systematically underdiagnosed, undertreated and underrepresented.

We've spoken a bit about why the 'hyperactive' element of this stereotype paints a pretty inaccurate picture of what many (possibly even the majority of) people's ADHD looks like. But how about the other bits? Well, why don't we start with gender?

It's widely accepted that women with ADHD are systematically underdiagnosed, undertreated and underrepresented. The question is, by how much, and why?

Before we dive in, I want to flag that the language and information in this chapter aren't going to be as inclusive as I'd like when it comes to intersex, gender diverse and trans people with ADHD, because unfortunately the vast majority of ADHD studies, even those specifically looking at gender, make no mention of those who fall outside the strict categories of cis woman and cis man.

ADHD intersects with 'womanhood' in multiple ways. Cultural expectations are placed on women and girls that clearly impact anyone society perceives as female, as well as those who went through a cultural 'girlhood' regardless of their identity now. And then there are also aspects of the disorder that are defined by biological sex characteristics, and are therefore more likely to apply to those born with bodies closer to the female side of the spectrum.

At first I assumed I'd be able to separate out the two, adjusting my language to include different groups as needed. But the issue is that research into the 'female' presentations of ADHD is in its absolute infancy, and for the majority of the time we just don't know with any degree of certainty which aspects of the disorder are caused by culture or biology or both. So including or excluding gender diverse people in the results of a study that makes no mention of them would mean me taking a wild guess at what causes that aspect of ADHD.

As a result, for most of this chapter I will only be referring to 'girls' or 'women' because, unfortunately, the research simply won't let me be any more specific. But please know that I understand how vastly inadequate this terminology often is.

Where are we?

It's generally – but not universally – accepted that ADHD is more common in males than females. When researchers pick out a random group of people and screen them for ADHD, they find there's usually a male to female ratio of a little over 2:1 throughout childhood and 1.6:1 among adults.[1] Now, there are a couple of complicating factors that potentially cast doubt on these ratios, but even if we just accept that boys are twice as likely to have ADHD as girls, we still have a problem.

Because that 2:1 ratio tells us how many girls *should* be diagnosed with ADHD, not how many actually *are*. When we look at studies that source their subjects from the 'clinical population' –

meaning the population of people actually clinically diagnosed with ADHD – those male to female ratios stretch out as high as 9:1.[2]

Again, because not that many places actually keep track of **diagnosis** rates, recent population-wide statistics are hard to come by, but UK health records,[3] as well as some smaller European clinical-population-based studies and the European Network Adult ADHD, place the boy to girl childhood diagnosis ratio in the range of 4:1 to 6:1 (using data from the 2010s),[4,5] while at least one study from eastern Asia puts it around the 4.1:1 mark.[6]

And remember, ADHD is significantly underdiagnosed in general. When you consider how many boys we're missing in the first place, those numbers paint an even bleaker picture.

Things might be getting better, though, at least in a few lucky countries. For instance, between 1995 and 2010, Denmark went from a 7.5:1 ratio of newly diagnosed school-age boys and girls, to 3:1. And from 8.1:1 to 1.6:1 in adolescents.[7] But even if every country around the world fixed their gender ratios of new ADHD diagnoses tomorrow, there would still be millions of adult women who have already fallen through the cracks, left to break the neurodivergent code by themselves, and trying to figure out what on earth went wrong.

So how did we get ourselves into this mess in the first place? Well, in true ADHD fashion, I've ordered all the things that are to blame in a nice, numbered list:

1. historical invisibility
2. widespread ignorance of female ADHD symptoms
3. the gendered social expectations placed on women
4. the fact that no one in this world is willing to talk about menstruation enough
5. and a healthy serving of plain old-fashioned sexism.

Let's get started.

Historically hyperactive boys

I was surprised to learn that some of the oldest historical references to ADHD-like conditions actually do acknowledge that girls can suffer from these 'morbid alterations of the mind' as well. Even way back in 1798, Sir Alexander Crichton described in his writings for the UK's Royal College of Physicians the attentional disorder he was seeing as 'giving him or her an unnatural degree of mental **restlessness**'.[8]

In Sir George Frederic Still's 1902 Goulstonian Lecture, which a lot of people consider to be the starting point of the scientific history of ADHD, he even estimated the gendered ratio to be around 3:1[9] – which isn't that far off the mark.

Fun fact: Crichton's original description of what in retrospect appears to be modern-day ADHD defined the condition as 'the incapacity of attending with a necessary constancy to any one object'. And, honestly, I think he kind of nailed it first go. He also suggests that the disorder is a consequence of the uniformity of the British education system and laments that 'the peculiar idiosyncrasies or dispositions of each individual are seldom sufficiently attended to'. Why didn't we just listen to him from the beginning?

Then again, while listing things that could distract those experiencing the condition 'to such a degree, as almost approaches to the nature of delirium', he included 'The barking of dogs, an ill-tuned organ, or the scolding of women.' So maybe not a total feminist hero.

Unfortunately, this gender-inclusive thinking didn't seem to stick, and although girls with ADHD were acknowledged in passing in most twentieth-century medical literature, they were rarely discussed, studied or treated as anything more than a curious aberration.

As a result, for more than two centuries, the vast majority of ADHD study has been done exclusively on male children. I didn't truly wrap my head around just how profound the ramifications of this were until I spoke to clinical psychologist Dr Ellen Littman, one of the researchers who has spent decades fighting in the trenches, trying to get the struggles of women with ADHD recognised.

'It's been a long, difficult road filled with, unfortunately, misogyny and gender **bias**,' she tells me. 'I've worked myself into the research organisations that are controlled by old white men, and some literally refuse to do research on females. And they have a lot of power, because whatever gets published in peer-reviewed journals, those are the facts in our universe.'

One of the core issues is that in those early years when the great minds of the mental health world were defining ADHD, they based their model and **diagnostic criteria** on what was easiest to see – the hyperactive little boy.

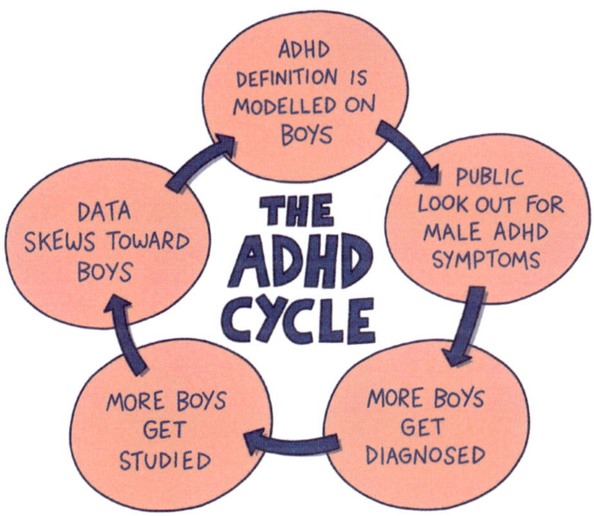

This dictated how ADHD was viewed by not just the medical world but the culture at large – so, of course, it was the disruptive, energetic little boys who parents and teachers were most likely to clock and send off to be diagnosed.

Thus, when the next wave of researchers came along, determined to refine our understanding of ADHD even further, guess what most of the pool of potential, officially diagnosed research subjects looked like?

'All of the studies are so skewed, and continue to tell us nothing about the girls who don't look like hyperactive boys,' Littman tells me.

And so the vicious cycle continued, with the male-centric model of ADHD reinforced again and again. Sometimes it feels as if this was the unintentional original sin of ADHD research, and we're only now beginning the slow, tedious process of untangling the knots it has created.

But, now that we are at least starting to recognise this mistake, why don't we have a look at what the last decade or so of research into female ADHD has uncovered?

Just a note: while there's next to no research looking into the intersection of both gender and race when it comes to ADHD diagnosis and treatment, it doesn't feel like much of a stretch to suggest that young girls of colour with ADHD would feel the compounded effects of both the gendered diagnosis and treatment prejudices, and the racial ones, which we'll explore further in the next chapter.

The inattentive elephant in the room

Right off the bat, I want to make it clear that there aren't two different ADHD disorders, one for boys and one for girls. Just as childhood ADHD and adult ADHD can look drastically different, so can the typical male and female presentations. It's all the same disorder, but a combination of biological differences, hormones and prescriptive gender roles mould the condition into different shapes.

If you'll allow me to drastically oversimplify and generalise for a second, the easiest way to describe the difference is that boys are more likely to externalise their ADHD symptoms, and girls are more likely to internalise them.

There are myriad reasons why this may be the case, but probably the most well-known piece of this gender puzzle is that girls tend to experience less of the hyperactive and impulsive symptoms, and more of the inattentive ones. Potentially 57 per cent of ADHD girls have **ADHD-I** (inattentive) compared with 47 per cent of the boys.[10] And, as we've seen, inattentive kids are already less likely to be diagnosed, with their symptoms often slipping under the radar.

You'll notice that 47 per cent of boys is still a huge percentage of people with inattentive ADHD, so please don't think I'm implying that girls and women are the only groups being failed by the system. This is another one of those ways that fixing the societal problems women face will also massively benefit men.

'There's lots of studies that show that both parents and teachers, and even primary care paediatricians, have drunk the Kool Aid,' Littman says. 'And so they're like, "Oh, these boys, they're really disruptive so we're definitely going to send them for evaluation." These girls who are just sort of daydreaming, they're passive . . . And so everyone agrees, "Yeah, they're weird," but they're not getting sent for referral or evaluation.'

Sometimes it feels as if this was the unintentional original sin of ADHD research, and we're only now beginning the slow, tedious process of untangling the knots it has created.

And remember, we didn't formally acknowledge the possibility of ADHD existing without **hyperactivity** until 1980,[11] meaning that for hundreds of formative years, half of all girls with ADHD wouldn't have met the criteria to be diagnosed (let alone studied) even if they did get the chance to be assessed.

Unfortunately, when discussing female underdiagnosis, people tend to both start and end with this inattentive explanation. As a woman with **ADHD-C** (combined), who honestly wasn't particularly quiet or unassuming in class and was *still* missed, it's always felt like this just couldn't be the whole story. And it's not.

Internalise that shit

Regardless of whether they have ADHD-I (inattentive) or ADHD-C (combined), girls still tend to internalise their symptoms more than boys, and even their hyperactive and impulsive symptoms look drastically different.[12]

While a hyperactive boy might be hyperphysical, running around and unable to sit still, hyperactive girls might be more hyper-emotional – with ecstatic bursts of joy and a tendency to dissolve into uncontrollable tears – or hyper-talkative – chatting someone's ear off about the things that excite them, and struggling to control the impulse to interrupt and to wait patiently with their hand up to be called on by the teacher.[13]

But as a society, we're not that kind to hyper-talkative, hyper-emotional little girls. In an article Dr Littman wrote all the way back in 2000, she noted that these young girls were often dismissed as 'silly', 'show-offs' or 'boy crazy'. And, god, does that 'show-off' line cut me deep.

We know that children are highly cognisant of and responsive to the restrictive and prescriptive gender roles in our society. Even though there's a big push to fight against these stereotypes nowadays, little girls understand that society wants women to be caring and soft and compliant, and not to take up too much space. From what I've seen of the world, girls are punished for being loud, disruptive 'show-offs' in a way little boys just aren't. But the little dreamer girl – the space cadet whose head is in the clouds – well, that's much more palatable. There's nowhere near enough research or data to say this definitively, but I don't find it too much of a stretch to suggest that we as a society may be subconsciously leading girls, with both carrot and stick, down the path of internalising and **masking** their ADHD symptoms, teaching them long before they ever step foot in a classroom which parts of their identity they need to hide in order to be a 'good girl', no matter their clinical **presentation**.

Even less is known about how societal bias affects ADHDers who are First Nations people or people of colour, especially the girls. But given the pervasiveness of racial stereotypes, it would make sense that the pressure to fit in and mask one's struggles would be even stronger.

Unfortunately, hiding in plain sight often comes at the cost of **self-esteem**. In general, Dr Littman says, 'Boys and men externalise these things and project blame onto everyone else. So they go, "I failed this test because it was a stupid test and the teacher doesn't know anything," versus a girl, who will say, "I failed this test, I'm so stupid, I didn't study enough, it's all my fault and I'll never get into college."'

This degradation of self-esteem is often compounded when class ends and lunchtime play begins, and those social-skills deficits rear their heads in a uniquely gendered way.[14] 'For boys, if you can all play baseball or football together then everything is fine, but for girls and women, where interactions are much more verbal and intimate, and about reading social cues that are subtle, ADHD girls have a terrible time, and are usually excluded and bullied,' Littman says. 'So they start, at a very early age, feeling pretty horrible about themselves.'

This is when we begin to see another vicious cycle form, with low self-esteem often leading to even further internalisation of girls' symptoms. 'They mask their symptoms as best they can, and they think that they've won if they can sort of – and you can't see the air quotes – "pass for normal".' Littman laughs, clearly not convinced by the whole idea of 'normal' to begin with.

Often girls and women with **undiagnosed** ADHD will attempt to compensate for their struggles with perfectionism. If the girl is bright, there may never be a report card full of bad grades that could cause concern for teachers and parents, and lead them to look deeper into the fact that she's struggling. If she can't focus and spends half her time distracted, she might just spend twice as long getting the task done. If she can't listen in class, no matter – she'll add an extra couple of hours of study to her afternoon to teach herself the content.

I'm saying 'she' here, but really, I do mean me. I know this isn't what ADHD is like for everyone, but especially near the end of high school, I became utterly fixated on the idea of doing well in the final exams and becoming dux of the school (or valedictorian, if you're in North America). I told everyone it was because I was desperate to get into law school, but I knew deep down that I didn't actually want that. What I wanted was something tangible that I could hold up to show my peers or the world and say, 'Hey, I might be weird and I'm pretty sure my friends all secretly hate me, but I am worth something.'

'Their experience still is just as painful,' Littman says. 'And no one will recognise that they need help.'

This habit of masking symptoms, combined with the fact that female versions of hyperactivity may be harder for a teacher to spot, means that the diagnostic practices of looking at someone's past or current school reports to confirm they displayed symptoms of ADHD prior to the age of 12 (one of the **DSM-5**'s key diagnostic requirements) may not be as reliable for girls,[15] which is a problem, given it's one of the most widely used techniques.

Complicating matters further is the fact that pretty much all the most popular clinical ADHD questionnaires barely reference internalised, emotional symptoms and **impairments** at all, so it's reasonable to assume that there are plenty of ADHD girls who might not meet the official criteria for diagnosis even if they were assessed.

But often it doesn't ever get to this point, because when someone does notice a girl is struggling, ADHD is rarely the first theory as to why.

Depressed, not distracted

One important aspect of the internalisation of ADHD symptoms is the tendency for the struggles a person is experiencing to be expressed through **comorbid** disorders such as generalised anxiety and depression – both of which appear to be more common among ADHD women than ADHD men.[16, 17]

Boys and men with ADHD are also at increased risk of comorbid anxiety and depression compared to the general population, but also tend to lean more towards externalised behavioural issues such as **substance abuse** and antisocial personality disorder.[18]

What often happens is that parents and teachers see something is wrong, the girl or young woman is taken to speak with a specialist, and they will take one look at her, see the stress she is under, how low her self-esteem is, how much she's struggling socially or academically, and diagnose her with anxiety or depression. If they learn she's restricting or bingeing foods, they might throw in an eating disorder diagnosis too.

Of course, these are all common ADHD comorbidities, but they're also just common conditions generally. So, without the telltale descriptions of the girl being 'disruptive in class' or 'unable to sit still', combined with the 'ADHD is for little boys' bias that the doctor likely subconsciously holds, it may never cross their mind that they should keep digging in order to uncover another diagnosis that ties everything together.

In case you wanted some real-world numbers to back up this claim, a survey from the US found that only 5 per cent of young boys were treated with antidepressant medications before receiving an ADHD diagnosis, compared with 14 per cent of young girls.[19]

I can speak from personal experience here, as I was diagnosed with anxiety long before anyone thought I might have ADHD. The low hum of my anxiety has been a part of my life since puberty, but I was first told it might be at the level of 'a disorder' towards the end of high school, around the time I became obsessed with becoming the dux of my year and utterly **burnt out** trying to get there. But despite my doctor writing me a prescription, I was too afraid to fill it (mostly because I'd heard that it made it hard to orgasm and, as a teen who had recently discovered how to do that, I wasn't about to give it up.)

But five years, three jobs and a couple of months of global pandemic lockdowns later, my mini panic attacks had become full-fledged ones and the periods of grey I'd become accustomed to transformed into deep, vast pools of black.

So, I decided I needed to chat to my doctor again about getting some extra help.

Taking my daily dose of anti-anxiety medication really did help smooth out the lowest of the lows and the highest peaks of panic (and thankfully the big O remained within my alphabet, unaffected).

But it didn't really touch the constant mountain of jobs and chores, or the voice in my head that shouted 'You're not good enough' during moments of quiet. I was still perpetually overwhelmed and prone to breaking down when things got too much. Life still felt way harder than it should, so that base level of anxiety didn't really ease.

I'd resigned myself to the idea that this was how I was always going to feel. But then, nine months later, I was diagnosed with ADHD. I had no idea this would happen, but starting stimulant medication helped turn the volume down on the constant wall of noise in my mind. I started to forgive myself for the things I messed up and started letting myself take breaks when I needed them. Then one week, maybe a year into my diagnosis, I woke up and realised that something was different now. I still got anxious, but I hadn't felt that constant hum of anxiety in months.

Some people even find that after starting ADHD treatment they can wean themselves off their anxiety or depression medication (under the careful guidance of a doctor), because they are now treating the root cause.

So far, this hasn't been my experience, but although I'm not utterly cured – and I still take my morning 100-milligram sertraline – being diagnosed with ADHD was like turning my anxiety thunderstorm into a spring shower. To the point where a few Fridays ago, my boss sent me a message saying, 'Hey can we chat on Monday?' and I actually still managed to have a good, relaxing weekend. Absolutely unheard of. (The chat ended up being some minor changes to how we should organise our files, so thank god I didn't spend hours crying over it like 2020 Matilda undoubtedly would have.)

Shark week . . . again

Another big factor medical professionals often ignore when they're treating people who have been through female puberty is the massive impact hormones and old Aunty Flo have on the condition.

Because the level of oestrogen in someone's system can impact their mood, their outlook, even the severity of their ADHD symptoms, it can totally skew how that person may appear to the doctor during their ADHD assessment, and may well mean they miss out if they seem a little too 'put together' (classic ovulating behaviour right there). Littman says that part of the problem we still face is that nowhere near enough mental health professionals are taking the time to ask the simple question, 'And when did you get your last period?'

Bias, pure and simple

The significant aesthetic differences in the traditional female ADHD presentation go a long way towards explaining why they're being so systematically missed by the schooling and medical systems, but we can't let our society off the hook that easily. The truth is, there's still a significant amount of plain old sexism at play, too. People in caring roles generally view girls as suffering less from ADHD-like symptoms and believe they will benefit less from treatment, even if their presentation is exactly the same as boys. How do we know this? Well, it was tested.

There have been a number of studies where teachers were given short descriptions or 'vignettes' of imaginary children whose behaviour was consistent with either ADHD-I (inattentive), **ADHD-H** (hyperactive/impulsive) or ADHD-C (combined), and then asked how likely they would be to approach the kid's parents and encourage them to seek further assessment. Each teacher got identical sets of vignettes, except the names of the children were randomly swapped between male and female.

Now, unsurprisingly, they were less likely to recognise the symptoms of ADHD-I in both boys and girls compared to the symptoms of ADHD-H or C, and viewed those kids with ADHD-I symptoms as being less impaired. However, within all three presentations, boys were still being referred for further assessment more often than girls, and teachers seemed to consider medication to be a less suitable option for girls, too.[20,21]

Remember, the descriptions of the kids' behaviour were identical, so it wasn't just girls expressing their hyperactivity in a different way that made them slip under the ADHD radar – it was simply the fact they were girls.

I should note that the results of the gender-bias studies mentioned above weren't totally universal. Two similar vignette studies concluded that symptom severity and ADHD presentation affected teachers more than gender.[22,23] But in both cases, teachers were still worse at recognising ADHD-I (inattentive). Thus, girls (who are more likely to have this presentation) are still less likely to be referred for treatment.

Interestingly, one of these studies that specifically showed a gendered referral bias against ADHD-C (combined) girls versus ADHD-C boys was conducted on primary school teachers in my home city of Melbourne, Australia, in 2009 – the year I was in Grade 6 – probably not much more than a couple of months removed from when my teacher called my mum to say I seemed to be interrupting in class more and ask was there something wrong.

I don't bring up these stats in order to place the blame on teachers. (I mean, parents also tend to underestimate the severity of hyperactive and impulsive symptoms in girls, while potentially overestimating them in boys.[24]) But I think it's important to recognise that in the current system, a huge weight of responsibility is placed on teachers to scout for and recognise symptoms of ADHD in children. Often they're our first and last line of defence, and yet we don't properly prepare them for it. In most places around the world, trainee teachers aren't taught how to spot the subtle signs of female inattentive ADHD, how to overcome racial and gender biases, or about the nuances of masking and hiding in plain sight. We just throw the teachers in at the deep end and hope for the best.

ADHD is the most common childhood **neurodevelopmental** disorder. There's probably at least one ADHD kid in every classroom. Surely university education courses around the world could spare a mandatory lecture or assignment or two to ensure every future teacher graduates with a correct understanding of it?

While no large ADHD-specific studies have addressed both gendered and racial referral bias as far as I can see, we know that in the US, African American girls are five times more likely to report being expelled or suspended than their white female classmates,[25] so it's plausible that even if an African American girl is hyperactive and acting out in class, teachers may be more likely to view this as a disruption requiring discipline than a sign of a kid who needs help.

The first to notice

Remember at the start of the chapter when I mentioned that there were still some question marks around that 2:1 boy to girl **prevalence** estimate for ADHD? Well, the thing is, when we move out of the realm of childhood diagnosis and into the adult world, where people have the ability to recognise the symptoms of the condition within themselves and proactively seek treatment, the gender gap in the rate of new diagnoses shrinks dramatically.[26]

There are a few potential explanations for this:

1. **Perhaps it's a simple course correction. Boys are more likely to be diagnosed young, so by the time you get to adulthood, the pool of undiagnosed ADHDers is disproportionately female.**
2. **Maybe there's something biological about women and those with female sex characteristics that makes ADHD more likely to persist into adulthood. We know that prevalence gender ratios (the population of people estimated to have ADHD overall, not just those who have been diagnosed) shrink from just over 2:1 in childhood to 1.6:1 in adulthood,[27] so that's not out of the question.**
3. **Perhaps it's because society places a larger executive-functioning burden on women (to care for husbands' and children's needs and run the household), and therefore the effects of ADHD continue to negatively affect women later into life, and thus they meet the DSM-5's requirement that symptoms clearly reduce a person's quality of life for longer.**
4. **Or maybe the way we've defined ADHD in children is still pretty bad at actually describing the way young girls experience the disorder, so it takes an adult ADHD woman to connect the dots for herself. That is to say, perhaps ADHD is actually distributed way more equally between the sexes than we assume.**

Honestly, it might be a mix of all four. But regardless of the root cause, it's clear we need to be making information about ADHD, especially the typical female and adult presentations, more widely known and accessible across the whole population. These numbers show that undiagnosed women with ADHD are eminently capable of recognising the symptoms of ADHD within themselves and are motivated to find the help they need – they just need someone to point out that they might need help in the first place.

So far left to go

If the ADHD gender balance does start levelling out in adulthood, why does the underdiagnosis of girls really matter? Well, because going undiagnosed is harmful in and of itself. This stuff doesn't go away when someone turns eighteen. It's not as if you can just run out the clock and suddenly troubled, undiagnosed girls will turn into fully functioning, healthy women.

ADHD children face these social and academic problems whether they're diagnosed or not, but without a diagnosis, they're left without an explanation for why they're struggling, and without treatments that have been repeatedly shown to drastically reduce their level of impairment.

'Our goal is early identification and intervention, because left unaddressed . . .' Littman says, pausing to find the right words. 'Well, I don't think I've ever worked with a woman who did not say at various points, "I am so stupid." These are people who are not in any way stupid.

'This is about your identity and labelling yourself in a very negative way, because it's very hard to undo those labels.'

Studies show that the low self-esteem and negative self-image ADHD girls develop in childhood persist into adolescence and well into adulthood, and remain more severe than in both ADHD men and non-ADHDers.[28] They have higher rates of anxiety and depression than **neurotypical** women their age,[29] are more likely to have persistent bipolar disorder and conduct disorder,[30] and are more likely to have become a teen mother.[31]

When girls move out of home, enter the workforce and perhaps start a family, the burden on their **executive function** keeps increasing, which leads ADHD women to feel a lack of control over their lives, as if they're constantly disorganised and have no agency or ability to fix the problems they are facing.[32]

We know that diagnosis and treatment help protect ADHD people's self-esteem.[33] We know it helps them function in school and at work and home and with friends. The sooner the treatment comes, the better our chance to mitigate the negative impact of ADHD on someone's life, and the greater their chance of achieving academic success and financial stability, and leading happy, successful, well-adjusted lives. We're not giving that chance to girls in the same way we are to boys, and both women and society as a whole are paying the price for that.

But, of course, when it comes to discrimination and inequality, gender is never the only factor at play. So it's probably time we talk about the other massive elephant in the room – ADHD's racism problem.

DIARY ENTRY

Grass shaped like a cow

I'm part of a local football club, and it's on the nights we have training that I can really feel the exact moment my ADHD medication wears off.

My coach will be giving instructions for some complicated round-robin kicking drill, and suddenly her words will begin to melt from English into that gibberish language they speak in *The Sims*. I'll notice there's a patch on the grass that looks kind of like a cow, and that will remind me that I need to buy oat milk next time I go to the supermarket, and actually now that I think about it, maybe I should be cooking more meals at home and trying to be healthier, and honestly I should exercise more, which I guess is a bit easier now that the footy season has started again and there's training twice a week, and, oh my god, I'm at training right now and I have no idea why everyone has started jogging to the other end of the pitch and why I'm jogging too and, wait, am I meant to be holding a ball or something right now?

To be perfectly honest, it probably doesn't help that, despite having been in the team for two full seasons now, I still don't actually know the rules of Aussie Rules. I just kick towards the goals and hope for the best.

In both training and real, competitive games, I'm going on context clues and vibes only.

Sometimes a teammate will notice my panicked, somewhat vacant stare, bump their arm gently against mine and say, 'All good mate, just follow me.' And 80 per cent of the time that little act of generosity is enough to get me back on track and help me work out what's going on.

It makes me wonder if all this time the sporty people have been onto something with this whole 'teamwork' thing.

7

How does race factor into this?

We've addressed the 'hyperactive' and the 'male' part of the ADHD stereotype, but what about the 'white' bit?

'First world problem'

A sentiment I've run into many times while talking with people about ADHD is that it's essentially a 'first world problem', a condition invented by wealthy countries obsessed with capitalistic success and achievement, which has then been exported around the world.

'Well, I reckon it's just, like, the modern world not letting kids be kids, y'know?' someone once said to me during a particularly unproductive conversation. 'You don't see a bunch of kids in Africa with ADHD, do you?'

There are several issues with this statement. Obviously there's the thinly veiled racism, but there's also the simple fact that . . . uh, yeah, you do. A **meta-analysis** of seven African countries (Nigeria, Sudan, Uganda, the Democratic Republic of the Congo, Kenya, Egypt and Ethiopia) found that the rate of ADHD in children and adolescents was between 6.81 and 7.62 per cent (depending on the type of diagnostic tool used),[1] which is pretty much bang on the global average of 5.9 to 7.2 per cent. (Just a reminder: this is how many people are estimated to have ADHD, not how many have actually been diagnosed.)

Although it's incorrect, I do understand why the perception of ADHD as a 'first world problem' is so prevalent. Wealthy countries are vastly overrepresented in the research and data. And, much like the vicious cycle that developed from only studying boys back in the day, this means our medical and cultural understanding of the disorder is almost entirely based on what it's like to have ADHD in Europe, the US, Canada and Australia – with maybe a few insights from the wealthier Asian nations such as Japan and Korea, if you're lucky. Even that statistic about ADHD **prevalence** in Africa only covered seven of the fifty-four countries on the continent, and yet it's the most robust data I can find.

It also doesn't help that the vast majority of resources for ADHDers – including this one – are written through the lens of someone living in a wealthy country. But even within those wealthy, well-studied nations, not everything is fair and equitable, because when it comes to diagnosis, ADHD has a serious racism problem, too.

Those who are part of a racial minority within majority-white countries find themselves at a distinct disadvantage when it comes to receiving an ADHD diagnosis or treatment in childhood. Unfortunately, having a detailed conversation about the intersection of ADHD and race is difficult, because this issue has received far less media and academic attention than the gender gap. As a result, we don't even have the type of intensive course-correction research that has occurred regarding ADHD women over the past five or so years.

To complicate matters further, the majority of racial data we do have comes from the US, which, as we saw in Chapter 1, doesn't necessarily make for a great globally representative ADHD case study. But despite the US's tendency towards overdiagnosis for some specific demographics in some specific states (i.e. boys in the South), the research we do have paints an extremely stark picture of racial disparity.

It was previously believed that ADHD just naturally affected Black people at a lower rate than white folks – that's even stated in the **DSM-5** – but more recent data suggests this likely isn't the case.[2] One 2021 meta-analysis showed ADHD prevalence rates may even be as high as 14 per cent among Black people living in the US. Part of the reason for this may be the strong **correlation** between ADHD and economic disadvantage – which Black families in the US face at a disproportionately high rate due to centuries of entrenched, institutionalised racism.

There are many complicated reasons why ADHD is so strongly associated with low socioeconomic status. Probably the most obvious link between the two is that the additional stressors of poverty and reduced educational support systems mean that kids whose brains already lean towards the ADHD-ish side of things may be more likely to tip over from 'having fairly benign **symptoms** of **inattention** or **hyperactivity**' to 'these symptoms seriously impairing their quality of life' and thus meeting the full **diagnostic criteria** for ADHD. More about this in Chapter 15.

The authors of this study theorised that racial marginalisation and discrimination, as well as racist microaggressions, may also exacerbate the symptoms of ADHD, which could also help explain this high rate.

And yet, when it comes to diagnoses, these big numbers aren't replicated. A 2014 study suggests that by kindergarten, Black children in the US are 70 per cent less likely to receive an ADHD **diagnosis** than white children, despite showing similar levels of ADHD symptoms.[3] Another study shows this disparity only shrinks to 50 per cent by the tenth grade (when students are around sixteen).[4] Children who spoke a language other than English at home were also significantly underdiagnosed, which presents barriers for many Hispanic children in the US as well.[5]

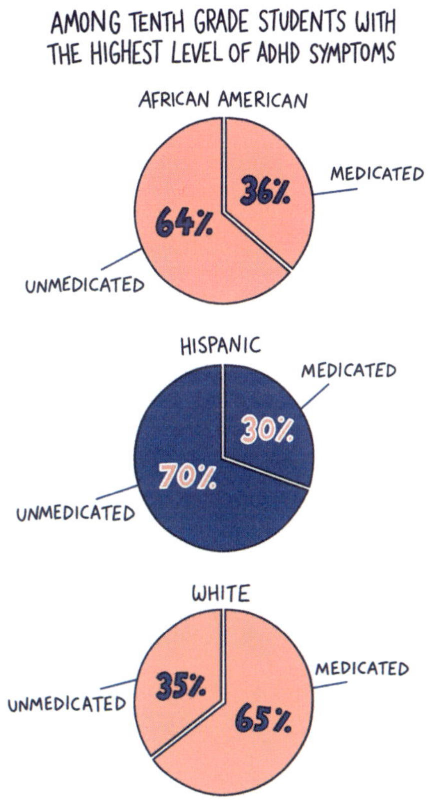

*Based on a US study looking at 4297 subjects across California, Alabama and Texas[6]

To make matters worse, even if a non-white kid is diagnosed, they're less likely to receive the highly effective medications used to treat ADHD. According to one study, among tenth graders with the highest level of symptoms, only 36 per cent of African American and 30 per cent of Hispanic kids who were diagnosed were medicated, compared with 65 per cent of white children.[6]

Bad kids?

One of the key issues here is that, at the end of the day, classroom detection of ADHD comes down to how a teacher interprets a child's actions, and this is where implicit or explicit racial **biases** are able to creep in.

To learn more, I talked to Dr Paul Morgan, an expert from Pennsylvania State University who has been examining the intersection of race and ADHD for years. He says that kids showing 'problem behaviour' tend to be sent down one of two paths, and race plays a significant role in determining which.

'Kids who are white are more likely to have those problem behaviours medicalised, so they'll get a diagnosis, or they'll get mental health support, whereas kids who are Black will tend to have those same behaviours criminalised: they'll be suspended from school, for example, or expelled.'

Morgan's work is centred on the US, but these patterns are replicated all over the world. Emily Johnson is a brilliant Australian artist, killer musician, recent **ADHD-I** (inattentive) diagnosis recipient and proud Barkindji woman. She tells me about how growing up as a student in the rural town of Broken Hill – and later, at an overcrowded high school in Inner Western Sydney – meant that teachers weren't looking out for signs of **neurodivergence** among the Indigenous kids. In fact, they were barely looking out for the Indigenous kids at all.

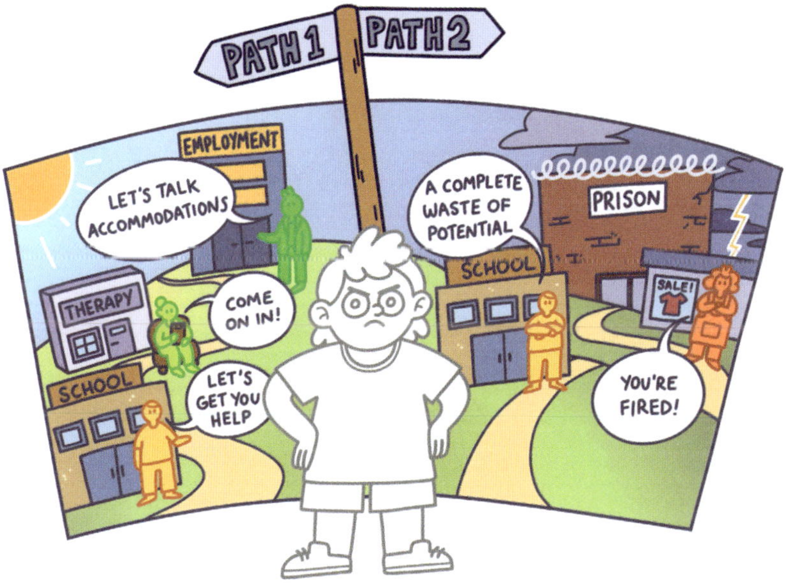
PATH 1
PATH 2
EMPLOYMENT
LET'S TALK ACCOMMODATIONS
THERAPY
COME ON IN!
SCHOOL
LET'S GET YOU HELP
A COMPLETE WASTE OF POTENTIAL
SCHOOL
PRISON
SALE!
YOU'RE FIRED!

'A lot of teachers just didn't know how to engage me. If I was interested in the topic, I would excel and then get bored because I finished my work, and then be disruptive,' she said. 'But for us Black kids, we were put in this category of, you know, "behavioural issues", and any frustration would just be seen as hostility, when actually I'm frustrated because I can't learn or concentrate.

'The attitude was, "Oh, it's just another Black kid being disruptive, they don't want to learn," whereas for the white kids it was much more like, "Oh, they're really struggling, so we're going to send them to the counsellor." I never got sent to the counsellor once, and I really was struggling too. But it was almost as if we were just in the "too hard" basket, as if they felt we were a lost cause anyway.'

Morgan tells me these 'two pathways' continue well into adult life as well. 'The kids that had their difficulties medicalised tend to continue on receiving mental health services, and those who had their behaviours in schools sort of criminalised can often end up more involved in the criminal justice system.'

We know that living with ADHD makes you more likely to drop out of school and less likely to find employment.[7] ADHD adults are also generally paid less, have worse health outcomes and have lower quality of life than **neurotypical** people. These are all barriers that people of colour already face to a greater degree, due to racial bias and economic inequality. Facing sustained exposure to discrimination and prejudice is also linked to higher rates of depression and harmful substance use – both things which ADHD people are already at an elevated risk for. ADHD people are also monumentally overrepresented in incarcerated populations,[8] which is especially worrying given the systemic over-imprisonment of people of colour in many wealthy countries such as the US, Australia and across Europe.

All of which is to say, not only are we denying ADHD kids of colour the treatments they need to succeed, but we're sending them out into a world where their condition will only compound the inequality they already face as a result of entrenched racism.

Understandable distrust

While you can draw a fairly direct line between racial bias and the dismissal of non-white children with ADHD symptoms in the classroom, Western systems leave non-white kids behind in other more subtle and complicated ways as well. One of the most widely discussed is the cultural barriers that influence many parents' understanding of and feelings about ADHD.

Much of the information for parents is written exclusively from a white, Anglo-European perspective, and for many communities this does little to instil trust. Until very recently, people of all races with mental health issues were in very real danger of being locked away in brutal institutions. So, while parents' anxieties about having their children diagnosed may be detrimental, that doesn't mean they're not logical. And this distrust is only amplified if, like Emily, your parents' entire lives have been shaped by the trauma inflicted by Western colonial systems.

Both of Emily's parents spent their early years on missions – government-controlled areas where many Indigenous people in Australia were compelled to live after being forcibly removed from their traditional lands, often with the express intent of converting them to Christianity and exploiting them for manual labour. Shockingly, the last of these did not close down until 1987. Emily's mother also lost her parents at a young age. Because she grew up at the tail end of the Stolen Generations era, governmental policy changes and bureaucratic red tape saw her bouncing between foster care and youth homes.

'Because of that, there's this real feeling that the government, the medical field, law enforcement, all of that is in the same kind of realm, like, the "outside",' Emily says. 'They don't like it if you're taking your personal problems and seeking institutional help.'

It's worth noting that despite the oppressive origins of missions, many Aboriginal and Torres Strait Islander people worked hard to transform these places into deep-rooted, Indigenous-led communities, and forged a strong sense of identity around them. So, it's not uncommon to see small townships and shires around Australia on former mission land.

Emily says that in her mob there's a big focus on talk therapy – discussing your problems with your family and the community, and working through it together. 'This is really great, and brilliant for everyday problems or even in dealing with my depression, just talking it all through. But at the end of the day, there's no talking through having a neurological disorder, having problems with the chemicals that affect your brain's functioning. So that has been a bit of a barrier, too.

'In the general population there's already a lot of mistrust about ADHD, but in my family there's this whole other layer. They were really worried about my safety. They feel that, you know, "Those Western doctors, they don't know about our people and what we've been through, and they're going to judge." And that worry is warranted, but it has been really difficult to navigate.'

The fact is, the way we think about and define ADHD is inherently linked to the Western medical model. There's something wrong with someone, so let's treat them and medicate them so they fit the system better rather than change the system to better fit them. That's not to say I believe medication isn't an extremely important part of ADHD treatment, or that we shouldn't be doing everything we can to communicate to all communities about how safe and beneficial it can be. But we have to be aware that this isn't a 'culturally neutral' system. It was built by white Western adults to treat white Western kids. That has ramifications.

We may be in a 'new era of ADHD awareness', but unless we make an effort to promote the voices of non-white ADHDers, acknowledge the legitimate concerns of marginalised communities, and put resources into ensuring our ADHD education and destigmatisation efforts are culturally informed, then at the end of the day we'll only be ushering in this 'new age' for those of us whom the system was already built to serve.

Luckily for all those who have previously been left behind – whether it be due to the way their condition manifests, their gender or their race – ADHD awareness and education have just become a lot more democratic, as the biggest voices in the neurodivergent space shift from a few select professors to social media creators with audiences in the millions.

The world of ADHD has changed. Now, the question is – what will be the ramifications?

Hobbies can hurt

DIARY ENTRY

Did you know people with ADHD are 50 per cent more likely to suffer accidental injuries?[1] That statistic often takes people by surprise, but it does low key make sense. I mean, how does one stop themselves from accidentally causing grievous bodily harm? By thoroughly thinking through one's actions before beginning a dangerous task. What do ADHD people have trouble doing? Thoroughly thinking through their actions before beginning a dangerous task. Especially if it's a craft project they saw on TikTok.

It's the middle of Melbourne's extraordinarily long COVID-19 lockdown in 2020. In fact, it's the single worst week to date. Case numbers climbing every day, thousand-dollar fines for leaving your house for non-essential reasons, and fear hanging thick in the air. So, naturally, I decide to spend the evening slicing though wine bottles to turn them into drinking glasses because it's all the rage online.

I order this little doodad from eBay that rests a wine bottle against a tiny blade so, by rotating it, you can create a light score mark all the way around. You then dip the bottle in boiling water, then iced water, then boiling water again, repeating until the shock of constant temperature changes causes a clean break all around. Sand it down and, voilà! You have a drinking glass, my friend.

I'm still living at home at this point, and yes, everyone in my house does tell me this is a terrible idea, including my partner, Anthony, who due to Victoria's 'intimate partner' lockdown exemption is camping out here for the night. But always the trouper, he helps me out anyway. We get through a couple of wine bottles and my confidence is up. I am an environmentally sustainable queen – no carbon-intensive factory-made glassware for me, thanks. There's nothing I can't turn into a drinking glass. So I decide to make some water tumblers out of small brown beer bottles, because how cute would that be?

We're sitting outside in the cold, dusky air as Anthony sands down a wine-bottle glass. I, having forgotten to put my protective glove back on, start twisting a beer bottle around, pushing it harder and harder to get the score line nice and deep. What hasn't occurred to me is that beer bottles are made with much, much thinner glass than wine bottles, and as I push, the glass gives way, shattering as my fist clenches around it.

Ouch.

I look down, unsure what's happened, and see blood gushing out of the back of my thumb.

'Ahhhhhh!' I shout, as realisation sets in. '*Ahhhhhhhhh!*'

'Oh my god,' Anthony says.

I jump up and start banging on the front door with my good hand.

'Use the spare key,' I hear my mum yell back, clearly in the middle of something.

'*I'm bleeding out!*' I yell in a moment of pure terrified dramatic ecstasy.

The door flies open and I sprint to the sink, leaving a trail of little red droplets in my wake. I run water over the cut to clear the blood and make the mistake of peering into the wound. I flick my eyes away in an act of self-preservation, unwilling to consider if the white I've just seen is bone. My attention then turns to trying not to pass out.

Unaware of just how serious the situation is, Anthony, Mum and Dad are all debating now.

'We should take her straight to hospital.'

'No, it's just a cut, it will be fine.'

'Maybe let's set a timer and see if she's still bleeding in five minutes.'

'If you're arguing about whether I should go to Emergency, it means I should go to Emergency,' I say, the quiver in my voice ruining what I thought was a pretty funny line.

So, Anthony and I hop in the car. No longer at risk of fainting, I insist that rather than the hospital, which will take all night, he drive me to the local clinic, because – and don't worry, I am ashamed of this – I don't want to miss *Bachelor in Paradise*.

I get the cut glued up and the doctor tells me that if it's still numb in the morning I should go to the hospital. It is still numb in the morning, and I do not go, because I have a feature story I'm really looking forward to writing. I clock in to work for the day and type that up, pausing as my hand starts to bleed again.

The next day, when my thumb is still totally numb, I know this is a losing battle. I have to go. Except, whoops! Now there's a COVID outbreak in the closest Emergency Department. So, with Anthony's help, I suit up with goggles, a plastic full-face screen, gloves and a double mask, and make my way in.

Everything goes pretty normally from here – I sit around for ages. They determine I've severed a nerve. I explain that my beer-bottle injury is way less drunken than it seems. I panic when a nurse tells me I might need to be off work for two months. I beg the plastic surgeon who will be operating to let me go back to work sooner. He says I can, but also that I need to 'think about my priorities a little'. I get the microsurgery the next day. I go home. I stay in bed, not even for a full week, and I go back to work.

But I did do one more little ADHD-esque thing, just to put the cherry on top of this undiagnosed disaster. When I first arrived at the hospital, I snapped a photo of myself – in my full COVID get-up – in front of the Emergency sign and popped it up on my Instagram story with the caption 'Hope I don't die, lol', and then totally forgot to update anyone any further.

In the days that follow I get several panicked and increasingly annoyed messages from people asking if I'm okay, and I seriously doubt I remembered to reply. Not my finest hour.

8

How did the internet know?

When ADHD videos started appearing on my TikTok 'For You' page, something felt intrinsically, profoundly right. Like that feeling you get when you're really upset and you don't quite understand why – then your friend manages to crystallise in one perfect sentence exactly what's going on in your subconscious brain. Watching people talk about adult ADHD made me feel seen in a way I'd never experienced before – but I wasn't quite ready to admit that to myself yet, let alone to the people around me.

After a week or two, when this neurodivergent niggling at the back of my brain started transforming into a full-blown 'I might have ADHD' theory, I began tentatively raising the possibility with Anthony, my parents and a couple of friends. None of them outright said I was wrong, but they didn't seem totally convinced either, and overall the light scepticism in their tone kept me from taking it any further. They're probably right, I told myself. It's a bunch of people making videos from their bedrooms. There's probably not all that much to it.

But the videos didn't stop coming, and the things they were talking about became more and more unnervingly specific.

I can pretty clearly remember the tipping point. I'd got distracted halfway through putting the supermarket shopping away, leaning against the kitchen bench aimlessly watching TikToks. Eventually I scrolled onto a video by one of the now quite familiar ADHD creators, who was talking about something called '**object permanence**' and why ADHD people struggle to remember things unless they're in their direct line of sight. I looked from my phone to the six jars of green olives that Anthony had purposely taken from their obscured shelf in the pantry and lined up along the counter to impress upon me how much I *had not* needed to buy them again during this week's shop. I looked into the shopping bag at my feet to see another jar staring out at me. 'Enough is enough,' I thought to myself. 'Things are just getting way too bloody spooky.'

When Dr Ellen Littman, the ADHD expert we met in Chapter 6, asked how I was diagnosed, I was a little reluctant to tell her.

'That's not embarrassing!' she said, when I finally spat it out. 'Those creators really are doing such fantastic work.

'First of all, there are a lot of people with ADHD who find reading burdensome. And they could be brilliant people, but they just haven't read a novel in years. So, sure, there are books and articles out there, but they're not reading them. Especially young people. Social media is the way they get information, all in small, quick chunks that you can process and hold on to pretty easily.'

And that's the thing, right? TikTok works really well at spreading ADHD information because it's an app that's extremely well suited to the ADHD brain. Better still, it's created a system where information is easy to stumble across. There's no barrier of actually getting your **executive function** together enough to think about ADHD, consider how it might apply to you, and proactively seek out resources.

Funnily enough, it was actually these specific characteristics of the app that led me to my current job, making short news-explainer videos for social media and specifically TikTok. At first I was just wanting to report in a way that scratched the fast-paced-content itch at the back of my brain, but turns out it's not only ADHDers who can benefit from relevant, educational content popping up effortlessly on their social media feeds. Who said nothing good can ever come from a malfunctioning mesolimbic pathway!

One of the creators I watched a lot during my ADHD incubation period was @Catieosaurus, aka Cate Osborn. I've interviewed plenty of social media creators in my time as a journalist, and it's always fun to see their professional set-ups in the background of our Zoom calls. Cate's was complete with a 'Catieosaurus' neon light glowing gently in the Atlanta afternoon sun.

She tells me that she never really intended to become an 'ADHD influencer'. She was just annoyed at all the videos of people's perfectly manicured apartments, so decided to spoof the trend, showing off all the 'Things in my ADHD home that just make sense'. 'I was like, "This pile of boxes that I've been walking by for six months, these dishes that I keep saying I'm going to do." I kind of roasted myself a little bit, and that video went super viral,' she said.

TikTok works really well at spreading ADHD information because it's an app that's extremely well suited to the ADHD brain.

'But a lot of people in the comments kept saying the same thing: "I've never seen anybody talk about having a house that looks like mine", "I've never seen anybody else talk about, you know, a 'doom pile' before."'

People were asking her about her organisation tactics, so she made a follow-up video. And before she knew it, she was talking to literally millions about a condition she wasn't even aware she had until she was well into her thirties.

'This rise in **diagnosis** we're seeing, I think it's just the perfect storm. With the TikTok algorithm and the pandemic, the fact that almost overnight, for almost the entire world, everyone's systems broke down. The things they've been hiding behind and **masking** behind, all of that went away,' Cate says. 'As people sat in their houses looking at TikTok, they started saying, "Wait, all of a sudden I can't do this. I'm struggling to get through the day." And I think a lot of people realised that they were neurodivergent for the first time.'

I tend to agree with her. Because, well, that's what happened to me.

Truth getting in the way of a good TikTok

While many I spoke to in the medical field were delighted that this perpetually underdiagnosed condition was getting more attention, some were also concerned about the unintended consequences of ADHD's new social media fame. Especially since many of the top creators, including those at the forefront of this evolving public conversation, don't have any sort of medical qualifications. 'The majority of the videos, over 90 per cent, were uploaded by non-healthcare professionals,' said Dr Anthony Yeung, a psychiatrist and fellow at the University of British Columbia, Canada. 'You get the sense that it's very much community driven.'

The paper he co-authored about the accuracy of ADHD TikToks is, as far as I can tell, the first-ever academic study looking into the online community, and it concluded that potentially half of these videos contained 'misleading information'.[1] 'A lot of the videos were simply talking about personal experience . . . but some misrepresented **symptoms** of other mental health disorders as being only specific to ADHD, maybe talking about treatments that haven't been studied for ADHD, or just describing things that weren't accurate,' he said.

While the study has yielded very interesting results, and has made headlines around the world, it is worth remembering that it only looked at the top hundred TikToks under the 'ADHD' hashtag, out of the millions of videos on the topic.

I reached out to TikTok, hoping to chat with someone about how they managed mental health conversations like this. But the notorious opacity of the corporate social media world struck once again, and I got a brief statement from a TikTok spokesperson instead. They said the app's community guidelines 'strictly prohibit misinformation, including medical misinformation that can cause harm to an individual's physical health', and that they have 'specialised misinformation moderators' and have partnered with fact-checking agencies globally.

'We love our community sharing their experiences, but we strongly encourage people to seek professional advice for any mental health or physical condition,' they said.

When I first read that statistic about misleading information, 50 per cent seemed far too high given how many great videos I had seen. I'm still not sure it's a truly accurate representation of the content on the app, but I must admit, as I've dived deeper into the scientific side of the ADHD conversation this year, I've realised that some of the most common terms used on social media in reference to ADHD can sound much more scientific than they actually are.

Object permanence

As you know, my light-bulb moment was discovering the ADHD brain's struggles with object permanence. I've forgotten wonderful outfits for years just because they fell off the hanger into the bottom of my wardrobe. Numerous bags of sad, dehydrated carrots have languished in the crisper because there was a head of lettuce on top of them. And I have 6 metres of fake grass in the boot of my car that I found on the side of the road a year and a half ago. (I still maintain that it would be fun to cover my car with it, but I covered it with a blanket to shield it from the sun at some point and only rediscovered the massive pile of faux turf during a recent clean-out.)

But there are a few issues with the experience I've just described:

- **It may well just be an average level of human forgetfulness.**
- **It hasn't been studied that extensively in relation to ADHD.**
- **It might simply not have anything to do with object permanence.**

'The term "object permanence" refers to a very core developmental aspect of someone's brain,' Dr Yeung says. Specifically, it's the ability of an infant to understand that something still exists even if they can no longer see, hear or touch it, and it usually develops around the eight-month-old mark. (This is why babies go wild when you play peekaboo with them – they genuinely think you are popping in and out of this corporeal plane.)

'It's actually not impaired in ADHD,' Dr Yeung continues. 'But because people with ADHD forget things, and they may lose things, you can kind of see how it's something that sounds quite scientific and kind of right-ish, right?

'What we found quite striking was that a video like that could easily be viewed 3 million times. And then if you look at the comments, you might see people typing, "Oh, wow, I didn't realise I lacked object permanence," and very quickly, it can become the "truth" or the "reality".'

Rejection-sensitive dysphoria

When TikTok taught me about **rejection-sensitive dysphoria** (RSD), it had a pretty profound impact on me. I was called 'overly sensitive' or told by teachers I needed to 'build resilience' as far back as I can remember. At twelve years old, I even put 'Learn to take things less personally' on my 'Goals for the year' poster on orientation day. The first mention of the term that I can find is in an article in *Attention Magazine* (a bimonthly publication from the US-based ADHD advocacy group Children and Adults with Attention-Deficit/Hyperactivity Disorder, or CHADD) by Dr William Dodson, a psychiatrist specialising in adult ADHD. He broke the emotional-regulation issues ADHDers face into three categories: overreaction, shame and guilt, and rejection-sensitive dysphoria. He stated that while the first two were commonly found among a number of disorders, RSD appeared to be 'associated exclusively' with ADHD.[2]

Dodson described RSD as an extreme emotional pain experienced by an ADHD person when faced with real or perceived rejection, suggesting it can be so 'primitive and overwhelming' that it can be difficult to find words to describe it. According to Dodson, around a third of ADHD teens and adults find RSD the most impairing aspect of their condition.

And I totally know what he's talking about. That lurching feeling, like you're a cartoon character who's just looked down after unknowingly walking off a cliff, seeing nothing but air beneath your feet. The rush of heat and that fuzzy feeling in the front of your face, your eyes going blurry as the embarrassment sets in. Or the desperation as you pore over a text or email, obsessively analysing the punctuation and tone. When you can hear your logical mind telling you this is ridiculous and you need to stop, but the sound is dampened by a thick layer of panic wrapped tightly around your brain.

But as relatable as his description may be, and as official as an acronym like RSD may sound, rejection-sensitive dysphoria isn't a clinical or diagnostic term – a fact that genuinely surprised me, given the sheer number of TikTok creators who talk about it as if it is.

While there's no doubt many ADHDers do struggle with emotional regulation,[3] and feel negative emotions particularly sharply, there's considerably less evidence to suggest that the way we experience rejection is unique to this condition. There hasn't been a huge amount of research on this topic, so the idea that this 'dysphoria' is caused by some core mechanism of ADHD isn't outside the realm of possibility – but perhaps it's more likely that rejection sensitivity is just a result of the battering many ADHD people's **self-esteem** receives while they're growing up. That doesn't make those feelings less valid or important, but it might change how we should go about addressing them.

And don't forget, ADHD rarely travels alone. A number of its common **comorbidities**, such as borderline personality disorder, also include heightened emotional responses, where sensitivity towards real or perceived rejection and abandonment is one of the central challenges. At least a portion of us could be mistaking the effects of another (**undiagnosed**) condition for the ADHD 'symptom' RSD.

ADHD paralysis

In one of the examples of a misleading video given in Dr Yeung's paper, someone describes a symptom called '**ADHD paralysis**', where the brain 'physically' won't let them do anything.

Once again, this was a little surprising, as 'ADHD paralysis' seemed like a pretty darn accurate description of my experience. But Yeung told me that the issue there stemmed from how broad and vague these non-clinical words can be. They can mean a lot of different things to a lot of different people.

I've seen 'ADHD paralysis' used to describe the feeling of being unable to make yourself just get up and do something, despite wanting to. Many use it when referring to an ADHD person becoming so overwhelmed by the mass of information they are receiving and the environment around them that they freeze, unable to make decisions or even think things through properly.

Other times I've seen people use the term when they have a task or activity that is scheduled for later in the day, and find that their brain goes into almost a holding pattern, unable to focus on anything else or get other things done until then.

Now, these are all things which I have experienced to some degree, and they aren't all that hard to trace back to **executive dysfunction**.[4] But where some of these TikTok creators go wrong is in describing them as if they are universal among ADHDers and unique to the ADHD experience – when plenty of these experiences could also be the result of anxiety, depression or a whole host of other conditions, too. Some creators even use them as pseudo-**diagnostic criteria** in those 'Five signs you might have ADHD' type videos.

But still, it's not like the term is strictly 'incorrect'. It clearly does reflect many people's experiences of the condition. It's just that it's more of a loose, cultural term than a strict, scientific one.

And the thing is, because the pool of known ADHDers has been almost solely made up of children for so much of the condition's history, there hasn't really been a community that was able to inject their own ideas and lingo into the conversation until now. Previously there were *only* scientific terms. Of course there's going to be a little friction as the cultural and medical worlds learn to coexist.

It'd be remiss of me not to point out that I've seen some fully qualified medical professionals saying some pretty dodgy stuff about ADHD on the app, too. (Often those with a helpful link to buy their self-help course or multivitamins in their bios.)

The 'cold hard science' of it all

One of the first bits of non-social-media ADHD information I was exposed to in my quest for scientific self-discovery was 'The World Federation of ADHD International Consensus Statement',[5] which, dry as its title may seem, is a pretty fascinating read. The World Federation of ADHD is a global consortium of ADHD experts who advocate for better education about and treatments for the condition. Back in 2021, they brought around eighty of their top academics together to compile a list of 208 facts about ADHD that can be backed up by large, statistically robust studies.

Obviously, plenty of really important aspects of the disorder don't make the list, purely because there isn't enough data out there yet, but there is something comforting about having these 208 pillars of (relative) certainty. However, going straight from the feelings-based, personal-experience-focused, neurodivergent musings of TikTok-ADHD-land to the reassuring but somewhat cold rigidity of the World Federation's Consensus Statement did make me feel like a child with divorced parents who each had vastly different opinions about how I should be raised.

I managed to speak with one of the main forces behind the Consensus Statement – the federation's president, Stephen Faraone – and, let me tell you, asking a man who regularly lectures at Harvard Medical School to tell me his opinions about TikTok does feel very strange indeed. But I simply had to know, did he think the popularisation of terms such as rejection-sensitive dysphoria was harmless? Or did he believe the conflation of pop science and real science is always dangerous?

'A lot of times, the traits that I see in social media refer to things that are related to anxiety and depression,' he replied. 'The problem with thinking it's just [part of] ADHD is that we want people to get treated for the right things. And somebody who has ADHD and is also depressed – they need to have their healthcare professional recognise that, so they can treat both.

'If people are listening to TikTok and it's telling them how to deal with ADHD, they can go down the wrong path. That's a bad thing. If it makes them go see a psychiatrist or, in the US, a primary healthcare person, then that's a good thing. Social media is good for activating people to act, but they have to act in the right direction to make it work.'

Changing the medical relationship

For better or worse, the mental health content and information on social media is fundamentally changing the relationship between doctor and patient. Dr Anthony Yeung told me that people often now come into his office after spending weeks or months online reading up about mental health conditions, potentially already with their own opinion firmly formed.

'It can be very difficult for them to meet me for two or three hours and for me to tell them, "I don't think you have this." That can be an incredibly jarring experience. I think it's something that some clinicians are running into a bit and struggling with . . . How do we match the expectations that someone might bring to the table already?'

Although this clearly complicates the work of mental health professionals, I can't help but feel hopeful about this shifting dynamic too. I mean, from a certain angle it's also kind of brilliant, especially for women, people of colour, queer folk and others who have spent decades fighting for the medical establishment to listen to them and take their concerns seriously. Being able to arm oneself with information when seeking a medical opinion is so liberating. For me, it was life-changing.

'Social media is good for activating people to act, but they have to act in the right direction to make it work.'

But I'm also not so enamoured of TikTok that I'm unwilling to admit there's plenty of ADHD information and other mental health information on the platform that could lead people astray.

False ADHD positives

Quite often for research purposes (and partially for procrastination purposes), I'll find myself on TikTok, typing 'ADHD' into the search bar.

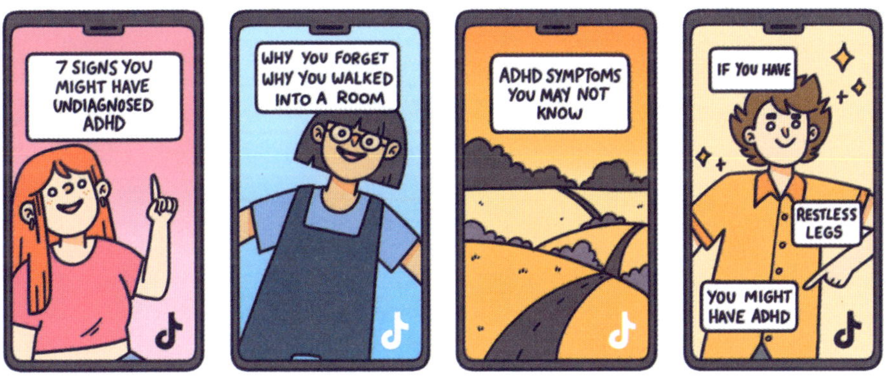
7 SIGNS YOU MIGHT HAVE UNDIAGNOSED ADHD
WHY YOU FORGET WHY YOU WALKED INTO A ROOM
ADHD SYMPTOMS YOU MAY NOT KNOW
IF YOU HAVE
RESTLESS LEGS
YOU MIGHT HAVE ADHD

But I'm always a little disheartened by the array of videos with titles like 'How to tell if you have ADHD' that only list 'zoning out a lot', 'forgetting why you walked into a room', 'random bursts of energy' and a few other equally vague or universal statements. Which, sure, may well be applicable to ADHD, but a title like 'How to tell if you're a little tired today' might be equally accurate. That one had nearly 500,000 likes, by the way.

I totally see how someone, if exposed to enough videos like this, could come to believe they have ADHD when they don't. But I guess I'm sceptical about the level of panic people seem to be feeling over this, because it's hard to see the inherent dangers of 'self-diagnosing with ADHD'. Because, for the vast majority of people, the step after self-diagnosis is talking to a doctor.

Even if someone doesn't have this particular condition, if they're relating to the traits of **inattention** or **impulsivity**, getting them in front of a medical professional who might be able to rule out ADHD and give them a proper diagnosis is still a brilliant outcome. Either that, or they start using some ADHD 'life hacks' to help them concentrate or improve their organisation and life admin skills. And I mean, that's still a good outcome, right?

Obviously, having a bunch of people running around claiming they have ADHD when they don't could delegitimise the seriousness of the condition, and that could be harmful in a broad, social justice sense. But it's not really the medical crisis that some news reports and think pieces would have you believe is currently unfolding.

A common argument is that the real danger of people self-diagnosing with ADHD is that it could lead to people **self-medicating** for ADHD, too. But I'm sorry . . . what? Do you think there are actually people out there convincing themselves they have ADHD, purposely deciding not to go to the doctor about it, and instead planning to buy a regular supply of dexys from their sketchy cousin for (literally) a hundred times the prescription price? The most infuriating thing is that self-medicating is genuinely a huge issue when it comes to ADHD – except it's not these apparent 'pretenders' making themselves a fake pharmacotherapy regime out of $10 backyard pills. It's people who have no idea they have ADHD snorting lines of coke because, for some reason, it seems to help them focus, or smoking weed every night so they can sit still and enjoy a TV show, or breathing in more vape smoke than oxygen at their home-office desk just to make it through the workday.

I'm even a bit hesitant to totally dismiss the internet-popular ADHD terms such as 'object permanence' or 'ADHD paralysis'. Because, despite their complicated relationship with the cold hard science of ADHD, they were genuinely the 'symptoms' that made it click in my head that I had this condition. They got me to that psychiatric consultation.

Cate Osborn, as it turns out, is similarly torn, coming from a background in academia yet acutely aware of how useful these terms can be as a shorthand for our shared experiences. 'I remember when I started talking about rejection sensitivity, so many people were like, "This is just trauma." And I'm like . . . yes. That's just what we're calling it. We gave it a name so we can all collectively talk about it.

'There's a reason why I don't use very academic language, and it's because that's not what this is for,' Osborn tells me. 'This is for the general population to learn, and to give them something to go to their doctor to talk about,' she says.

And despite his reservations, Faraone agrees these community terms can help drive the academic conversation, too. 'At some point, some of these social media memes that are coming out may well motivate researchers to look at it. You've got all these people talking about rejection-sensitive dysphoria, and currently we don't deal with it. But maybe we ought to study it and see what its causes are.'

Horrific small talk I can't escape from

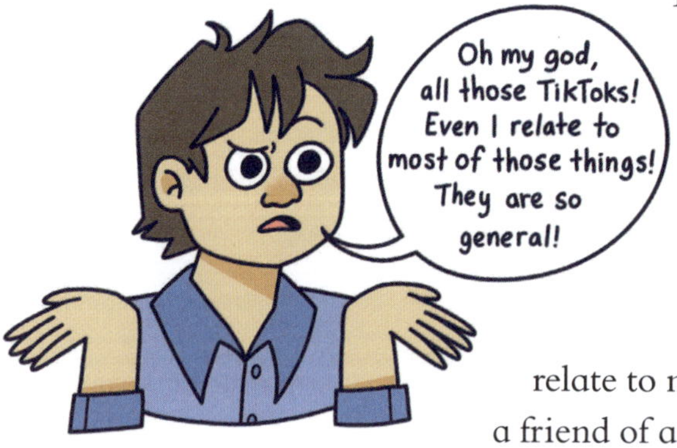

However, when people complain about TikTok's role in bringing ADHD back into the zeitgeist, the conversation rarely gets that deep. Instead, they are usually just worried that the app is 'making everyone think they have ADHD nowadays'.

'Oh my god, all those TikToks! Even I relate to most of those things! They're so general,' a friend of a friend tells me, unprompted, after I casually mention my diagnosis over Friday drinks.

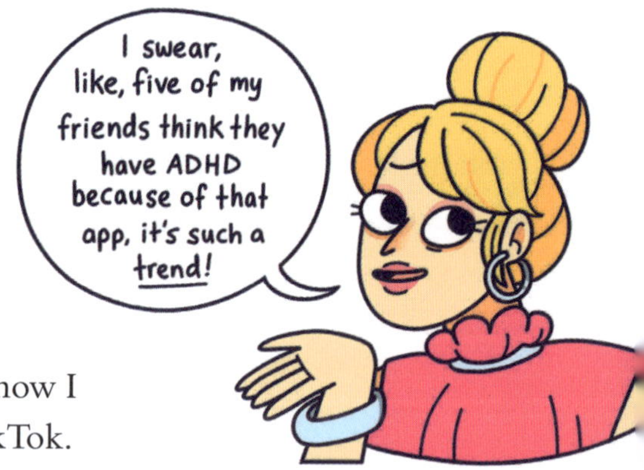

'I swear, like, five of my friends think they have ADHD because of that app. It's such a trend,' says a reporter from another paper at a journalism awards night, strangely immediately after telling me they loved my article about how I found out I had ADHD from TikTok.

'Social media is giving us all ADHD nowadays, though, we have such short attention spans,' says the semi-relevant TV host online.

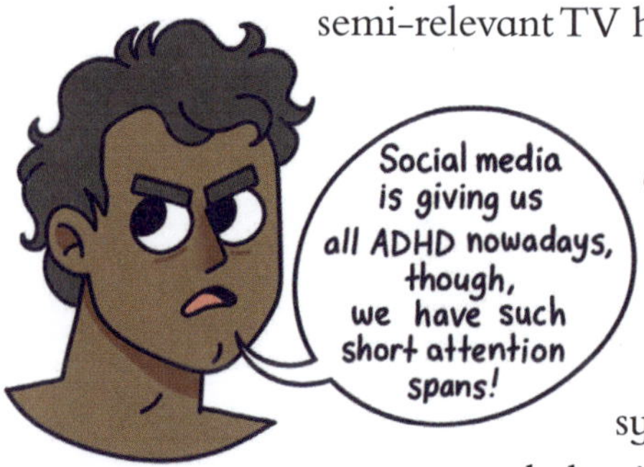

I'm genuinely so sick of having these conversations, so let me address this once and for all. Yes, there are some dodgy videos out there, but the reason most of the 'symptom' videos seem very general is that ADHD symptoms fundamentally are normal human behaviours, except they occur at a frequency and severity that has a significantly negative impact on one's life. No, it's not weird that five of your mates think they have ADHD now, it's just been aggressively underdiagnosed for decades and you're seeing the course correction. And no, social media is not giving people ADHD. If anything, undiagnosed ADHD might be giving people a social media addiction.

ADHD symptoms fundamentally are normal human behaviours, except they occur at a frequency and severity that has a significantly negative impact on one's life.

'It's so strange when people see others identifying with symptoms and think that's somehow a bad thing,' Osborn says. 'But if going on ADHD TikTok and learning how to fold your laundry more efficiently, or organise your mail, or whatever it may be, helps you get through the day, helps that person feel less alone, less like a fuck-up and less like they're broken and less like their whole world is burning to the ground – why the fuck do you care?'

Osborn is right. There's a vast number of people out there looking for help. It's not TikTok's fault that this is the place where we first properly learnt about ADHD, it's the fault of decades of racist, patriarchal medical research, an educational structure that – by and large – only views mental health conditions through the prism of classroom disturbances, and a sustained campaign of anti-medication propaganda convincing the public that ADHD diagnoses are a dangerous fad to be avoided at all costs.

Believe me when I say that I desperately wish I hadn't found out one of the most fundamental things about my brain on the goddamn dancing app. It's nobody's dream to have a few lines of computer code designed to sell your attention for profit be the first one to notice you have a lifelong, potentially life-ruining neurological condition. But the fact of the matter is, I'm so unbelievably glad it did.

'There's nothing that prepares you for the first letter that says, "I chose not to kill myself because of your content,"' says Osborn.

'I try to treat it with the greatest of respect and the most compassion and kindness that I can, because it's . . .' She pauses. 'It's a gift to get to do this every day. And it's one I take so seriously.'

While it's clear, yes, that the ADHD-TikTok ecosystem is filled with half-truths, questionable conclusions and occasional outright bad-faith actors, ultimately I feel like the 'dangers' and 'harm' are kind of small in the broad scheme of things. No, it's not great if someone misunderstands how a certain brain function relates to ADHD. Yes, it's bad if vague 'How to tell if you have ADHD' videos make ADHD look more trivial than it is. Yes, a few people may mistakenly think they have ADHD when they don't, and, yes, they might even waste a few hundred bucks talking to a doctor just for the doctor to tell them they're wrong.

But these risks are all so theoretical, while the benefits of having this online community and this public conversation are as tangible as they come. It means people finally understanding themselves, finally getting the help they need, and finally starting to right the wrongs that centuries of misogyny and racism have embedded so deeply into our world of mental health. There's no doubt in my mind that these silly little ADHD videos are genuinely saving people's lives.

part two

living

Not ADHD enough

Yesterday a friend told me they're not convinced I have ADHD because I'm so 'high-functioning'. It's not the first time I've heard this, but for some reason it hit me so much harder this time, and I've been staring at a blank screen all morning, trying to figure out why I can't stop crying.

I won't pretend I've had the toughest possible experience with ADHD. Since uni I've been able to cultivate a career for myself, and obviously writing a book isn't a privilege available to everyone with this condition. I'm high-achieving in a number of areas, I'm not going to deny that. But that 'high-functioning' label still bothers me.

Partially it's because I'm acutely aware that, although I've worked hard to get where I am, truthfully, my success has just as much to do with me accidentally winning the genetic lottery as it does pure merit. Our society likes to hold up intelligence as some moral victory, but I did nothing to earn that advantage in life. While it's true intelligence almost certainly had the adverse effect of helping to hide my ADHD from view, causing me to grow up without some key supports, it also allowed me to scrape by despite my attention deficits. Sure, I couldn't listen in class, but 90 per cent of the time I could work out what was going on from the snippets I did catch. It can be very easy in the adult ADHD community to romanticise all ADHDers as some kind of eccentric savants, but people of all intelligences have ADHD. Plenty of them don't have this buffer, and experience much worse life outcomes. That's not some sort of cosmic justice, it's just luck.

I was also born into a middle-class family, with parents who had the time and ability to create a structure that allowed me to thrive, reminding me to do homework, getting me to appointments on time, and encouraging me to pursue the things I was passionate about. We weren't wealthy, but I grew up never knowing the stresses of food or housing insecurity, and when it came to my final years of high school, I could forgo part-time work to focus on my studies because we didn't need that additional income to get by.

I grew up in a big enough city that I could still live at home while attending university, meaning that parental scaffolding continued throughout the entirety of my formal education. When it came to picking my career, I was able to wholeheartedly pursue the thing I was passionate about – journalism – even though the industry is renowned for its job insecurity, because I knew that even if I failed miserably, my family would be able to support me while I got back on my feet. Plenty of people with ADHD have no choice but to pick the safe option, and counterintuitively end up underperforming or struggling in their career because it's so much harder for us to focus on work that doesn't excite us.

And then I got lucky once again. By bloody random chance, when I was twenty-one, I was heading into a TV studio at the ass-crack of dawn on New Year's Day to appear as a guest reporter. And I was paired with exactly the right super-organised, generous and kind producer who said yes when I asked him out for a coffee after the show. We fell in love and moved in together, and his innate caring and generosity provide so much support and structure in my life.

Countless random factors, social phenomena and crossroads moments in my life could have made me what one might call a 'low-functioning' person with ADHD. I just accidentally skated past them.

But there's also the fact that I don't always feel 'high-functioning'.

When I'm so incapacitated by a day's work that I shut down, unable to move from my bed. Or when I'm desperately counting the number of antidepressant tablets I have left, trying to work out if I've already taken them today or if I just imagined I had. When I cry thinking about all the projects and career paths and goals I want to achieve, but feel as if I'm utterly stuck and my brain will never let me better myself. When I'm screaming in my head, begging my mind to let me get even one piece of work done for the day and I still can't manage it.

I didn't feel high-functioning when I broke down at my former doctor's office after being told I'd been put on a probationary list, no longer allowed to book appointments in advance because I'd missed so many. Nor during the countless hours I spent growing up, praying to a higher power I didn't even really believe in, begging them to forgive me for being such a selfish, horrible person. I didn't feel high-functioning during the teen years I spent feeling like a little alien watching from afar as the girls around me managed to navigate life with mysterious ease that I could never understand.

So, sure, the negative impact of my ADHD probably doesn't immediately jump out when you look at my résumé, but I still feel it every day.

I guess the truth is, I'm crying because I had hoped that upon learning about my ADHD, my friend would look back on my life, realise I'd been grappling with all these invisible struggles, and then see where I am now, and see my successes and my achievements in a new light – finally understanding how much it took for me to get here. Instead, it felt as if they looked at where I am now and used it as evidence that those struggles never existed.

I know this isn't what they meant. I know it was coming from a place of love and wanting me to see myself in relation to my talents, not my deficits. I also know not everyone looks at the prospect of being diagnosed with a psychiatric disorder in the fairly destigmatised – even positive – way that mid-twenty-year-olds who grew up on the internet do.

I know all of that. I just didn't expect it to hurt so much.

Perhaps it's because I'm still fighting to reconcile it all in my brain, too, and my friend accidentally expressed my secret deep, dark fear aloud.

9

What happens now?

The fear

It's a weird thing to admit, but I spent the first few months after my **diagnosis** utterly petrified I might have made the whole thing up. That the psychiatrist got it wrong. That I knew too much about the **symptoms** of ADHD going in and just said all the right things so I could pass the ADHD test. That somehow I faked it, and this had all simply been a convenient excuse to make myself feel better about being lazy and disorganised.

This fear grew into a secret, immobilising shame that I carried around with me each day. But after speaking with dozens of other people who were diagnosed as adults, I've come to learn that this is a shockingly common experience – especially among women, for whom imposter syndrome is already so pervasive.

This is only my armchair hypothesis, but I think a big reason why people begin to worry that their ADHD is fake or artificially exaggerated after their diagnosis is that human brains are just naturally really good at pattern recognition – and suddenly we now have a pattern to look for.

Before I became aware of the symptoms of ADHD, there would be maybe ten or fifteen micro-incidents in my day where I would misplace something, or get distracted, or lose track of time. I'd go 'Hmph', scold myself slightly, then move on and forget all about it.

They weren't linked in my mind. But once I learnt about my ADHD, I started connecting the dots. I would get distracted reading about whether polarised sunglasses actually protect your eyes while I was meant to be writing an article on the tourism industry. 'Probably ADHD,' I started to think. I would forget to call my partner back, even though he had called me twice. 'Classic ADHD.' I'd see a YouTube video of someone recommending the classic science fiction series The Hyperion Cantos, and I would spend the next three hours researching every bit of that universe's lore – and oh, wait, **hyper-focusing** is an ADHD thing, too. Every time I messed up, I'd gouge another neurodivergent notch in my subconscious tally. Suddenly, my entire day was utterly consumed by the sheer 'ADHD-ness' of it all, and it felt like I had gone from zero to one hundred in a flash.

'That can't be right,' my subconscious told me, 'therefore I must be faking it.'

It also didn't help that at the time I was diagnosed, our society was (and still is) in the grip of a reactionary backlash over this new wave of people discovering their condition, with heightened cultural suspicion over people 'faking' their ADHD. I've been forced to justify my own experience at cafes, in bars, at a child's birthday party, even live on radio after literally having been invited to talk about how ADHD is misunderstood in adults.

This is extremely difficult to confront day in, day out – especially when you're still trying to work through your insecurities about this life-changing news. Even with a formal diagnosis in your back pocket, it's hard not to internalise the idea that ADHD might be a craze and you're just one of the suckers that got caught up in it.

What's me and what's the ADHD?

But the confusion doesn't stop there, because while I was convincing myself that I was faking it, I was also petrified that ADHD would utterly consume my life. The more I learnt, and the more dots I connected, the more I realised just how many aspects of my personality were shaped by the condition. It's hard to describe how destabilising it can feel to realise that the core of who you are – elements of your personality that you love and cherish and are proud of – are actually, well . . . symptoms.

I always liked that I hated being alone – I thought it meant that I was a deeply social person who thrives on community and kinship. But what if it's just that my brain has a chemical imbalance that makes me excruciatingly bored when not constantly being stimulated?

The more I learnt, and the more dots I connected, the more I realised just how many aspects of my personality were shaped by the condition.

I always liked that I was able to chime in with a witty joke even in the most inappropriate of circumstances – I thought it was a testament to my comedy chops. But what if I do it not because I'm funny, but because I struggle with **impulse control** and don't absorb social cues the same way other people do?

I liked that I was constantly picking up hobbies or getting engrossed in a new topic – I thought it made me spontaneous and inquisitive. But what if it's an expression of my malfunctioning **prefrontal cortex**'s inability to properly regulate my attention?

Knowing that these parts of me might be connected to ADHD didn't necessarily make me like them less, but it did make them feel less 'mine'. In fact, I felt less 'mine' all over.

When I was thirteen, my mum's car got broken into while parked in the street outside our house. It wasn't anything dramatic – they just yanked out the spare change compartment and rifled

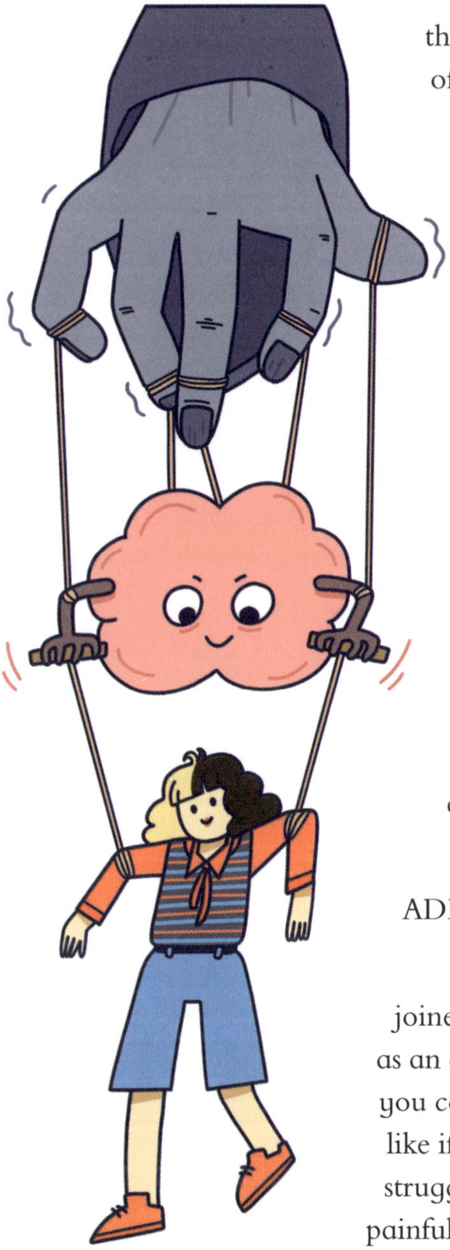

through the first-aid kit, stealing half a packet of home-brand paracetamol. But still, it felt so disconcerting the next morning, sitting in the car knowing a stranger had been there.

For a while after I was diagnosed, that's kind of how I felt about my own brain. Like there had been a secret stranger in my head all these years, a puppet master dictating what I did and how I acted. And now that they had been found out, I was left sitting in the car again with everything feeling different.

Where does ADHD stop and where does it begin? Does it encompass my strengths and my weaknesses, my interests, my emotions too? Did it even affect my career choice, seeing me gravitate towards a high-pressure environment with daily deadlines and an ever-changing array of things to research?

For a while, it was hard to find a part of me that ADHD hadn't touched.

Shortly after that, the grief began, quickly joined by a tinge of anger. Because when you learn, as an adult, that you've had ADHD your entire life, you can't help but wonder what it would have been like if the system had been built to recognise your struggles all those years ago. And there's a much more painful question lurking just below this one: Who would I be, and what would I have achieved, if I never even had ADHD to begin with?

In those early months after my diagnosis, I had this image of a 'Matilda without the ADHD' burnt into the back of my brain.

She was skinnier, and healthier, with clothes that were never wrinkled and hair that never frizzed. She lived in a perfectly tidy, beautiful house, with journalism awards crowding her dust-free shelves and money flying into her bank account. But the most unbearable part was how happy she looked – not weighed down by constant fatigue and frustration at herself for not living up to her 'full potential'.

Truthfully, this image of myself wasn't entirely born when I learnt I had ADHD; she has always sort of been around. But before my diagnosis, she was the goal – the person I believed I was only a long, relaxing holiday and an ultra-efficient day-planner organisation system away from being. After I was diagnosed, she became the person that I 'should have' been. The future that I was owed, until my own goddamn brain ripped it away from me.

This is of course all bullshit. ADHD or not, I would never have lived up to other Matilda's standards. No human could. Still, there's a grief in accepting that the struggles you are going through aren't just a 'phase' or a 'rough patch'. In accepting that this is simply who you are.

For a long time, the prospect of letting go of this 'perfect' version of myself was too painful, so she stuck around as a mean, taunting ghost.

But, slowly, over many, many months, her grip on my mind and **self-esteem** began to weaken. She began to feel less and less real, until eventually, the idea of saying goodbye to her didn't feel like a loss. It felt like a wonderful relief.

There is no me without ADHD

It was then that I realised I had to stop thinking of myself as 'someone who has ADHD' and start living my life as an 'ADHD person'.

This is known as 'identity-first' language, and it's a concept that has developed in the past decade or so within the broader **disability** advocacy space. So, for example, one might say 'disabled person' or 'autistic person' rather than what many people initially assume to be the more politically correct–sounding 'person with a disability' or 'person with **autism**'.

Now, this conversation is in its much earlier stages when it comes to ADHD – possibly because the initialism makes identity-first language more grammatically difficult. But neurodivergent and disabled communities can learn a lot from each other, and, at least for me, calling myself an 'ADHD person' or an 'ADHDer' feels far more empowering.

By definition, **neurodevelopmental** disorders, such as ADHD and autism, fundamentally affect the way our brains have developed. They shape our minds and our emotions. They are a foundational part of us. So, really, it doesn't make sense to think of my ADHD as some stranger living in my brain that could be removed and leave the normal 'me' behind. ADHD doesn't define me, it's not the entirety of who I am, but it does play a part in every thought I have. Just as my gender does and my race does and my socioeconomic class does. I'm moving through the world as an 'ADHD person'.

So, yes, I was – and to some degree still am – grieving the person I could have been if I didn't have ADHD. But I've now come to recognise that this person wouldn't actually be 'me' – and I care so much more about being 'me' than being a bit more successful or having a tidier house.

Everyone's circumstances and experience of ADHD are

different, and it's okay if feeling this way simply isn't realistic for you. There are still plenty of days when I can't bring myself to feel like this either.

But, speaking purely for myself here, I've found a lot of freedom in making a deliberate, concerted effort to stop endlessly pondering the possibilities of 'what could have been' and take stock of the bits I love about myself the way I am. The things I would never want to give up.

No, but really, am I faking it?

I don't want to pretend that I've somehow got this all worked out, or that I'm utterly at peace with my diagnosis only two years in. In fact, the paralysing fear that I might be faking it and that I'm using my diagnosis 'as an excuse' for my deficits is devilishly hard to shake.

I had to stop thinking of myself as 'someone who has ADHD' and start living my life as an 'ADHD person'.

I know so many people who are going through this, and objectively, it's not hard to see why. After years of swimming in trauma and shame, self-inflicted or otherwise, it's only natural that we would be suspicious of a life raft appearing out of the blue that allows us to forgive ourselves. Self-forgiveness is probably a brand-new concept. It certainly is for me.

But emotions aren't facts, and just because you might feel guilty about having an explanation for your deficits doesn't mean that explanation is wrong. You may just have been a good and talented person all along.

You've earnt the right to be happy about that, and you owe it to the younger version of yourself, who spent all those years struggling, to accept the life raft and forgive them, too.

The other day I plucked up the courage to tell Anthony I was worried I might be faking my ADHD. He looked me dead in the eye, gestured to the pile of unfolded washing sitting next to me that I'd started doing an hour earlier, and the monstera-pattern long-stitch cushion-cover kit that I impulse-bought while going to the shops for bread the week before that was now occupying my hands instead, and laughed.

And, at least for now, that look of utter bemused disbelief from someone who knows me so well is enough for me.

The guilt of burnout

DIARY ENTRY

It's self-indulgent to talk about writing a book within that book, but I'm about halfway through the process and I think this book might be destroying me. My ADHD has never been worse. And all the while I'm writing about ways to manage ADHD better, I have absolutely no energy to do any of it for myself.

When I got busy, things started falling through the cracks. Suddenly I was playing catch-up in my life again. And the weight and pressure of that just made those cracks widen further. I've let so many people down. I can't even bring myself to open messages from friends, let alone call people to talk about ADHD for the book.

I yelled at my mum on the phone today for asking about my plans for work. I was sobbing and throwing out the words 'I'm so fucking tired. I just want to rest. I just want to have a day off', while holding my hand so tight against my eyes that thousands of moving grey dots appeared in the darkness of my eyelids.

Last week I messaged my primary school teacher to see if she would speak to me for the book about what I was like in class as a kid. She graciously agreed and then I totally forgot. She waited for thirty minutes in the staffroom after school before she messaged me, 'I'm going to have to go, can we do it some other day?'

I saw that message appear and scrolled up to see, 'Hey, are we still on for today?' and 'Hey, just wondering what time you were planning to get here.' And there I was, sitting in the office in the city, with the crushing feeling of, oh my god, I've done it again.

I lost my AirPods for a month because I never checked the work group chat to see my colleague posting that he'd found some in the studio.

I cancelled on a friend last minute because I realised I was double-booked.

I've rocked up to work late the last five times I've been into the office, and didn't have the mental capacity to just play it cool, instead telling my boss a hundred different excuses about the trains being delayed and drawing more attention to it.

I haven't been swimming in weeks. I haven't gone jogging in months. I haven't called my grandma back. I haven't transferred my share of an Uber ride to my co-worker. I haven't sent experts thank-you texts for speaking with me. I haven't cleaned up the ever-growing pile of clothes in my room.

I feel as if I leave a trail of inconvenience in my wake and the longer it gets, the less I can bear to even try to rectify it. ADHD has a way of making you feel like a bad friend, a bad daughter, a bad granddaughter, a bad colleague. It makes you reliant on other people's capacity to forgive.

I'm pretty sure that, for me, ADHD is why one minute my life and mental health can seem totally fine, and the next they fall into utter shambles. If I get seven hours' sleep I'm fine, but if I get six and a half I'm a mess and chances are I'll break down crying in the middle of a workday. I'll forget my meetings, burn my dinner, be rude to Anthony. And then the anxiety and guilt will keep me up at night even though I'm desperately tired.

The moment I become overworked, the same thing happens. The moment I get a cold. The moment I have a disagreement with someone. I feel like I'm constantly walking a tightrope.

And I just want to be tough. I want to be like all the US presidents you hear about who sleep four hours a day and still manage to run a country.

I wish I never saw that stupid inspirational quote, 'Find a job you love and you'll never have to work a day in your life.' I *do* have a job that I love, but I still feel every minute of work in my bones.

What I'm coming to understand, though, is that having ADHD means I need to do a whole host of extra things every second of the day just to seem 'normal' and keep my life together. I'm concentrating on not interrupting the person I'm speaking to. I'm forcing myself to focus on their words even though the lightbulb is flickering behind them. I'm going through a list in my head of everything I need to do and can't forget, over and over and over again so it doesn't disappear.

Multiple times an hour, I find myself adrift and I have to thread a vast expanse of thoughts through the head of a needle just to figure out what it was I was doing again.

I'm only just starting to comprehend what people mean when they talk about 'masking' one's ADHD, and the fact that I've been doing it, too. It's like my brain is carrying an extra 20-kilogram bag around on its back. No wonder I wear out more quickly when the incline gets steeper.

But, I'm trying to get to the point where, when I'm burnt out, I no longer double my pain by hating myself for being exhausted in the first place. I'm not doing a great job of it right now. I feel bad, I feel weak, I feel like an inconvenience.

But typing this has made me realise that maybe this is one of those times when it's important to take my own advice. Perhaps the solution here isn't reading another peer-reviewed study, as if the opposite of failure was 'pushing through no matter how much it costs you'. Maybe what I need to do is give my brain a break, sit down with a hot chocolate, eat something more nutritious than stale corn chips, and watch an episode of *Gilmore Girls*.

I have a feeling the world might feel a lot better on the other side.

10

How do I live with it?

If you reached late adolescence or adulthood by the time you were diagnosed with ADHD, chances are you've found a sort of slapdash, higgledy-piggledy system that allows you to mostly get by in life. I certainly have.

I've never been able to keep a consistent diary, so I tried to get good at remembering everything that was happening and everywhere I needed to be for the upcoming week of my life, and if I forgot something, which I almost always did, I would just hope that my mum or my sister or my boyfriend would text me and remind me. This has got me pretty far, but it's also resulted in a heap of missed doctor's appointments, a ton of missed work opportunities and a bunch of disappointed friends and family members waiting for a birthday text that was never coming.

I constantly struggle to get work done when a deadline isn't looming, so I've become really good at forcing myself to work while in a panic – busting out a thousand-word article an hour and a half before the deadline – but consequently being unable to calm myself enough to properly read my work before hitting submit. They were good articles and I would still sort of get them filed on time, but doing this also earnt me a reputation for being a bit sloppy, because from the outside it seemed as if I couldn't be bothered proofreading. I like to think this hasn't impacted my career too drastically, but I just don't know. Doors may well have closed because of it.

I find it really hard to remember to reply to my friends' text messages, so I've developed a big list of excuses about 'my inbox being flooded with work stuff' or 'not getting the notification' that I sheepishly type three days or three weeks or three months later. It gets the conversation back on track, but I sometimes wonder how many moments of my friends' lives I've missed because of it, how many times they might have needed me and I wasn't there, or worse, how many times they never bothered to reach out in the first place because they knew I couldn't be relied upon.

There are plenty of ways to survive as a neurodivergent person living a life built for neurotypicals, but I'm sick of it. I want a life that works for me and my brain. Pardon the 'girl boss' coffee-mug slogan, but I don't just want to 'survive' any more, I want to thrive.

So I set out to find out what really works (at least for me) when it comes to the day-to-day business of living with an ADHD brain.

How do you get there?

Now, you've probably noticed there's one glaring issue with the idea of simply changing the way you live your life to help mitigate the **impairments** associated with ADHD. Purposely setting out to make, and then maintain, major organisation-based life changes is exactly the kind of sustained, laborious task that's really difficult to complete when you have ADHD.

This is what frustrates me about the majority of 'Tips for living with ADHD' articles you find online. Either they're written for parents of ADHD children and are therefore totally reliant on **neurotypical** adults steering the ship, or they're all things that would require immense, continuous **executive-functioning** capacity. Telling me I need to 'keep my home and workspace tidy' to increase focus, and 'use a planner to keep on top of things' isn't that far away from telling me to 'get more organised' by 'being more organised' and 'improve my focus' by simply 'being able to focus more'. One of these articles literally listed 'stay on task' as one of their brilliant hacks. Amazing! Wow! Why didn't I think of doing that?

I'm sorry to break it to you, but buying an expensive planner to write down all of our events and to-do lists probably isn't going to cure us of our **neurodivergence**. Chances are we won't even get to day two of writing in it. Quick fixes like that are for those blessed with executive-functioning capacity to spare. Getting your shit together when you have ADHD is a much broader, slower and far less linear process. But it will probably be a much more rewarding one too.

Telling me I need to 'keep my home and workspace tidy' to increase focus, and 'use a planner to keep on top of things' isn't that far away from telling me to 'get more organised' by 'being more organised' and 'improve my focus' by simply 'being able to focus more'.

Obviously I'm no expert – I'm not even wearing pants right now (not because it's comfy, but because I genuinely can't bear the idea of finding them in the tottering pile of clothes next to my bed) – but when it comes to living with ADHD as an adult, I like to divide my tactics into three categories:

1. **the habits and routines we can adopt to reduce ADHD symptoms (the topic of this chapter)**
2. **the systems we can create to work with our brain on its own terms (discussed in Chapter 11)**
3. **the fights I've simply decided to let ADHD win (see Chapter 12).**

All three are equally important, but let's focus on the first one for a second.

Obviously a big factor in reducing your ADHD symptoms is getting on medication. I'll cover this in detail in Chapter 14, but I want to talk about the non-pharmaceutical stuff first. Taking medications won't suddenly mean you don't have ADHD, and they won't eliminate your symptoms either. They're just one of the tools you may need to help you get your shit together, and while they're a great one, they can never be your only one. To quote a popular adage in the ADHD world, 'Pills don't make skills.'

Stop soldiering on

In the first year after being diagnosed with ADHD, I was so excited about every productivity hack, innovative morning routine or tip to 'heal' my ADHD that I'd throw myself into it full throttle. Then two or three days later, I'd be so exhausted and mentally stretched that I'd end up collapsing, giving up on my brand new 'habit' and feeling terrible, frustrated and 'unhealable'.

But now, in my more educated, more proactive second year, I've figured out that a lot of these systems were never aimed at reducing my symptoms, they were just training me in how to push through the **executive dysfunction** no matter the emotional cost. Those tips like 'Never put something down, put it away' or 'Tell yourself that you aren't allowed to stand up from your desk until 4 pm, no matter how much work you get done'.

I'm not saying there's no place for these 'force yourself' tactics – they're definitely in the ADHD toolbox. I'm just not sure we should be reaching for them so often. I know I can *force* myself to work when I really need to. I've written an entire article while genuinely worrying that I'm going to break my computer because I keep crying into the keyboard. But I also know that I'm absolutely empty after I do that. Even if it's a less extreme example than this, pushing and pushing and pushing still costs me something deep down that an extra hour of sleep and a quiet afternoon won't fix. I don't believe it's ethical to suggest using these tactics for everyday tasks.

The goal has to be to make living with ADHD less exhausting, so it's easier to complete the task in the first place. And the good news is, there are actually ways to do that. The bad news is, they are going to therapy, eating healthily, getting enough sleep and exercising regularly.

I know. I was fucking devastated when I found out too.

Making it easier for Ethel

Remember your friendly executive-function lady, Ethel? Well, as far as I can tell, besides medication, the main thing you can do to reduce the impairment caused by your ADHD is make her life easier.

Ethel wants you to go to therapy

One of the most frustrating things about poor Ethel's job is that so much of her precious time is wasted dealing with all those 'anxiety' memos that keep filling up her inbox. As we know, living with ADHD has a way of making that mental health paperwork pile up fast. How is Ethel meant to be on top of reminding us to brush our teeth and turn the stove off when she's filing away yet another form that reads 'I'm a bad person because I didn't get enough work done today' or 'He didn't text me back because he can see that deep down I'm rotten and selfish and terrible'? That's where therapy comes in. To slowly but surely reduce that emotional strain on our brain, and, as a happy **side effect**, make us feel better and happier in the process.

A couple of different therapy styles have been suggested for ADHD, but the one generally considered to be the most effective is **cognitive behavioural therapy (CBT)**, with **meta-analysis** showing that it can moderately reduce ADHD symptoms in adults.[1, 2] The crux of CBT is learning to separate the objective facts of what's happening from our subjective interpretations of them and our emotions. For example, if an old friend doesn't wave back when you wave at them from across the road, CBT would notionally help you not immediately assume it's because they hate you, and instead recognise that it was a busy street, they looked a bit stressed and preoccupied, and maybe they just didn't see you. CBT for ADHD tends to focus on the thought patterns that impair our ability to get things done, such as feeling like we're a failure if something isn't perfect or feeling defeated if we struggle to get things right.

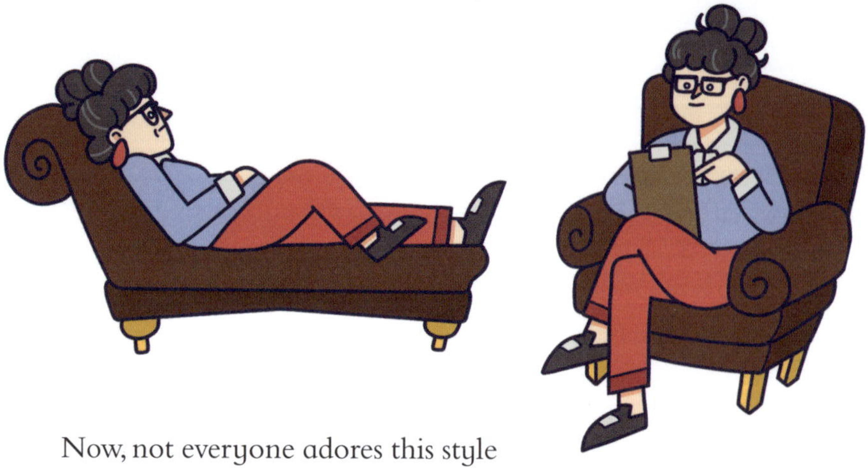

Now, not everyone adores this style of therapy, finding it invalidating, or feeling it teaches them to intellectualise their feelings rather than actually feel them, so I'm cautious about outright recommending it. My experience with CBT has been positive, but that doesn't mean it's for everyone, especially given how wide the range of ADHD psychological **comorbidities** is. So don't be afraid to try out different psychologists or approaches until you find a therapy plan that works for you.

But regular therapy sessions, even once every couple of weeks, aren't economically feasible for everyone. They're not economically feasible for me. I wish I was chatting to my therapist way more often, but at the moment I'm making do – and have arranged my spending so that therapy is among my top priorities after stuff like 'food', 'housing costs' and 'funky earrings that I order online when I'm a little tipsy'.

But even beyond correcting your impairing ADHD symptoms and treating your comorbidities, it's worth remembering that suddenly finding out you have a condition like this as an adult is a bloody massive, earth-shattering event. It will almost certainly have stirred up a great deal of memories and trauma and probably grief. It's not fair on you or your Ethel to expect the two of you to deal with that alone.

Therapy is also the thing I recommend most frequently to my friends who are stuck on Australia's (presently) ridiculously long wait lists for psychiatrists willing to diagnose adult ADHD. You might not be able to get your hands on the medication for a while, but while you wait you can still do a huge amount of work towards getting your mind in order and learning to forgive yourself.

While it's by no means a replacement for therapy, another service offered is ADHD coaching. Coaches focus on practical skills and organisational systems as well as providing a form of external motivation to help you actually put these methods into place (basically because you don't want to rock up to your next session and have to admit you haven't even attempted them).

When I saw a coach, for example, I wanted to get better at taking my medication regularly, getting to sleep earlier and being more reliable at replying to emails and messages. I really enjoyed the strategies my coach taught me, some of which I'll cover later in the book, and it was nice to be able to tell someone that I struggled to remember to take a pill even if it was right in front of me, and for them not to look at me with confusion or concern.

I went a handful of times, and would have liked to continue but, I won't lie, it was a decent whack of cash – around $100 per session – with no government or insurance subsidies. I'm not sure I could have justified it financially if I didn't feel a responsibility to at least try it for this book. Luckily, the coach I saw focused on setting me up with the tools to continue on my own.

Also, be aware that ADHD coaching is not a regulated industry, so quality isn't guaranteed. There are psychologists and counsellors who offer ADHD coaching as part of their services, but people in this line of work aren't necessarily medical professionals. Many are more like life or career coaches. Among this group, some will have completed formal training and be accredited with an organisation such as the International Coaching Federation. Others will just be winging it.

The ADHD coach I saw wasn't a therapist, but was recommended by my psychiatrist, who said many of his patients found a lot of value in her services, so I had some reassurance she'd know what she was talking about. But if you're going in blind, it's probably worth asking exactly what training they've done and what professional organisations they're a part of, and looking for any reviews online before you fully commit to an expensive session.

Also keep an eye out for social media influencer–type coaches who are charging exorbitant amounts.

Ethel wants you to exercise

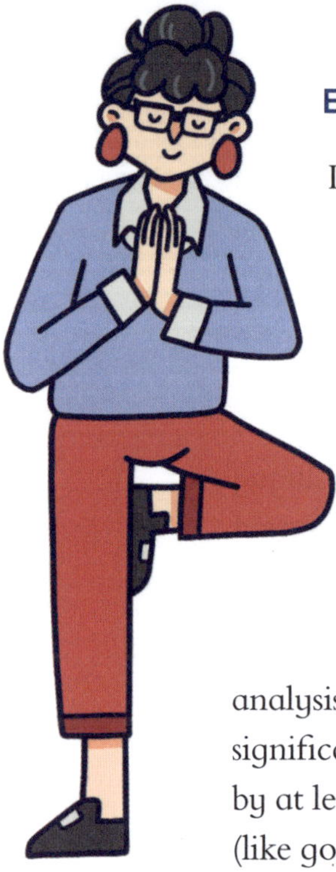

I hate that I'm about to write this, but exercising – getting your heart rate up, or at least getting your body moving – is an important part of reducing the impairing symptoms of ADHD.

While the science world isn't at the point of universal agreement just yet, a decent crop of studies show the positive benefits of exercise for ADHD symptoms, and plenty of doctors even prescribe exercise to their patients, either to complement the effects of medication or as an alternative if pharmaceuticals aren't viable. A recent meta-analysis looking at ADHD children concluded that exercise has a significant positive effect on executive function,[3] which is backed up by at least one small study looking at the benefits of acute exercise (like going for a run or doing a workout) in ADHD adults.[4] Two other meta-analyses found more modest[5] or inconclusive results[6] in reducing ADHD symptoms, but the latter did show a significant reduction in anxiety and depression, ADHD's frequent comorbidities.

Combating feelings of anxiety and depression is a massive part of the ADHD battle, and there's no disputing that exercise is a brilliant treatment for this.[7,8] I won't get too bogged down in the details, but the words 'significant', 'essential' and 'comprehensive body of high-quality evidence' tend to get thrown around a lot in studies about exercise's effect on general mental health. So, just like therapy, exercise and physical activity are mostly about making us feel better generally.

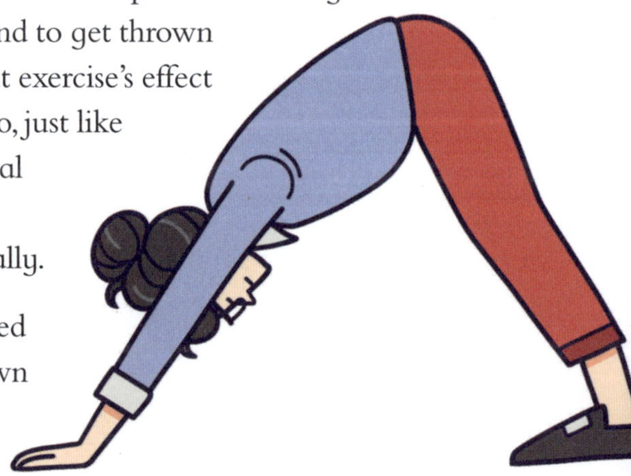

If we feel good, refreshed and awake when we sit down to work, study, do chores, or socialise with family and friends, then it's way easier for our poor little overworked Ethels to focus on the important stuff, rather than deal with all the dense paperwork that comes flying in when we haven't been outside in a week and our bodies begin to merge with the couch. Obviously in the throes of a severe mental health flare-up this isn't always going to be feasible, but as a form of general emotional maintenance, it's invaluable.

'Well, that's all well and good, Matilda,' I hear you say, 'but how does an ADHDer actually make themselves exercise in the first place?'

Because I viscerally hate exercising so much, I was about to write that I'm probably not the best person to ask, but perhaps that actually means I'm one of the best. So, here's how I manage to force myself, kicking and screaming, into moving my body.

First, it's important to remember that ADHD brains naturally have a harder time weighing the cost of short-term pain against long-term gain. So simply knowing that if you do this every day for weeks you're going to start feeling happier or healthier probably isn't the powerful motivator it might be for a neurotypical person.

Rather than focusing on those long-term benefits, we need to find types of exercise that provide implicit rewards – meaning the act of doing the workout is pleasurable in and of itself. We need to set up explicit consequences – meaning we have to do the annoying workout in order to avoid something slightly more annoying. And we need to integrate these rewards and consequences into our routines – meaning we eventually start doing them without having to consciously bully ourselves into it. Let me give you some examples.

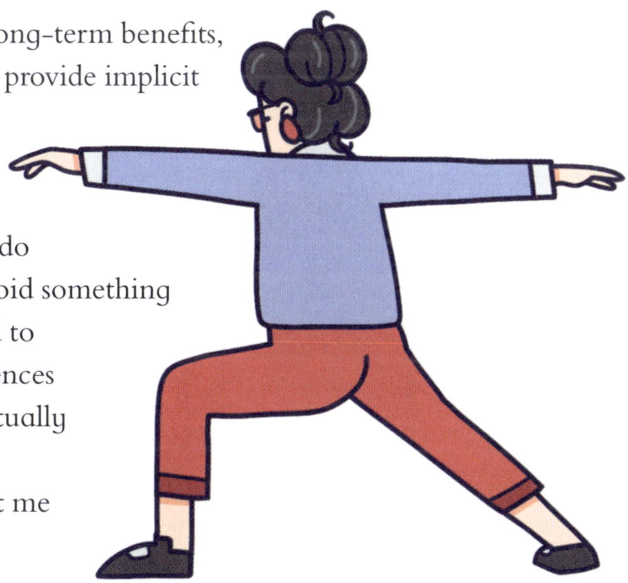

Over the past year, I've managed to find three types of exercise that I find bearable: riding my bike to work, swimming and playing in a local football team.

Implicit rewards: These are forms of exercise that bring me pleasure beyond the endorphins they release in my brain. I ride to the office because I like being out in the fresh air and I find it really helpful to have forty minutes to listen to the radio (quietly and only in one earphone, to ensure road safety) before I start my day's work. I like football because I enjoy having a place to go and socialise with other women, and my teammates have become good friends who I want to hang out with even if I'm exhausted at the end of a workday. And I like swimming because it's calming and refreshing, and I get to use the funky workout features on my smartwatch.

Explicit consequences: If I don't ride my bike fast enough to actually get my heart pumping, then I'll be late to work. If I don't show up to footy because I can't be bothered, then I'm letting the team down (despite being by far the worst player on the field), and if I don't try hard enough when I'm at training, then I'll get embarrassed by how slow and unfit I am, and my coach will look at me with disappointment in her eyes. And finally, the pool I go to is attached to a little sauna, and it feels like some sort of blasphemy to enter a sauna without actually getting into the water first, so if I don't swim then I don't get to steam, and that's a sad state of affairs.

Integration into routine: Riding my bike into the city is a means to an end, literally. It's part of my day-to-day life. I don't have to actively decide to exercise, I just need to get to work, and exercise is an accidental part of that now. Footy training and matches are always at roughly the same time on the same days, and, importantly, on a schedule I can't control. It's consistent enough that I can remember not to schedule anything at the same time (usually), and I can't just 'put it off an hour' or 'do it tomorrow', which almost always ends up meaning 'never'. Swimming is less perfect on this front, but when I get into the routine of going at night, taking a book to read in the sauna (one that I don't mind if it falls apart due to the steam), hopping in the shower back home and into bed, then I tend to do it pretty consistently and, importantly, unthinkingly. Unfortunately, when things get busy it tends to be one of the first things to go.

For me, the key to getting exercise done is to take away the moment when I have to actively decide to do it. I've created situations where I'm dragged into it whether I like it or not. And ninety-nine times out of a hundred – when those reward chemicals eventually do hit – I'm extraordinarily glad that I did, and relieved that I didn't have the chance to talk myself out of it.

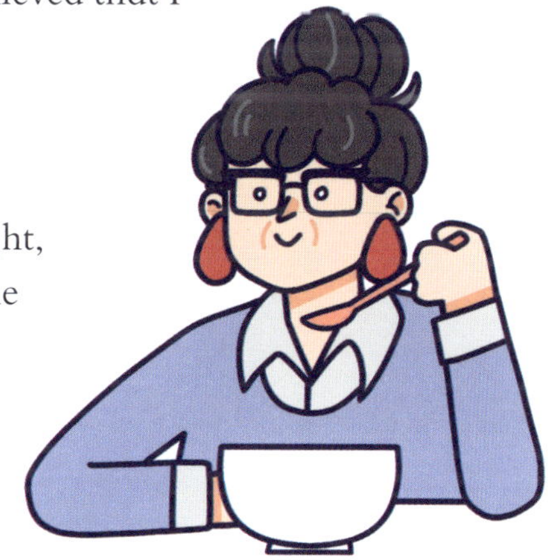

Ethel wants you to eat a healthy breakfast

Talking about ADHD and diet can be pretty fraught, because for decades naysayers have argued that the disorder is simply caused by kids eating too much sugar or processed foods.[9] This concept is still so prevalent that it makes it hard to even google what foods you should be eating to help with ADHD symptoms, because the top search results are dominated either by misinformation or by articles disproving said misinformation. So, let's get this out of the way quickly before we move on to the useful information.

It is true that there's a significant association between having ADHD and consuming an unhealthy diet – shying away from fruits and vegetables and going hard on fats, meats and foods with added sugar.[10] We also know that young people with ADHD are three times more likely to be medically classified as 'obese', and 2.5 times more likely to have type 2 diabetes,[11] which are both at least partially influenced by diet.

But while plenty of studies show a **correlation** between unhealthy eating and ADHD, there's little to no evidence to suggest that the food causes the disorder. Rather, ADHD can make it harder for us to resist highly pleasurable, cheap and convenient junk food. The condition may impair our ability to maintain the organisationally intensive and time-consuming work of preparing healthy meals every day. And it can negatively impact our socioeconomic status, which in turn can make nutritious food financially inaccessible. It seems more logical to conclude that it's the condition that causes the diet. But that isn't to say diet doesn't affect the condition at all. In fact, there are some fairly simple dietary changes we can make to help our brains a little and make our symptoms more manageable.

Whether we're ADHD or neurotypical, the food we eat is linked to our ability to focus. In particular, studies have shown that eating breakfast can improve cognition in a variety of ways, including the ability to maintain attention.[12] So when people say 'Breakfast is the most important meal of the day', they're especially talking to people like us.

In fact, it's even more important given some of us are probably about to take medication that will significantly reduce or even eliminate our appetite for the next ten or so hours.

This side effect of stimulant medication can make it super tempting to try to fix fatigue with a fast cup of coffee and get on with our day, never feeling a twinge from our stomach. But just because we don't feel hungry doesn't mean our body isn't, and this will impact our mood, our energy and our ability to focus. This is why I try to take my medication immediately after eating breakfast – sometimes I keep them on the dining-room table for that exact reason.

The ADHD advocacy organisation CHADD recommends breakfasts high in proteins and complex carbohydrates, from plant sources such as beans, veggies, whole grains and rolled oats, or from animal sources like eggs, milk or (although my vegetarian sensibilities cringe to admit it) lean meats.[13]

No one is at their best when their Ethel is running on fumes, and ours are so flustered to begin with that we can't afford for them to lose productivity because we forgot to grab a nut bar and an apple on our way out the door.

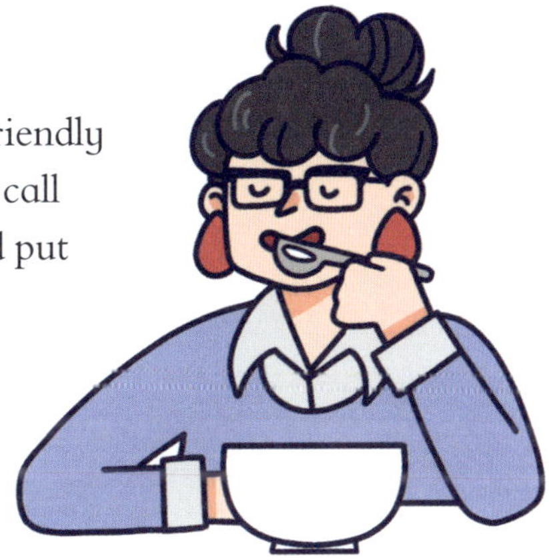

I've taken to trying to incorporate an ADHD-friendly breakfast into my life by utilising something I like to call 'the velociraptor diet'. This is when you wake up and put a couple of eggs on to boil, do your other morning chores while you wait, then peel them, chuck on a little butter and garlic salt if you're fancy, and sit there and eat a bowl of eggs like the fucking prehistoric scavenger you are. In the name of complying with the velociraptor way of life, these eggs must be from a proper free range farm. (Sorry, I don't make the rules.) Also, eggs are somewhat high in cholesterol, so you shouldn't do this absolutely every day – we don't have prehistoric stomachs, after all.

That being said, there are *plenty* of mornings when even a velociraptor breakfast is too much preparation for me. This is why, if you're cooking dinner, it's a great idea to make enough for tomorrow's breakfast as well. And when even chucking leftovers in the microwave is too much, a banana, some crackers and dip or some shredded cheese shoved in your mouth as you're bathed by the cold, judgemental light of your fridge will suffice. These aren't optimal, they're not going to yield the best possible results, but something is still way better than nothing. So if that means three cold spring rolls and a few squares of fruit-and-nut chocolate, then all power to you.

Also, try to eat a proper, nutritious lunch. I know it's hard, but it will help prevent you crashing and **burning out** at the end of the day. I'm slowly getting better at this – setting an alarm on my phone and even occasionally packing my lunch the night before. But just in case I fail, I now keep a bag of cashews or almonds in my desk drawer at work. (If you are out and about during the work/school day, you can keep this in your backpack or car glove box.) Try to do better than this back-up plan whenever you can, but again, if, like me, you're still in the 'taking what I can get' stage of ADHD-life, the goal is 'done', not 'perfect'.

The ADHD world is also filled with people telling you to take their specific vitamin mix or dietary supplement to help ease the condition's symptoms. But I'd take all such assertions with a grain of salt, because the evidence for these miracle fixes is pretty limited. (Also worth taking note of: online ADHD personalities who have their own supplement range in the background of every video.)

There's some indication that getting more omega-3 fatty acids might help marginally,[14] so that could be an option. Vitamin tablets might also be useful for filling in the nutritional gaps if you're struggling to maintain the type of diet CHADD recommends. (That's what I use them for.) But ultimately, your body has a much easier time absorbing vitamins from food than supplements,[15] so generally eating well will probably do more for you than any expensive tablet. Also, you should check with your prescribing physician before starting on supplements, because vitamins can affect your medications.

Actually, that brings me to my last piece of breakfast advice. If you're taking an amphetamine-based stimulant (such as Adderall, Vyvanse, Dexedrine, etc.), high levels of gastrointestinal acidifying agents in your system (i.e. things that make your pee more acidic), including vitamin C, may seriously reduce your body's ability to absorb the medication, make you pee it out faster and potentially reduce the amount of time its effects will last.[16] That means it's probably best to avoid supplements containing vitamin C (ascorbic acid) an hour before and an hour after you take your meds.

When it comes to vitamin C–rich or highly acidic foods and drinks, it depends on the exact type of amphetamine stimulant you take. (For example, the information document for Vyvanse says having a glass of OJ straight away is fine, but short-acting dexamfetamine tablets warn against it.[17, 18]) So it might be worth chatting with your doctor about this next time you see them.

Do still include vitamin C in your diet, though, otherwise you could end up developing scurvy.

Ethel wants you to sleep well

Before I started researching ADHD, it never occurred to me that there are people out there who can just trust that they will go to bed at the right time every night. Like, 'Oh, I have an early start tomorrow, I'll go to bed an hour early.' And not, 'Fuck, I have an early start tomorrow, let me pray to Cthulhu that the stars align and I can manage to find the willpower not just to go to bed at the right time, but to actually go to sleep.' Every night of my life is like flipping a coin to see if the universe has blessed me with the self-control and emotional balance necessary to get a good night's rest. But unlike flipping a coin, the results are far from fifty-fifty.

Regularly getting a good night's sleep is an integral part of the whole reducing your negative symptoms and improving your life thing.

As I mentioned in Chapter 4, sleep issues can significantly worsen the symptoms of ADHD,[19] so it's pretty obvious that regularly getting a good night's sleep is an integral part of the whole reducing your negative symptoms and improving your life thing. But, unfortunately, the ADHD gods decided to make this really bloody hard for up to 85 per cent of us.[20] So how do we fix it?

Well, simply recognising that we have to prioritise sleep is a big step. Before I was diagnosed, I'd sometimes stay up into the wee hours of the morning finishing everything that I hadn't completed for school or work. But then I would barely sleep, which meant I would barely get anything done the next day and suddenly whoops, would you look at the vicious cycle I've created. Learning just how interconnected ADHD and sleep are has made me realise that I can't rely on this tactic any more. Which is a shame, since I think I genuinely do work best in the middle of the night. It's the great envy of my life that Anthony regularly manages to do a full day's work with only four or five hours of snoozing under his belt – but even the idea of attempting that terrifies me. I've just had to accept that we're built differently, and I need seven hours minimum.

I've also learnt that my brain takes a long time to wind down. If I finish writing or doing extra work after 9 pm, there's no chance I'm getting to sleep before midnight. This is frustrating, as it means I simply have fewer potentially productive hours available in the day. But the alternative is being desperately sleep-deprived and having zero productive hours the next day, so it's an accommodation I have to make.

So now that we've accepted that we need it, the next step is figuring out how to actually get this mythical 'full night's rest'. The best way to increase your chances of getting to sleep when you actually want to is by practising 'sleep hygiene', which basically means going to bed and waking up at the same time every day. Obviously this is easier said than done, but many people find it helpful to have consistent night-time routines. I'm not great at this, but lately I've been trying to make a nice herbal tea as a quasi-ritual to signal the start of the 'wind-down' process. Then I'll put on my Oodie, prop myself up in bed with some pillows, lay my weighted blanket over my lap and play some *Legend of Zelda* on the Switch until my eyelids start feeling heavy.

Now, I think technically, in the name of good sleep hygiene, you're not meant to do anything in your bed besides sleep and have sex (and I assume you could probably even relocate that last one if you have a comfy enough couch). But this suggestion isn't on the cards for me at this bed-loving point in my life (and honestly sounds a bit like neurotypical nonsense). So I ignored that idea and went looking for some more concrete fixes.

At least anecdotally, I've heard a lot of ADHDers talk about the 'sleep of the dead' phenomenon, where you sleep restlessly for the first half of the night and then for the last few hours plunge into a deep, deep slumber from which it's extraordinarily difficult to wake. Sure, an alarm will make you sit up, but if your head accidentally touches the pillow after you turn it off, then *bam!* it's two hours later and you're late for work. Or perhaps you do get up at the right time, but the first few hours of the day are then clouded with an unshakeable zombie-like fog.

My main issue with mornings is that 'normal me' and 'waking-up me' have aggressively different motivations and attitudes to 'being on time'. I can set five different alarms, and that AM bastard will turn every one of them off. I can promise myself a thousand times over that I'm going to get into the office an hour early that day to get some prep done, and yet that morning gremlin continues to disregard my wishes.

If you take stimulant medication for your ADHD, one trick I've learnt is to set a second (or sixth) alarm for an hour before I'm meant to wake up, take my ADHD medication then and then fall blissfully back to sleep. By the time my normal alarm goes off, I'm raring to go. Also, yes, this does contradict my advice to eat breakfast before taking your meds, so I tend to switch between systems depending on the vibe of the day. In a perfect world I'd have a high-protein muesli bar on my bedside table to make sure I'm at least eating something before the appetite suppression kicks in – but I haven't reached that elite level of efficiency just yet.

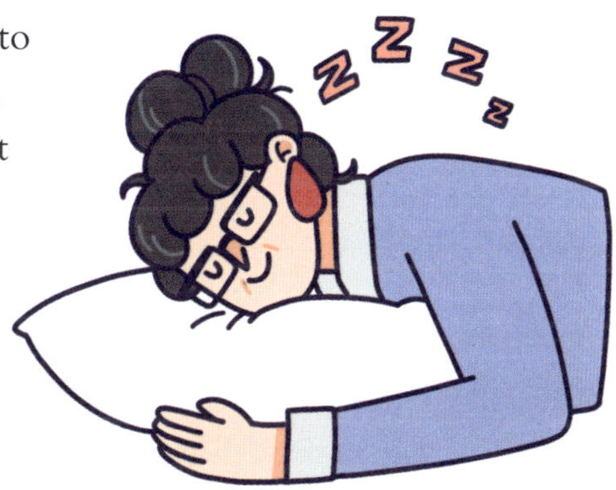

Obviously, plenty of our sleep issues are caused by simply not having the executive-functioning capacity to get ourselves to bed on time, or not being able to quiet our brains, but this might not be the whole story. In Chapter 4, I mentioned that a decent whack of

ADHDers potentially have issues with a delayed **circadian rhythm**,[21] meaning the simple comfort of 'being sleepy when it's bedtime' isn't guaranteed. But there are potentially some fixes for that as well.

One fairly popular and reasonably effective option[22, 23] is to take **melatonin** supplements (but please talk to your doctor first, especially if you're already on ADHD medication, because when used incorrectly or for too long, melatonin has been linked to depression). I've found melatonin incredibly helpful. It's not a miracle fix, and I'll still have nights staring at the ceiling on occasion, but it's really great for speeding up that eyes-heavy, mind-empty, acute feeling of tiredness when I need to rip myself away from my phone and put effort into going to sleep.

If melatonin isn't for you, there's another (admittedly less robustly researched) tactic, that's either very funny or extremely *Black Mirror*–esque, depending on how you see it. It's buying a sunrise online. Hear me out.

Basically, one way to potentially get our circadian rhythm and our melatonin-release schedule back on track is to beat our brains over the head with the fact that the sun is up by using something called 'morning bright-light therapy'. For half an hour first thing each morning, you chill out with your face 60 centimetres away from a super-bright (at least 10,000 lux) lamp usually used for seasonal affective disorder. Two studies on ADHDers showed a significant improvement, both in bringing their circadian rhythm forward and reducing ADHD symptoms in general, for the weeks they used bright-light therapy.[24, 25] But while the results were promising, the study sample sizes were small, so there's no guarantee it will be worth the cash splash.

I believe part of the morning-light therapy process is meant to include limiting your exposure to blue light at night, too, meaning no screens or phone in bed. But given my brain's night-time tendency to become consumed with the crushing reality that I will one day die when it's not constantly distracted by technology, I went for the alternative technique suggested by one study, which is wearing blue-light-blocking glasses from 4 pm onwards.[26] I ran my own extremely small science experiment on these two tactics for a few weeks and my conclusion was . . . yeah, sure, I think it helped a bit. But, god, it's hard to remember to put on those glasses at 4 pm.

So, those are the four main pillars of reducing the intensity of our ADHD impairments. Achieving this lifestyle is still a difficult (potentially lifelong) mission, but hopefully, even with little, incremental improvements, we will start giving our Ethel some room to breathe. She's earned it.

Now we've gone through all the ways we can help our brain fit our world, it's time to talk about how we can make our world fit our brain. And I have brilliant news: this is where the life hacks start.

11

How do I hack it?

One of the best things about learning you have ADHD is realising that once you let go of the idea of what's 'normal' or 'the proper thing to do', there are so many ingenious, helpful and fun ways to make your life more ADHD-friendly.

So welcome to 'all the fun stuff'. We're talking life hacks, we're talking to-do lists, we're talking a complicated system of different-coloured bracelets to help remind you to brush your teeth in the morning. And if by any chance your natural disposition is not to be as excited about this kind of thing as I am, fear not – I'll spell out all the benefits so you simply won't be able to resist.

But as joyous as ADHD tips and tricks can be, the first and most important one is not to overload yourself. One or two new ADHD systems are fun; eight or nine all at once is a recipe for overwhelming your **executive-functioning** capacity rather than improving it. It's probably best to try a couple of things out, see if you can get them integrated into your routine, and once they become second nature think about adding a couple more.

The next big hurdle is pride. A lot of the systems and habits I'm about to describe could be viewed as a little childish or embarrassing – especially if you're in possession of an annoyingly judgemental inner monologue. But the fact of the matter is, ADHD brains respond really well to fun things, so to make your world more ADHD-friendly, you kind of have to accept that you'll be making it more playful, too. And there's no point denying yourself something both whimsical *and* productive just for the sake of feeling like a 'proper' grown-up.

And one last thing before we launch into the hacks – while some have come purely from my own personal experience, most are things I've picked up from others along the way. Friends, medical professionals, TikToks, tweets, comments in ADHD Facebook groups (the only reason I go on Facebook nowadays), or the random woman I sat next to on the train who was talking loudly on the phone about her 'brain dump' list. Many of these hacks have been floating around the ADHD community for a while, which makes crediting the original creator (if one exists) extremely difficult or downright impossible, but I've endeavoured to do so where I can.

Okay, let's go.

Make it impossible to ignore

One thing I struggle with in day-to-day life is remembering. This isn't just forgetting events that should be written in my calendar, like hairdresser's appointments and entire lectures I've agreed to deliver to university students about the use of TikTok in the modern journalism landscape. I also have a lot of trouble keeping track of what I'm meant to be doing in the medium term, like taking out the bins, removing the spanakopita from the oven before it burns or putting in my annual leave request.

I'm not good at spontaneously remembering to do something I've mentally flagged for later, so I need external cues to ensure the thought pops back into my head. I'll try to jot down the important things in a notes app on my phone, but then I never check it. Or I'll text my boyfriend asking him to remind me, although this requires an extremely patient boyfriend, which I've been told is not a universal commodity.

Lots of people use phone alarms for this, but I tend to struggle with:

1. remembering to actually set the alarm
2. setting it but then having no bloody clue what it's for once it sounds
3. just turning off the alarm and never thinking about it again.

Instead, I need something that will remind me again and again until that goddamn task is done.

And the solution? Just putting something random on the ground in the middle of the room. If there's something important for me to do in the medium term, I take an object that would be weird to have in the middle of the floor and I leave it there. Then every time I come into that room, see the thing and, heaven forbid, have to step around it, I'm motivated to do the task just so I can pick the thing up. Need to pay the electricity bill this morning? Candle in the middle of the dining-room floor. Good luck forgetting now. Need to pack your laptop charger for your work trip, but can't yet because you're still using it? Deodorant can on the hallway floor. No letting your computer die on this flight. It's a great system – just don't use anything edible if you have dogs.

One or two new ADHD systems are fun; eight or nine all at once is a recipe for overwhelming your executive-functioning capacity rather than improving it.

Chore charms

Using this same 'constant reminder' principle, I also utilise a chore charm system. I didn't invent this, and it's hard to pinpoint exactly who did, but it's been used widely by people all over TikTok.

The basic concept is that you have a bunch of chunky, stretchy bracelets with a little jangly tag attached (I use keyring tags), each listing a chore around the house you need to do on a weekly or monthly basis. Things like 'wipe down the stove', 'water the living-room plants' or 'throw out all the mouldy food in the fridge'.

Each room has a different jar with its unique chores in it.

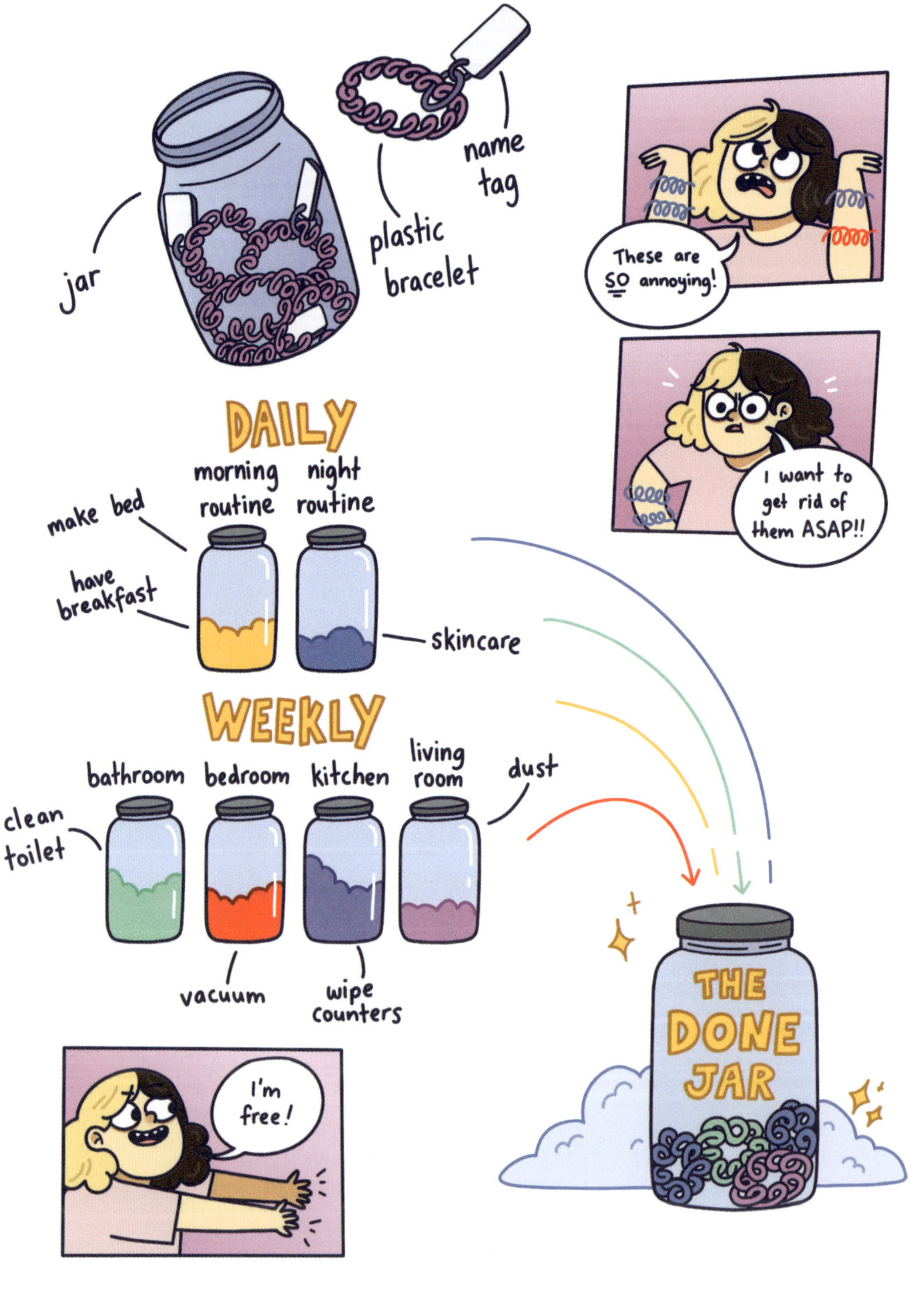
jar
plastic bracelet
name tag
These are SO annoying!
I want to get rid of them ASAP!!
DAILY
morning routine
night routine
make bed
have breakfast
skincare
WEEKLY
bathroom
bedroom
kitchen
living room
dust
clean toilet
vacuum
wipe counters
THE DONE JAR
I'm free!

Whenever you have time to do housework, pick out three or four of the bracelets from the jars (or however many you want) and put them around your wrist. Here's the important bit: you're not allowed to take the charm off until you've completed the chore written on it.

When you're finished, you chuck the bracelet in a big empty jar labelled 'done' and, notionally, by the end of the week you will have filled it and finished all your chores. Then you can empty it back out (leaving the monthlies in there till the end of the, you guessed it, month) and start again. If that sounds overwhelmingly difficult, don't worry. I don't think I've ever actually filled the 'done' jar. It's more of an aspirational goal.

This system has a couple of big benefits:

- **Once you make the charms, it takes away the complex executive-functioning task of figuring out what chores you need to do every single time.**
- **You get a little hit of dopamine and satisfaction when you finally get to take off the bracelet and chuck it in the 'done' jar.**
- **The rattling of the tags on your wrist is not only a constant micro-reminder of what you're meant to be doing, but it's slightly annoying, so you're motivated to get the chore done, and fast. (This might be a bit of a turn-off if you have sensory sensitivities, especially if you're also autistic, so you could consider using tags made out of cloth or another soft material to avoid clanking.)**

The chore charm system is really handy for cleaning, but I've found myself adapting it for my morning routine, too. I have a separate 'morning' jar with every step I need to complete to get ready for a workday – 'make the bed', 'have breakfast', 'put on deodorant', 'brush teeth', 'do skin care', 'take medication', etc. It's not so much that I think I'm going to forget these things (although I regularly do), but with my habit of drifting off course when I'm sleepy (read: accidentally sitting on my bed in just a towel after a shower, scrolling on my phone), this system helps keep me on task. It means I'm constantly thinking about what's next to do and how I can get those bloody bracelets off my wrist as soon as possible. I can see how the outsider might think it childish, but I get to host my own little game show every morning where I race against the clock to defeat the bracelets. Waking up to that level of fun and whimsy is totally worth it for me.

This system does require a good few hours to set up – writing and finalising your list of chores, labelling every tag, washing old jam jars, etc. I recommend watching a bunch of videos about it online and then harnessing your excitement, allowing that to morph into **hyperfocus**, ordering everything online in a fit of passion, and busting out all the prep work in one afternoon while you steadfastly ignore the need to vacuum.

Break the fridge rules

When it comes to ADHD, never underestimate the power of rearranging your home so that you can physically see the things you need to remember. And this is especially true when it comes to food.

I have a really hard time remembering to use my fresh fruit and veg before they go off. I'm simply never going to be the kind of person who can go, 'Oh, well, if I remember correctly I bought an eggplant seven days ago, therefore I should craft a meal around said eggplant tonight to avoid it rotting.' (I have no idea how long an eggplant lasts in the fridge – that's part of the problem.)

It will only occur to me to cook with an eggplant if I open my fridge and see an eggplant. But my crisper drawer is really deep, meaning I can only really see the top layer – perhaps 20 per cent of the veggies in there. But then I saw a few ADHD Instagram accounts suggesting I rearrange everything so my veggies live in the door of my fridge, where one might usually put condiments, so I can't help but see them every time I open it up. My condiments have now been relegated to the crisper, the theory being that you never base your ideas for a meal on a condiment – as you cook, you remember what sauces or pastes you need and specifically go into the fridge to get them – so there's no need for them to occupy valuable, easily visible space.

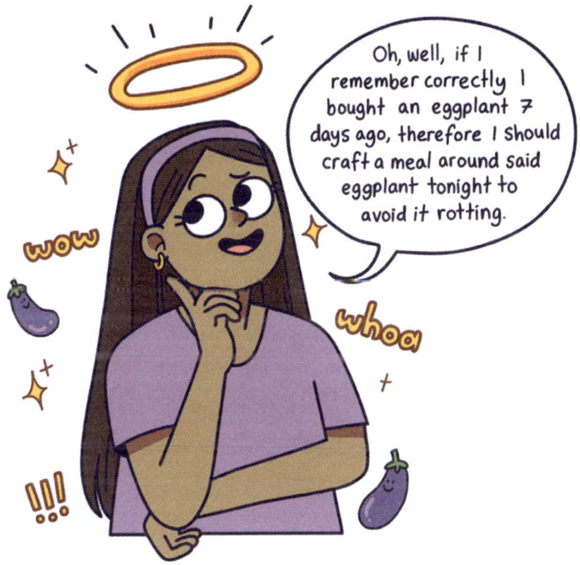

Then I put everything perishable – cheeses, tofu and containers full of leftovers – on the shelves closest to my eye line, where I can see all the way to the back (due to my short stature, these are the middle two). And anything that's going to last longer – pickles, butter, etc. – I put on the bottom shelves, where my view is obscured. I did this before Anthony and I moved into an apartment with just the two of us, so the last step was remembering, 'Oh shit, I live with roommates,' and sending a message to the share-house group chat asking if they were okay with me rearranging things, in a tone that implied I hadn't already done it. And the system worked great! My food waste was down, my vegetable consumption was up and my roommates were (thankfully) fine with it.

Staying on track

So, once you've remembered all the things you need to do, how do you actually get them done? Well, your tactics will vary drastically depending on whether you're trying to get a lot of little tasks done in a row (like doing the chores at home), where your time-management, planning and task-switching abilities will be put to the test; or you're trying to get stuck into one mega job (such as sitting for several hours to do your tax, submit invoices, study for an exam or write reports for work), where you'll need to sustain intense focus, avoid distractions and maintain motivation.

Let's go with the string of little tasks first.

Keep your brain busy

Cleaning, cooking, shopping and all the other minutiae of life are kind of boring, and it can be hard for us ADHDers to tear ourselves away from doing something fun, like watching TV or crafting a little cardboard hat for your cat to make him look like an elf. So bring some fun with you. Subscribe to a great line-up of podcasts, get an audiobook app, find some YouTube video essays you really like, and listen to them while you do all the dull life tasks.

This also helps bridge that gap between, say, folding the washing and moving on to vacuuming. For me, that's the most dangerous time for my productivity – I'll either sit down and accidentally lose all motivation, or become so consumed by trying to plan my next move that I end up paralysed and overwhelmed. The chore charms help massively with this, but so does filling up some of that extra space in my head with a good audiobook – it leaves less room for the anxiety to bounce around, and I can slip more easily into autopilot rather than focusing on all the wrong things.

This isn't just a helpful tip for me, it's utterly imperative. I used to feel really guilty that I required constant entertainment, as if it was a failure of character. But no, it's just what I need to get the job done. There's no shame in that.

Body doubling

One interesting quirk of ADHD is that a lot of us find it extremely useful to have someone else in the room when we're trying to complete a chore. This is known as '**body doubling**', and there are a bunch of reasons it can help:

- **It makes us feel accountable for staying on task, because the person will notice if we end up sitting on the floor googling the downfall of the Roman empire for an hour.**
- **Their presence is a physical reminder of what we're meant to be doing, so even if we do get a little side-tracked, as soon as we see them we can pull ourselves back to task.**
- **They can encourage us to keep going and not to leave that frustrating final 10 per cent undone.**
- **Dealing with the day-to-day complications of life is kind of scary, so it can be comforting to feel like you're not in it alone.**

I often find myself asking Anthony to come and sit on the bed while I clean up my clothes. He doesn't even need to talk – he can be on his phone or getting things done on the computer – I just need a warm body there. This is true for regular work as well as housework, which is why some ADHDers find they prefer physically being at their place of employment to working from home.

If you don't have someone who's physically able to be with you, you can always video-call someone – perhaps another ADHDer who's trying to get stuff done too – and you can be each other's double. There are even websites that will pair you up with a stranger for this very purpose, although this is a bit too high-pressure for my liking.

For longer-term tasks, you could try a more traditional 'accountability partner' – a friend or a trusted work colleague, or maybe a favourite aunt who will check in on you every week or month or whatnot, to ask how much progress you've made on your chosen project. This motivates you to get stuff done so you actually have something to report back to them. Even better, if you can find someone with a similar goal, you can check in on each other.

One-stop shop

The other danger zone when completing a string of tasks is all the things that can distract you along the way. You're never going to rid your home or workplace of all distractions (we have ADHD, we'll find something), but you can reduce your exposure to them by limiting the travel time between the steps of a task. I'm not talking about car trips and highways here – I literally mean that I'll have a way better chance of getting the sheets changed if I don't have to walk past a comfy couch on my way to get a pillowcase.

So put things where you're going to use them. It sounds simple but it's honestly revolutionary. Here are a few examples.

Medications

I constantly forget to take my medication because I'll take the pills out of their bottle, pop them on the table and stand up to go get a glass of water. Spoiler alert: that pill isn't going to be taken for hours, and, oh no, it's a long-acting stimulant so if I take it now I'll never get to sleep tonight.

My solution was purchasing a water bottle online that has a days-of-the-week pill organiser built into the side. This way, once a week I can load up the compartments with my medications and vitamins, fill her up with water, pop it on my coffee table or by my bedside and huzzah! A two- or three-step process becomes one step, and therefore much more likely to be completed.

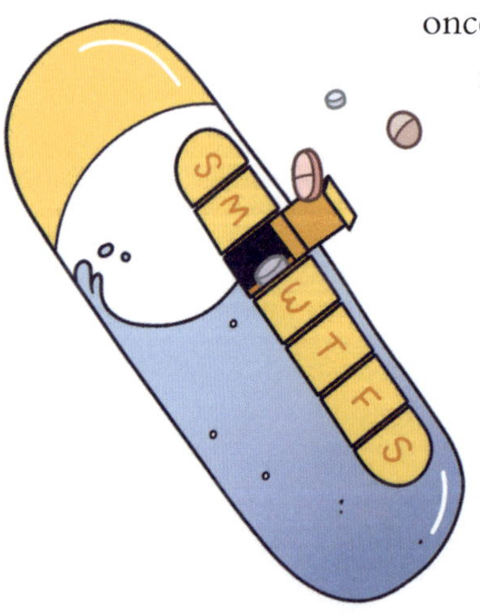

The issue with this particular set of ADHD hacks is that they often involve buying things. The pill organiser cost me about $18, which luckily I'm able to afford, but not everyone can. So, wherever possible, I'll try to include a low- or no-cost alternative. Like, for this one you can also literally just tape your medication box to any old water bottle. It doesn't have to be pretty to be functional. But if, like me, a little capitalist demon sometimes sneaks into your body and convinces you that you need to buy something to feel whole again, these things are at least a productive purchase that still provide that 'there's a package making its way to me' rush of dystopian joy.

Cleaning

I try to put a little rubbish bin in every room of the house, as well as next to my desk, meaning I don't have to get up and ruin my workflow by popping chewing gum or a wrapper in the rubbish. Of course, any old box or container can serve the same purpose.

I've also endeavoured to have a set of cleaning products, sponges and paper towels in each room where I might use them. That way, if I see the bathroom mirror is dirty, I just reach out, grab everything I need, do the whole job and put everything away without ever having to leave the room. These can be the cheapest no-name brands, by the way – remember: 'done', not 'perfect'.

Out-of-the-house essentials

I try to keep a little notebook, pen, mints, sanitary pads, a muesli bar, a day's worth of medications and a phone-charging brick in my handbag at all times, so I only need to worry about my keys and my phone when I'm heading out the door. (And a wallet, I guess, if you still use cash or physical cards.) Eventually, I'm aiming to get a set of these essentials in every handbag so I don't even have to move them across, but that's a goal for another dopamine-filled day.

Getting the big stuff done

Now on to the mega tasks. For me, the hardest part by far of doing intensive, mentally challenging work is getting started – because unlike physical tasks and chores, I can't get that extra stimulation from a TV show or a podcast playing in the background. I have to dedicate my whole brain to something that isn't fun . . . and that's a pretty hard sell for poor little Ethel up there. So often I need to ease us into it, aka tricking myself into focusing – a vital skill to have in your adult ADHD toolbox.

Bamboozling your brain

I know it sounds counterproductive, but in those dire 'impossible to get started' moments, my go-to tactic is to put on a podcast.

I'll press play on the episode then move the phone just out of reach so I can't subconsciously grab it and start scrolling. Then I start work while still trying to listen to the podcast – which might not be that conducive to clear thinking, but that's kind of the point. It means that for those first crucial minutes, I'll still have the 'fun' kind of stimulation that my brain needs to stop desperately begging me to find some other source of stimulation. But now that I've eased myself into actually getting started, I slowly begin focusing more and more on the work and not the words I'm listening to. Eventually, the podcast will become sort of an annoyance, and I'll naturally want to turn it off. And like magic I will have managed to switch my brain into focus mode without even realising, and the podcast can go off.

Fake it till you make it

I'll let you in on a little secret. If you pantomime as a productive person and commit hard enough to the bit, you just might end up being one.

This isn't always easy, but if, for example, I'm working from home, I try to wear work clothes, shoes and all. If I need to get things done in the morning, I sit at my desk rather than on the couch (although I don't stay like this all day, as you'll see in a second). If you're going to be out and about, packing your lunch in the morning, grabbing a coffee from a specific shop before you clock on or wearing jeans rather than tracksuit pants to your university lectures can be part of your 'work mode' ritual.

Another popular tactic I've seen online is not taking off your shoes when you get home from work and keeping them on until you've washed your food containers, packed your lunch for the next day, done a chore or two, cooked dinner, picked out tomorrow's outfit and put your dirty clothes in the wash. (I assume if you're wearing pants, you do have to take off your shoes before that very last step.) Basically, you can't put your feet up on the couch while you have shoes on, so you don't risk simply collapsing. That being said, if you really need to collapse, I'd suggest just taking off your shoes and doing it. Washed food containers aren't worth utterly exhausting yourself. But this can be a handy tactic for higher-energy days.

I need to reiterate, however, that these ways of tricking yourself into productivity are a tool to be used when truly needed; they shouldn't be the crutch that you lean on every time. Putting your energy into being healthy and happy and naturally better equipped to get things done is a much more sustainable source of productivity. But if you really do need to push through and get that to-do list done, there are always shoes.

Brain dump

Getting started is one thing, but maintaining that intense level of focus is a whole other beast.

Part of eliminating your distractions and detours is understanding what causes them in the first place. A lot of the time I'm getting diverted from the work at hand because I think of something I have to do, I simply can't trust myself to remember

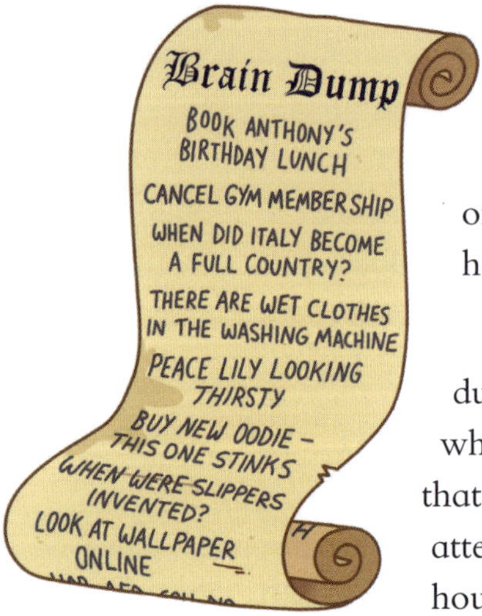
Brain Dump
BOOK ANTHONY'S BIRTHDAY LUNCH
CANCEL GYM MEMBERSHIP
WHEN DID ITALY BECOME A FULL COUNTRY?
THERE ARE WET CLOTHES IN THE WASHING MACHINE
PEACE LILY LOOKING THIRSTY
BUY NEW OODIE – THIS ONE STINKS
WHEN WERE SLIPPERS INVENTED?
LOOK AT WALLPAPER ONLINE

it later. In a very real way, it's now or never.

Sometimes this impulse to just 'get it done' is a good one for people with ADHD, but it's not always that helpful when you're mega-tasking.

I've managed to handle this by using my 'brain dump' space – a Word document I keep open at all times where I write down every important thought or task that pops into my head. This way I only have to divert my attention for a couple of seconds rather than minutes or hours, and I don't have to feel anxious about my thoughts floating away into the ADHD-ether. If you aren't in front of a computer all day, a note on your phone or a little notebook can work wonders too. But tie a pen to the notebook with a string or ribbon to make sure it's always there when you need it.

The main challenge with this system is actually remembering to go back to your brain dump list later and action those things. Maybe I should add 'check the list' to the list, too.

The Pomodoro method

Another popular way of sustaining concentration is to break up your mental marathon into lots of little sprints and rests, using something called the Pomodoro method. This is a productivity technique created by Francesco Cirillo in the late 1980s, where you structure your work into medium-length bursts with short breaks in between. Broadly, it involves the following steps:

1. **Decide what you're going to do.**
2. **Set a timer for 25 minutes and do *nothing* except your chosen task until the alarm goes off.**
3. **Set your timer for five or ten minutes and take a short break, where you can check your phone or make a cup of tea.**
4. **Repeat this pattern two more times.**

5. **Take a longer break, usually 20–30 minutes.**
6. **Start again.**

This system is extremely popular in the ADHD community and it works wonderfully for a lot of people. However, I'm not one of them. As I said, for me, getting started is the hardest bit, so stopping every twenty-five minutes just means I never really get into the flow of things. Instead, my brain tends to work in extended bursts of several hours, with significant breaks between.

I'm sure I'd benefit from a bit more structure to my days, but honestly, the rigidity of the Pomodoro method and other similar techniques fills me with anxiety, and I end up feeling like I'm failing before I've even begun. But if it works for you, then use it!

Climbing the habit hump

One of the truly frustrating things about ADHD is that the **executive dysfunction** most people with the condition experience means the majority of these tips and tricks will work best if they become an almost automatic habit. Unfortunately, ADHD also makes it exceedingly difficult to do something consistently enough to form a habit in the first place.

So how can we get over this hump?

Habit stacking

In the world of behavioural science, there's a popular concept known as '**habit stacking**', which involves purposely creating a mutual association between something you already instinctively do and something you're more likely to forget to do. I think **neurotypical** people use it to remember to take their vitamins or get fit or whatever, but it's also a super useful way for ADHDers to inject some organisational admin into our lives.

For example, because I have a lot of trouble using a planner or diary, I've begun trying to train myself to check and update my Google Calendar when I sit down to eat. In fact, as I'm grabbing the food, I repeat in my brain 'calendar, calendar, calendar' to really drive it in. This ebbs and flows in effectiveness for me, but I have had a couple of good month-long runs. And when it's going particularly well, I add another step: when I sit down to eat, I check my calendar; and then, when I check my calendar, I reply to any texts. This also has the added benefit of confining those omnipresent anxiety-inducing tasks, like replying to people, to three neat five-minute blocks a day, and helps alleviate some of the 'Oh my god the whole world is crashing down on me all the time' panic. Notionally, you could end up having your entire morning or night routine stacked, but I'm nowhere near that level yet.

Other stacking options could include:

- **Checking your emails every time you go on public transport.**
- **Doing the laundry every time a new episode of your favourite podcast is released.**
- **Putting your clothes away before you have a glass of wine at night.**
- **Taking your medication straight after you get dressed. Then making your bed once you take your meds.**
- **Calling your grandpa when you put away the food you just bought from the supermarket.**
- **Going for a walk around the block when your cat starts begging for food at 4.15 pm every single night even though he bloody well knows he gets fed at six.**

Again, this requires being able to form the habit in the first place, so don't be too down on yourself if you find it difficult (I certainly do); however, it's relatively painless to keep trying to implement stacks in your daily life.

You can apply the stacking principle to physical objects as well – attaching something you might lose to something you can't live without. For instance, I constantly misplace my keys, but I usually know where my wireless earphones are because I use them a lot. So I bought a case with a keyring attachment to combine those bad boys. I now know where my keys are around 70 per cent of the time.

Don't break the streak

Another way I've been attempting to implant good habits into my routine is by using what I like to call 'the Duolingo method', named after the language app that tries to get you to keep a streak of consecutive learning days by creating a false sense of urgency, thus motivating you to go back to the app at least once every twenty-four hours. Well, you can create your own version of this for pretty much any habit. Simply print a whole year's calendar on a single page, tie a pen to it, stick it on your fridge and cross out every day you successfully implement the habit. (If you don't have a printer, just buy a cheap calendar next time you're walking past a discount store and use that weird page at the back with the whole year on it.)

For me, the joy of seeing every one of those little boxes fill up, and the fear of having a blank box staring back at me, is almost enough motivation in and of itself, but you can also write little rewards at the end of each week or month if you want that extra push. Maybe seven days earns a chocolate bar of your choosing, sixty days means buying that nice notebook you saw, a hundred is a trip to the zoo, and a whole year is, well, you better believe you're getting yourself roller skates. (Although I'm not sure many of us ADHDers made it through the COVID-19 lockdowns without buying ourselves skates already.)

So as not to become too disheartened by a failed day staring at you all year, you can also create a 'buy-back' system with other tasks you've been avoiding. So if, say, I actually finish doing my tax return, then I get to fill in three of my missed days on the habit tracker.

Making your brain happy

By this point, our brain has really been putting in the hard yards for us with all this productivity and focus, so it's important to reward it from time to time. Sometimes the best way of getting your brain to work the way you desire is to give it what it wants. And what it wants is little things to fiddle with.

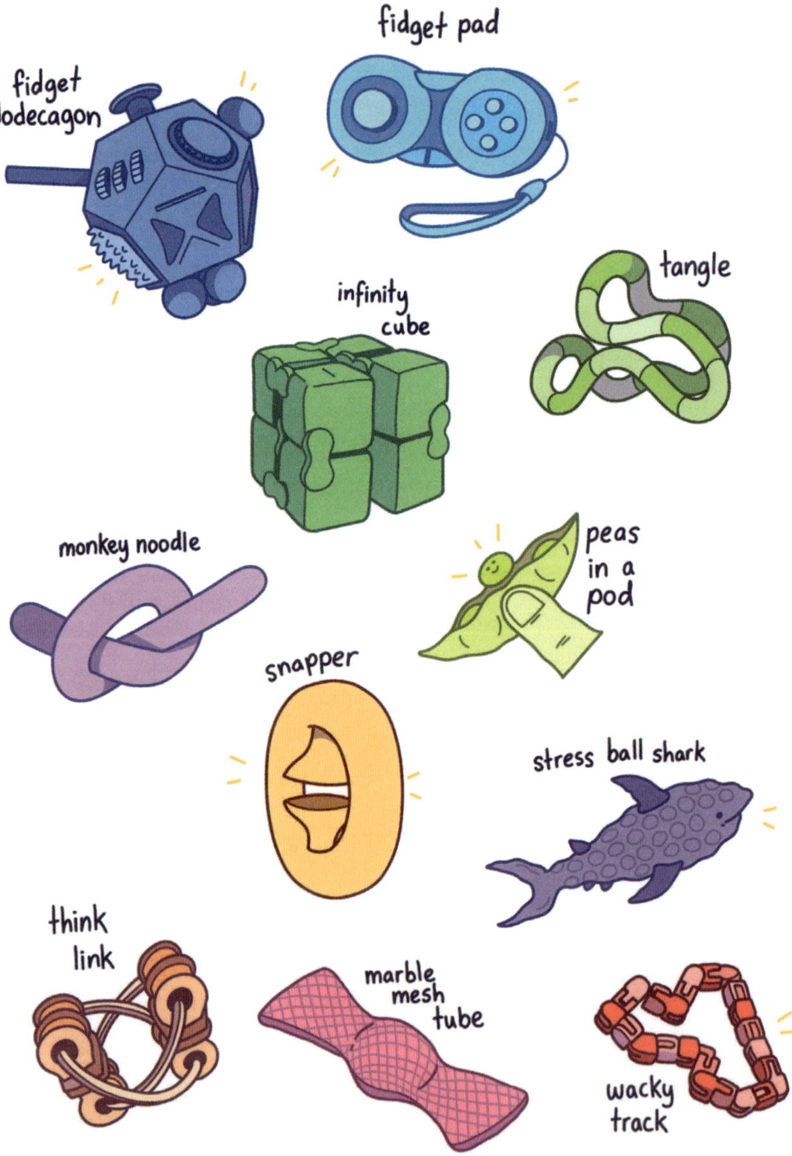

Fidget toys

ADHD people, especially those of us with hyperactive **symptoms**, love to fidget. I always need to be doing something with my hands, whether it's ripping up paper, fiddling with my earrings or cracking my knuckles. And when I have to keep still, I find it *way* harder to focus. Given my job involves me focusing really hard for extended periods of time on what the person I'm interviewing is saying, while also not making a bunch of weird tapping or ripping sounds that will carry over from my end of the phone call, this can be a bit of an issue.

At first the idea of 'fidget toys' seemed a little bit childish to me – not helped by the fact that, at the time of my **diagnosis**, they were the massive fad among primary school students. But a misplaced expression of ego isn't a good enough reason not to do something that will be beneficial for one's brain, so I went online and bought a cheap bulk package of different fidget toys that now live in a little drawer under my desk.

Any time I'm not actively typing, I'm fidgeting. Squeezing shark-shaped stress balls full of water beads, tying knots in stretchy rubber tubes called 'monkey noodles', flicking a little switch on my fidget dodecagon, moving a marble up and down in its mesh enclosure. I love all of them. I even keep them in my handbag now for hyperactive emergencies. If you've ever seen me appear on TV via video link, please know that I had a wacky track just out of shot.

Sit on the floor

Remember how I said I don't stay at my desk all day? Often I work better sitting on the ground. Some people say this is all about engaging your core, activating more of your muscles and putting yourself in some form of active rest. I'm not sure about all that. I can't find too many studies to support it, but what I can say is that I do most of my best work on the floor. In fact, my optimal position is flat on my tummy, firm pillow under my chin and arms stretched out to the laptop in front of me, but I'll probably go on some kind of physiotherapist watch list if I actually recommend this ungodly working position. (I even lie on the floor at work when it gets towards crunch time some days, but obviously this only works if you have an office job – plus a workplace that's unusually accepting of ADHD needs/a person's general idiosyncrasies.)

Even if you're less computer-bound than I am, try changing things up a bit. Take calls while going for a walk, sit on an inflatable exercise ball rather than a chair, move around as much as your environment will allow. Basically, don't get too bogged down in how things are 'meant' to be done, and whenever it's culturally and physically safe, do what works best for you instead.

Fighting the overwhelming monster

Feeling utterly and completely overwhelmed is a pretty central, and shitty, part of ADHD, and while I haven't cracked the code on avoiding this altogether, I do have a couple of tips on how to make that avalanche of clutter and unfinished admin a little easier to deal with.

The clean basket

Full disclosure, this one didn't work for me, but it might for you.

No matter how many times I promise myself I'll get better at it, I've never been able to simply put clothes away as I go, which means dauntingly large piles of clothes tend to accumulate in my room. So I bought an extra laundry basket, this time for clean clothes. Because, while taking something off after a long day and hanging it up is hard, taking something off and just chucking it in the 'clean' basket rather than on the floor pile is a pretty easy change.

The problem is, our cat loves peeing on laundry. Don't ask me why, he has a beautifully clean litter tray – I assume it's just a nice little treat for him. So I had to buy a clean clothes basket with a lid. Unfortunately, with the lid on, the contents of this basket suddenly became extremely easy to ignore and forget about, resulting in a bunch of crinkled-up, invisible clothes accumulating in there indefinitely. I even bought a replacement shirt once because I assumed I'd lost my original shirt, only to find it months later at the bottom of my brilliant ADHD-innovation basket. But, hey, if you don't have a cat with the same taste for linen, perhaps this is a good option. Also, chucking everything on a chair achieves the same thing. It's mostly about confining the mess to one manageable spot.

You can apply this 'confine the chaos' mentality to other parts of your home, too. For instance, having a designated area on the dining-room table for dumping all the bits and bobs you don't have time to put away right now, and clearing it on the weekend.

When faced with a big house-tidy, I divide the chaos with a 'macro' cleaning stage, where I do nothing but move every object into its correct room. That way, I have a number of small piles where every object is only a couple of steps away from its correct home, and each stage from then on feels more manageable.

An ADHD-friendly to-do list

Obviously, to-do lists are a very important part of every ADHDer's life. It's vital that we take the load off our **prefrontal cortex** by putting our thoughts down in writing rather than trying to carry everything in the forefront of our minds.

But not all to-do lists are created equal, and sometimes seeing the vast list of everything that needs doing can be more daunting than motivating, so we end up paralysed again, unsure where or how to start.

The ADHD coach I had a few sessions with (see Chapter 10) taught me an ingenious way to structure a list on particularly overwhelming days – although it does take a bit of extra prep time. First you sit down and vomit every single thing you can think of onto a page. Every task, no matter how big or small or urgent: just get it down.

I recommend doing this on your computer or phone, because the next step is to put everything on that list in order of priority – with whatever will have the most catastrophic consequences if it doesn't get done in the next couple of hours at the top. This might be paying your overdue phone bill or writing the university essay that's due tonight, or it could be as simple as letting your friend know if you're coming to drinks. Regardless, if it needs to get done now, it goes to the top. If it would be good to get the task done today (maybe stacking the dishwasher), it sits in the middle. And if you could put it off till tomorrow or next week (e.g. mending your ripped cardigan), you can pop it down low.

When you have your ordered list, go through it one more time and break everything down into chunks you can reasonably achieve in twenty-five minutes or less. 'Paying the phone bill' might just be one block, but 'writing the essay' might be broken down into 'read an academic paper', 'review lecture notes', 'plan out structure', 'write introduction' and so on. Give it a quick once-over to see if anything has changed priority now that's it's all been broken down, and you're good to go.

Suddenly you have a straightforward, logically ordered plan for the rest of your day. Just start at the top and see how far down the list you can get.

Scary hour

ADHD involves a lot of delaying. Sometimes something important needs doing but it feels too overwhelming, or we're scared we'll do it wrong, or we're embarrassed we haven't done it sooner. And so we don't do it. And it keeps getting worse and worse and more overwhelming and more scary and more embarrassing until it just becomes impossible.

I have genuinely forgone a payment of hundreds of dollars because I didn't know how to send in an invoice and it was too complicated to figure out, and then I got so embarrassed I hadn't done it that I just tried not to think about it, and then suddenly a year had passed and I didn't even know if I was still allowed to ask for it. And I'm really not in a financial position where I can afford to let money like that slip away. It was just that scary.

It's vital that we take the load off our prefrontal cortex by putting our thoughts down in writing rather than trying to carry everything in the forefront of our minds.

But then I listened to the podcast *Dear Hank and John* – hosted by brothers Hank Green (the dude from SciShow and TikTok) and John Green (the dude from Crash Course and the author of every book fifteen-year-olds were obsessed with in the mid-2010s) – and Hank mentioned that every week he has a 'scary hour'. He takes everything he's afraid of doing – all those scary emails and bills and phone calls – and dedicates a single hour to getting them done.

The idea is that then the spooky tasks aren't haunting you for the whole week, because you know you don't have to deal with them till scary hour comes round. And with that weekly deadline in place, they don't get the chance to turn from 'a little bit stressful' into 'full-on terrifyingly demonic'. Of course, you could adapt it to once a day or once a fortnight, or make it a 'scary ten minutes after lunch' or 'scary afternoon', depending on your needs. I've come to adore scary hour, and now each Friday when 3 pm rolls around – that's spooky time. (Also, I still haven't submitted that invoice yet. It's been, like, two full years now. Do you reckon it's too late?)

Scary hour is for the things that really do need to get done – whether they're exhausting or not. But one of my biggest revelations in learning to live with ADHD isn't discovering how to fight every battle all the time – it's been figuring out which battles actually aren't worth fighting in the first place.

12

Which battles are worth fighting?

The thing about all the tips, tricks and tactics covered in the preceding chapters is that even if you implement every one of them perfectly, chances are you'll still have ADHD.

While it's been incredibly important for me to try to make my brain suit my world and my world suit my brain, one of the most crucial parts of reducing the burden of my ADHD has been accepting that there are just some things I'm never going to be good at. My life is probably never going to look like a **neurotypical** person's, my brain is probably never going to look like theirs either, so what's the point of constantly punishing myself for not fulfilling the vision of 'who I should be' that I crafted before I had all the relevant information? I have to learn to appreciate and accept the person who actually exists. I'm still working on it, but I'm getting closer.

My life is probably never going to look like a neurotypical person's, my brain is probably never going to look like theirs either, so what's the point of constantly punishing myself for not fulfilling the vision of 'who I should be' that I crafted before I had all the relevant information?

Towards the end of my first officially diagnosed year, I found a TikTok account, @CallMePaulHollywood, run by another woman in her early to mid-twenties, Ksa Curry. She'd also just got her neurodivergent news and was making a series of videos called 'Battles I have decided to let ADHD win'.

'First up, we have grocery lists,' she deadpans in one clip. 'These are impossible. I refuse. I go to the store, I follow my heart. Do I get what I need? No. Do I get the one thing I went there for? Absolutely not. Is there anything to be done? Also no.'

The videos are light and funny, mostly functioning as a way of gently teasing herself about being forgetful, and yet they've had a profound effect on how I think about life.

In that first year, I felt as if my goal was always 'winning' against my ADHD, because I assumed that was what you were meant to do. If you have a disorder, you do whatever it takes to stop it from affecting your life, right? But when I saw those videos, it was the first time it had ever occurred to me that I could just ... not.

So, I reached out to Curry, who was kind enough to jump on a call with me (once we'd figured out the time difference between Melbourne and the American Midwest).

'I started looking at the different resources and how people deal with ADHD, and it honestly kind of super turned me off, because there were all these hacks that were basically telling people who exist with a neurodivergent brain to just live as if you don't,' she says.

'There are definitely some battles that come with ADHD that I have to fight – ones that are for survival and for the sake of communication. But there are a lot of battles that I just don't have to have. And I honestly think that most of the hacks that I find are for the battles we don't need to fight.

'So, yes, it's a joke. But I also really do believe it.'

And clearly this sentiment struck a chord, with hundreds of thousands of people sharing Curry's posts.

I ask her why she thinks the series was so popular and she says, 'When it comes to neurotypical people giving advice to people with ADHD, I think there's a lot of us who have been invalidated for a really long time, and I think there's a lot of anger. For me, just being able to say "Fuck that ... no, I'm not going to do that" and joke about it felt really validating. And it turns out a lot of other people feel the exact same way.'

Not to get all 'waving the red flag' on you, but this idea of productivity as the ultimate moral virtue is a tool of capitalism. It's convenient for us to think of 'laziness' as evil, because that makes us better workers. And because capitalism is so intrinsically woven into our lives, this 'virtue of productivity' leaks into things like having a tidy home, keeping a neat planner, remembering to eat healthily and basically every other aspect of day-to-day existence. I wasn't doing chores because they would make my home feel nicer, but because deep down it felt like being messy was a sin.

'There are definitely some battles that come with ADHD that I have to fight – ones that are for survival and for the sake of communication. But there are a lot of battles that I just don't have to have.'

I might never be able to pack for a holiday without forgetting two or three vital things. I might never remember that we already have olives at home when I'm at the supermarket. I might never be able to correctly estimate the amount of time it takes to walk to the train station. These things might be frustrating, but the world isn't divided into *organised* people and *bad* people.

That's not to say there aren't consequences for not planning properly or being unproductive. But put it this way: if I do have to confront some sort of divine moral arbiter when I shuffle off this mortal coil, they sure as hell aren't going to punish me for leaving my wet clothes in the washing machine for too long. It's genuinely okay.

It's not a moral failure to constantly lose your keys.

It's not a moral failure to find exercising incredibly boring.

It's not a moral failure to let your phone die all the time.

It's not a moral failure to need a podcast playing to get to sleep.

It's not a moral failure to reply to that email a little late.

We don't have to put these ADHD systems into our lives because we're obliged to 'learn our lesson' or 'atone for our sins'. We should choose to do it because it's probably going to increase our net level of happiness. If something just isn't worth the fight and won't drastically negatively impact those around you, then you don't actually have to engage with that battle.

I'm still trying to truly, deeply internalise that message. But in the moments I do, it's extraordinarily liberating.

What's the goal?

With the growing acceptance that my ADHD doesn't make me a 'bad person' has come the realisation that my goal doesn't have to be to 'heal' or 'recover' from my condition.

I know that technically you can. If you get to the point where your **symptoms** no longer negatively impact your life, then you notionally graduate out of the **diagnosis**. But I don't really like that we define ADHD solely by its associated **impairments**, and I don't buy the idea that your brain magically goes back to being neurotypical once you remember all your doctor's appointments for a year or something. Honestly, the thought of trying to 'cure' my ADHD is really scary. I've only just managed to get comfortable with the idea that I actually have this condition. I feel like working towards getting rid of it is a sure-fire way to plunge myself back into a pit of despair and grief.

But if we aren't trying to 'defeat' our ADHD, what's our goal in all of this? Once we fix our home and our health and our sleep and all the rest, what do we actually want our lives to look like? I really recommend sitting down and writing out a list, because you might be shocked at what makes the cut.

Here are some of the points on my list:

- **To no longer think of myself as lazy, clumsy or thoughtless.**
- **To rebuild the self-worth I lost from all the years of thinking those negative things in the first place.**
- **To find a way to stop being so constantly tired and burnt out, learn to take the time off I need and no longer feel guilty for not being able to work forever and never take a breath.**
- **To get to sleep at the time I intend to get to sleep at least 60 per cent of the time. (We've got to be realistic, guys.)**
- **To have my actions reflect the kind of friend, daughter, sister and partner I want to be.**
- **To recognise when fear, anxiety and the general sense of being overwhelmed are sneaking up on me, and learn ways to work through paralysis and take back control.**
- **To forgive myself when I don't always live up to all of these goals all the time.**

It was only after writing this list that I realised most of these weren't even directly related to the official ADHD symptoms. That's another reason why 'healing' my ADHD will never be a useful goal for me. Sure, there are things I want to achieve in order to improve my **executive functioning** and make my life easier, but being forgetful is so much less damaging to my life than hating myself for being forgetful.

Amphetamines and a profound capacity for self-forgiveness, baby!

Work in progress

So, after months of life hacks, chore charms, behavioural science and high-protein breakfasts, how did I actually go at the whole 'getting my shit together' thing? Well:

- **I have my bedtime set on my phone as 10 pm, despite never once being in bed, let alone asleep, by then.**
- **Every night I promise myself I'm going to get up early enough to put makeup on for the morning meeting at work, and yet every day I scramble in at 8.58, brushing my bed-head knots out with my fingers, hoping no one notices the bags under my eyes.**
- **I decided to work out every evening to get my heart pumping and my mind clear, and I stopped after the second day.**
- **I posted a video online that more than 5 million people watched about the chore charm bracelets I use, and then got overwhelmed and went months without touching them again.**
- **I've got a calendar to mark off my streak of 'good organisational habits', and this month is spare and sporadic at best.**
- **I've never taken a multivitamin in my life without my mum reminding me when we chat on the phone.**
- **The plant just to the right of me is going yellow, yet I know if I get up to water it I'll never finish writing this.**

All of which is to say, I feel like a bit of a fraud writing this book, trying to tell you how to live with your ADHD when I'm still working it out. But then again, I feel like more of a failure when I read article after article and book after book from people who seem to have it all figured out.

Because that's the thing with this condition. You don't just 'fix' something once. You're constantly repairing things then breaking them again. Adopting habits and abandoning them. Learning to love the gym and then forgetting about it. Building bridges and then burning them.

But every time you change your life, every time you sit down and decide 'today's the day', you pick up something new. Sure, 90 per cent of your efforts might crumble by the end of the month, but if you're lucky, a little something will stick.

So, let's look at that list again:

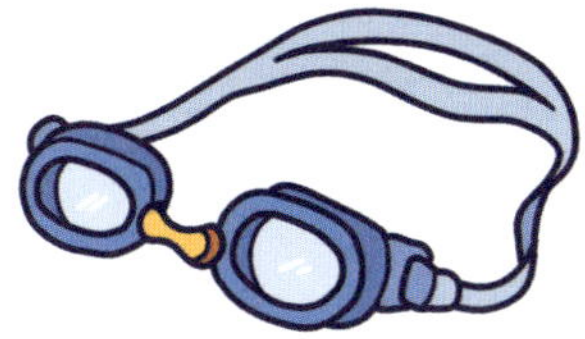

- I've never got to sleep at 10 pm, but in my attempts to, I've stopped drinking coffee after 2 pm on weekdays.
- My morning routine hasn't gotten to the point of having my makeup done before the daily conference, but I do manage to eat a high-protein breakfast almost every day.

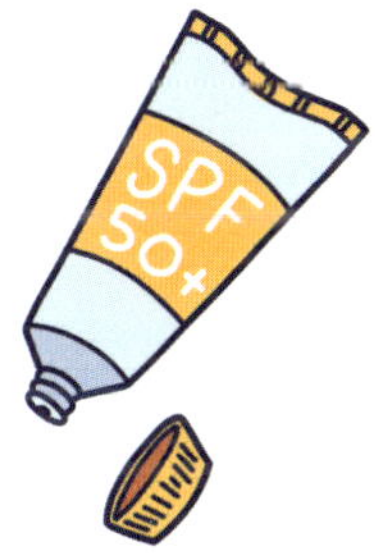

- I don't work out every evening, but I have learnt to take myself for a swim when I need to shake off a stressful day.
- I didn't touch my chore charms for months, but I did remember to put on sunscreen at least two-thirds of the time.
- I may not have ticked off all my 'good organisational habits' in a while, but I do check my Google Calendar more often, and it's saved me from missing four appointments this month.

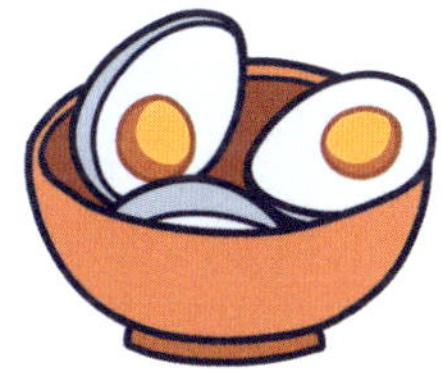

- I've never remembered to take a multivitamin, but I haven't missed an antidepressant pill in weeks.
- My plants might not be as big and lush as they could be, but I've kept them alive and growing.
- I still feel like a bit of a fraud – but I kept writing this book.

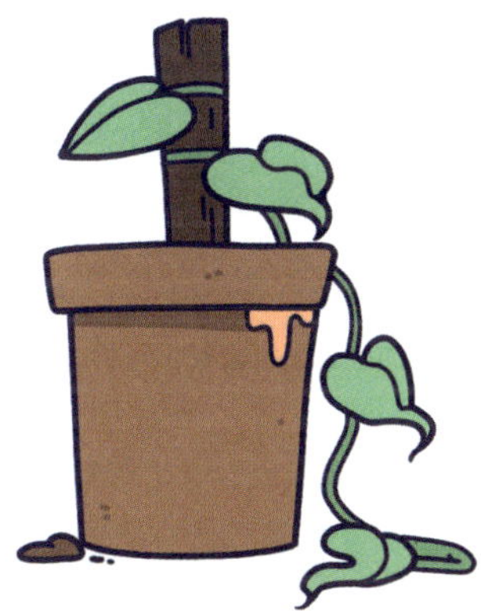

I'm learning how to forgive not only my past self, but my present self, too. With ADHD, if you're aiming for perfection, you're going to be disappointed. Even if you're aiming for 'way better', you're probably not going to get there in one fell swoop. You need to learn to appreciate the little wins, the little habits you pick up almost by accident in your crusade for a better life. Because although I do kind of feel like a failure for not being able to 'cure' my ADHD in the name of science and tell you all the secrets to a perfect neurodivergent life, I'm considerably better off than when I started.

And I'm going to keep getting better and better, even if my successes are just accidental by-products of my failures.

DIARY ENTRY

The logistics fairy

So, I told you before about one of the worst days I had during the process of writing this book – but it's important to share what happened the next morning, too. Because it's genuinely one of the kindest things anyone has ever done for me.

When I woke up, still feeling a little raw, I saw a call from my sister, Perrin. And I'm not going to lie, I did ignore it at first, terrified that she would require me to make a decision or do a task of some kind. But she called again, as, after twenty-five years, she's cottoned on to my idiosyncrasies.

'Hey, Mat. Mum said you had a bit of a rough one,' Perrin said.

'Yeah, I'm just kind of over it, you know . . .' I replied.

'Yeah, I get it,' she said, pausing for a second. 'Is there anything I can do to help? Can I, like, do a supermarket shop for you, or cook you some dinners to put in the fridge?'

I paused for a second, too. I was close to saying, 'No, I can handle it all. Thanks though.'

I was ashamed to admit it, but the truth was, I genuinely couldn't handle 'it all'. It's just that a supermarket shop and cooking weren't the things I was struggling with. But instead of shrinking back into my shell, I said, 'Can you just, like, deal with all the family stuff?'

'What do you mean?' she asked.

'Well, Nana texted like four days ago about her birthday and I can't figure out how to say I can't come, and Kieran messaged me and needs my address to send the save-the-date for his wedding, and I opened the message so he knows I saw it but it's now been like two days. And I can't buy birthday presents and I can't explain to people why not, and I can't deal with the logistics, you know? It's just too hard.'

I understand how utterly ridiculous all of that may sound. These are things that would take two minutes to complete. They were objectively the easiest tasks on my to-do list. This is clearly not what she was expecting, but she didn't go, 'Wait, how is that hard?' or 'Are you sure that's what you need?' or, worse still, 'Just do it right now while you're on the phone with me, it will take ten seconds.' She said, 'Okay, I'll sort it out,' and then she did.

She called Nana, texted our cousin Kieran, bought the presents that needed to be bought and texted me how much I owed her. She was my buffer for logistics while I got through the rough patch, and it was such an unbelievably generous thing to do. She even remembered to mention I'd need a vegetarian meal for the wedding.

And then, a few days later, without even asking, she texted me a list of things she knew Mum and Dad might want for Christmas, because she was getting presents sorted early this year and thought it might be stressful for me to have to come up with ideas. 'If you're happy with that, I can order them and you can transfer me.' I tell you, I nearly cried. I love my sister so, so very much.

ADHD doesn't always make sense to the outside world. What's easy and what's impossible are based more on emotion and mental load than actual complexity or time required. So, quite often, the help that neurotypical people will offer might not really hit the mark, as well-meaning as it might be.

If you're a non-ADHDer reading this in the hope of understanding how you can help your ADHD loved ones, that's how you do it. You ask them what they genuinely need, and listen to them when they tell you.

13

How do I live with other people?

As I reach the three-quarter mark of this year, I've been thinking more and more about what my life would look like if I just dived all-in and lived exactly the way my ADHD brain wants me to.

If I had no commitments and no one relying on me, I'd stay up till 3 am every day, sleep in till noon, reply to emails all in a big batch once a month, clean the house exclusively in unbelievably intense two-hour bursts every couple of weeks, randomly show up at friends' and family's homes on a whim, and probably spend far too much money on lava lamps. If there were no consequences for living like that, I'd probably feel a lot less pressure in my day-to-day life. I'm not saying my ADHD would no longer be a problem, but I reckon around a good 70 per cent of the **impairments** would vanish.

But obviously I can't live like that – not just because there would be personal consequences, but because I have loved ones who I need, and want, to construct my life around. I want to show up for them. I want them to be happy and content and to feel loved. And unfortunately, my condition sometimes makes it harder for me to do that.

Throughout most of my life – and I imagine this is a familiar feeling for many ADHDers – I've had little points of tension with the people I love where, much to my disappointment (and theirs), I've consistently let them down. I knew messiness made Anthony anxious, but I couldn't keep our room clean. I knew it was important to my mum and dad that I offered to help clear the table instead of sitting on the couch watching TV, but I never seemed to notice when people started getting up and moving. I knew my friend Andrea needed me to text her back more, but the anxiety of having to engage in a conversation when I was exhausted was too much for me.

Exactly how do you navigate those important relationships – with family, friends, long-term partners – or even the intricacies of dating when you're staring across the ADHD divide?

Family

A fascinating aspect of being diagnosed with ADHD as an adult is that some of the most fundamental relationships in your life – the ones with your family – require a retrospective rewrite.

Raising an ADHD kid can be hard. I've never had to try it myself, but I think that's a fairly safe assumption. And it only makes things more complicated when no one has any idea that **neurodivergence** is even involved. All kids are challenging occasionally: not cleaning up after themselves, causing the family to be late, forcing their guardians to stay up past 1 am pasting pictures of Galapagos giant tortoises on a poster for the assignment they left until the very last second.

But with (secretly) ADHD kids, this might not be behaviour that just resolves itself as they get towards their teenage years. From an outside perspective it simply seems as if they aren't growing and learning from their mistakes the way the other kids are. They're not taking responsibility for themselves. I mean, fifteen-year-olds are always going to be arseholes, but like, seriously, this one doesn't seem to be considering their parent's time and needs at all.

Of course, it's frustrating for the parent on a basic level – but I assume there's a deeper pain there, too. It's their job to help teach their children all the skills they'll need in life, but somehow it seems they haven't managed to do that. There's guilt that they're failing as a parent. There's fear about how their kid will cope when they're not around to bail them out any more. And there's worry that their child isn't going to reach the potential they can so clearly see in them. These feelings can weigh a relationship down – something an ADHDer, who's likely already keenly sensitive to rejection and criticism, is bound to pick up on, at least subconsciously. This tension can build and build, with clashes becoming more and more common.

But the good news is, quite often an ADHD **diagnosis** – even if it's well into the kid's adulthood – can help lighten that load. This is certainly what happened in my family. But I figured that, given how much was on my mind at the time, I might not be the best authority on this, so I asked my mum to jot down some of her memories that have been recontextualised since the news of my neurodivergence broke. Here's what she said:

You were bright, inquisitive, funny, often loud and exuberant, forgetful, restless, kind, and just a very sweet kid. Someone once told us that you were joie de vivre – that you had come into our lives to make sure we didn't take ourselves too seriously. And this is true.

But if we knew then what we know now, there were lots of markers – you constantly fiddling with the saltcellar when we were out at restaurants (and, yes, there were lots of incidents where it spilled onto someone's dinner because you'd loosened the top), the huge pile of wet and mildewy towels in your bedroom, the inability to remember a thank-you note for a present or the permission slip for an excursion. I can't tell you how many school jumpers, vests, hats and bathers were lost over the years (and that was expensive!). And, in particular, your lifelong battle with sleep.

So when you, as an adult, showed me the **symptoms** of ADHD, I was shocked because all of those things we'd thought were 'just Mattie' were clearly part of the condition.

It makes me profoundly sad to realise that the things you struggled with had eroded your **self-esteem** and that, with a diagnosis, we could have done something about it. (Although, to be honest, in the early 2000s there was such a stigma about overmedicating children that I'm not sure we would have taken advice about medication if we had received it.)

Lately, I've been thinking about what is you and what is the ADHD, and the conclusion I've come to is that they're indefinable. The aspects that make you wonderful are also the things that make your life hard, but there's no separating them, so the solution is just to love the whole person you are.

(I tried to cut out that bit at the end where my mum was just being nice to me, but she made me put it back in.)

When I was first diagnosed, I was quite scared to dive into these in-depth conversations with my parents. I was worried that in my euphoria of realising that I wasn't a 'bad kid' – a label they never actually gave to me, and told me multiple times growing up wasn't true, but that still somehow managed to wiggle its way into my brain – I'd create a huge well of guilt and regret in them. I hadn't really unpacked the impact the disorder has had on me, so I was worried it would come across as me telling them that they were somehow 'bad parents' instead of just people who didn't know the whole story.

But as the year has gone on we've been discussing it more and more, wading deeper into the difficult waters of 'what could have been different'. My parents have been beautifully open to these discussions; however, I know many of my ADHD friends have been met with defensiveness and even denial that they have the condition altogether. Obviously this isn't a brilliant reaction, but it's also not hard to imagine why their parents may have responded in this way. No one wants to think they missed something so vital and made their child's life harder. They were probably doing their best – and the idea that their best still wasn't enough may just be too painful to consider. So while these retrospective childhood discussions have brought me so much healing and growth, and I highly recommend pursuing them if you feel safe to do so, I understand that this simply isn't going to be possible for everyone.

I've said before that a huge part of 'treating' your ADHD is really about going over the history of your life, recognising the times where you've needlessly blamed yourself or been blamed for things that were out of your control, and forgiving yourself. But another aspect is also recognising that the people who blamed you were just as in the dark as you were. When you suddenly learn that your life could have been different, it's only natural to ask, Whose fault was this? And our parents are often the simplest answer.

But ten years ago, ADHD, especially the inattentive **presentation** (and well, any version of the condition in girls) was vastly misunderstood and overlooked. Ultimately, noticing a pattern is a lot harder if no one ever tells you that you should be looking for one.

If I'm being perfectly honest, even if my parents had known I had ADHD, I probably would still have developed self-esteem issues through school, friendships and a hundred other things that are just trickier for those of us who grow up neurodivergent. My parents weren't the be-all and end-all. They were simply humans who were trying their best.

Also, it might be worth keeping in mind that, because of the highly **hereditary** nature of ADHD, one or both of your parents might have a case of jittery brain, too. As far as I can tell, this isn't the story for either of my parents (and believe me, I've forced them to take all the online tests), but it's pretty darn common. It might even be part of the reason they missed your symptoms. Because to them, that was totally normal behaviour.

One of the classic stories you hear is the adult woman finding out she has ADHD when she takes her son in for an assessment and relates a little too much to what the doctor is saying. Which is to say, you're reading this book as the parent of an ADHD child, you might want to give the **DSM-5**'s **diagnostic criteria** for ADHD (at the back of this book) a little once-over. There's a chance you'll find some of those symptoms surprisingly familiar.

Friendship

Making new friends is difficult for everyone, but having ADHD can throw up some pretty unique challenges. Following social cues and norms isn't always the easiest for us, but even beyond the initial conversations there's the simple fact that it's hard to establish a deep, ongoing connection with someone if it's a significant struggle for you to remember to actually stay in contact.

While I'm lucky enough to have some very stable and wonderful friendships, I also know there are a lot of people out there I probably could have been mates with if I hadn't left them hanging. So many suggestions to go for a walk or grab a coffee or have dinner that I've either forgotten to reciprocate or given up trying to organise at the slightest hurdle. A lot of this is about **executive dysfunction** and forgetfulness, but there's also an element of trauma in there, too. Friendship was really hard and painful for me as a child. It is for a lot of ADHDers. We were constantly faced with social rejection and feelings of being an outcast, so it's not surprising that starting new friendships as adults is a scary prospect, and why backing away the moment we feel we've made a mistake often seems like the easiest solution.

But ADHD **impulsiveness** can be a pretty powerful tool for forging relationships, too. One thing I really like about myself is how easily I can click with people, going from a light chat to a mutual, heart-wrenching confession session over the course of a party. I used to shame myself for being such an 'open book', wishing I could just stay mysterious or keep others at arm's length, but I've come to learn that a lot of people out there crave that connection – and my openness (intentional or not) often acts as the invitation they've been waiting for.

This is how I found my best friend Andrea, a five-foot-eleven Norwegian goddess and all-round glorious human being. When we first met while working on our university newspaper, our internalised misogynistic urge to view any other accomplished women as our competition got to us, and for approximately five days we resented each other deeply. Then we got paired up on a podcast project, went to dinner afterwards and were crying in each other's arms confessing our deepest secrets by the time the first round of dumplings were served. We've been inseparable ever since.

Well . . . we try to be.

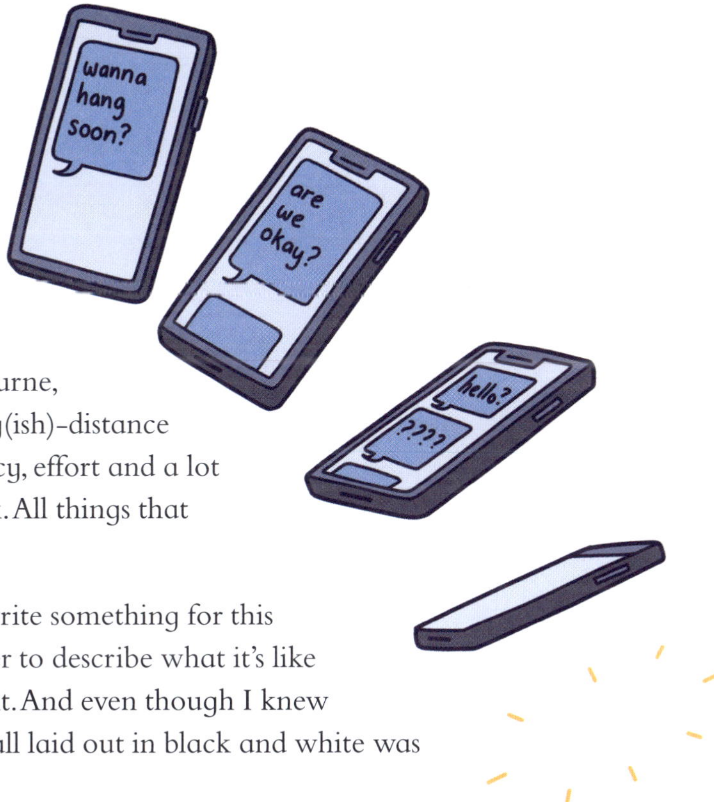

See, Andrea is now one of best podcast producers in Australia, which unfortunately her bosses noticed and made her move from Melbourne, where I am, to Sydney. Long(ish)-distance friendships require consistency, effort and a lot of remembering to text back. All things that I really struggle with.

When I asked if she'd write something for this chapter, I specifically told her to describe what it's like for her on the days I go silent. And even though I knew what was coming, seeing it all laid out in black and white was devastating.

I remember one specific time when I sent a string of messages. I think I first complained about one of my family members back in Norway trying to make me feel guilty for living overseas. The next day I told you I'd finally booked a counselling session to deal with my lingering eating disorder. The next said I had fought with my partner. Although you clearly didn't mean to discard my messages, you didn't reply for a week.

I finally decided to just text you, like, via SMS as if we lived in the 90s, and asked if you'd deleted your Messenger app, and within twenty-three seconds I got a frantic call from you, vehemently apologising. You felt *horrible*. And, yeah – I was a little bit hurt. But I know this is very much a common thing for people with ADHD, just forgetting to do something.

And, in the past year with your writing, I'm learning more and more about what it's like for you actually living with ADHD. It's changed my understanding of some of the things you do. But also, hey, that goes both ways. You've learnt to understand me over the years too. That's what friendship is, baby.

It hurts to know I've hurt people, but part of living with ADHD as an adult is accepting that as much as our condition does explain our behaviours, it doesn't rid them of consequences or responsibility. We need to take this on board and use it to grow, rather than trying to ignore it or potentially even retreating from important relationships so we don't have to deal with our feelings of guilt.

So now, when Andrea needs support, to vent or maybe is just dying for a chat, she'll call me instead. If I'm busy and I say I'll call her back, but then forget, she'll just call again. And calling works brilliantly for me. I can chat while I'm cooking or walking or cleaning or shopping, and it actually helps me get those tasks done because my mind is focused on the conversation, not on the million and one distractions. Which means I now find myself calling her all the time as well.

Because I was able to put forward a solution and she was accommodating enough to adapt to my needs, our friendship is closer than ever, and we probably talk to each other more now with 878 kilometres between us than we did when we were both in the same city.

Part of living with ADHD as an adult is accepting that as much as our condition does explain our behaviours, it doesn't rid them of consequences or responsibility.

It's easy to overlook the importance of friendship – especially when life feels so hectic, especially when your brain isn't great at remembering people when they're not right in front of you, and especially when it's an area where you've been burnt before. But it's worth pushing through the discomfort and having the hard conversations, because the reward is having people in your life who deeply understand you.

Also, don't forget that while, yes, ADHD can sometimes make it harder to be the kind of friend you'd like to be, it's probably also part of what drew your mates to you. We're interesting people to be around! Don't underestimate just how much that counts.

Dating, etc.

When people talk about romantic relationships and ADHD, the conversations often revolve around navigating life at home and the day-to-day challenges the condition can exacerbate in a long-term relationship. Something that's less discussed is the way the condition can make getting into a long-term relationship difficult to begin with. The symptoms of ADHD don't just suddenly go away when it comes to your romantic life. In fact, it might bring them into even sharper focus.

ADHD brains are desperate for stimulation, and what's more stimulating than 'the chase'? The dance of dating, having sex with a new person for the first time, learning about their lives and world and family, and, like a little romance detective, slowly solving the puzzle of who they are. With that much excitement, it's easy to become obsessed with someone and, without even realising it, accidentally allow them to slip out of the realm of 'actual human being' and into the land of '**hyper-fixation**'. From the outside it might not look the same as that time you decided to get really into rock climbing, but falling in love with a person is a dangerously enticing hobby.

The issue with someone becoming your hyper-fixation is that – just like with waking up at the crack of dawn to scale a 9-metre indoor cliff face – eventually that well of beautiful stimulation will run dry. The excitement will wane, but unlike the rock wall, the person at the other end of your hyper-fixation has the capacity to be extremely hurt by your sudden lack of interest.

This isn't a universal ADHD experience, but it is a fairly common one. That's not to say that no relationship can outlast our hyper-fixations. But when that rush does inevitably end, we shouldn't panic. It doesn't mean the relationship is suddenly doomed, just that it's time to take a breath, assess the person for whom they really are, and

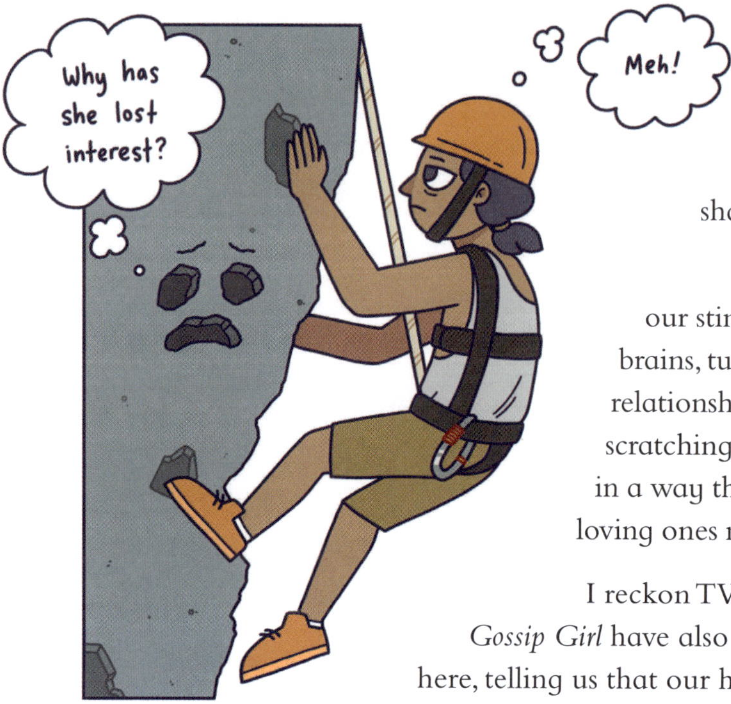

figure out if they were a hobby or someone we want to share all our hobbies with.

Unfortunately for our stimulation-starved brains, turbulent, fiery, volatile relationships also tend to keep scratching that 'excitement itch' in a way that stable, supportive, loving ones might not.

I reckon TV and romcoms and *Gossip Girl* have also set a bit of a trap here, telling us that our heart or our soul, not our brain, always 'knows what's right', and that if we suddenly get the urge to get back out there, find someone new and start that rush all over again, this is 'our heart sending us a message'. Maybe that's the case for **neurotypical** people, I don't know. But for us, there's a decent chance that it's our under-functioning **mesolimbic pathway** talking to us, not our hearts. I'm not saying you should slog it out in some boring, unfulfilling relationship no matter what, but we shouldn't mistake that perpetual sense of inner **restlessness** common to many ADHDers as a sign that someone isn't right for us or that the relationship is automatically doomed.

It's also not just the 'excitement' factor that might lead ADHDers to avoid emotionally intimate relationships. '**Rejection-sensitive dysphoria**' (see Chapter 8) may not be an official clinical symptom, but plenty of people with ADHD do feel rejection in an acute and painful way,[1] and this can make dating a more intense and painful experience, because the possibility of repeated rejection is part of the package. In fact, a study of around five hundred university students from China and the US even showed a **correlation** between the severity of ADHD symptoms and a person's fear of intimacy.[2]

On top of that, many of us are grappling with low self-esteem and, because of the **emotional dysregulation** that often comes with ADHD, are far too used to being told we're overreacting. This may well leave us vulnerable to partners with controlling, narcissistic or abusive tendencies. It's not yet been extensively researched, but at least two (moderate-sized) US studies showed a correlation between the severity of inattentive symptoms and higher rates of psychological abuse victimisation.[3]

Unfortunately for our stimulation-starved brains, turbulent, fiery, volatile relationships also tend to keep scratching that 'excitement itch' in a way that stable, supportive, loving ones might not.

It would be remiss of me not to mention that people with ADHD can be perpetrators of abuse as well as victims. So, it's also extremely important that we reflect on how emotional volatility and issues with **impulse control** are affecting our behaviour in our relationships. Having a neurological condition in no way excuses abusive behaviour, but it does provide a treatment pathway to help ensure this doesn't happen again. If you're worried you might have fallen into these sorts of patterns, you owe it to everyone in your life to seek help and find ways to correct them.

Long-term love

Let's say you do find the right person. You get over the hyper-fixation hump, you see them for who they are and you love them for it. And, wow, would you look at that, they love you too. Suddenly you're in a long-term relationship, you might even be living with them, and now it's time to figure out what it means to share your life with someone as an ADHDer.

Anthony and I had already moved into a share house together when I was diagnosed, and I distinctly remember coming into the lounge room after my psychiatric assessment and seeing him sitting on the couch. He turned and looked up at me and smiled in that loving way that always feels like home to me, and I thought to myself, 'Sucked in, motherfucker. You can't get annoyed at me for leaving all my clothes in a pile now. That shit is medically exempt.'

We've since moved out of the share house and into a tiny little apartment that's all our own. This was wonderful, but moving into a home with only three rooms total has come with some challenges.

Anthony doesn't have ADHD. In fact, forcing him to take some of the same online tests and seeing how drastically lower his scores were than mine was one of the factors that helped convince me I needed to get formally assessed. A heap of great things can come out of these 'one of each' relationships, but I won't lie, they can also be difficult to navigate.

Of course, I'm only one half of this dynamic, so I figured I needed to get Anthony's take too.

Maybe it's sort of like I'm the 'manager' and you're the 'do-er'. Like, I handle most of the keeping up to date with bills and remembering events and writing shopping lists and stuff – and you're more in charge of deciding, 'Hey, let's buy an apartment' or 'Let's adopt a cat' or 'Let me re-caulk the whole bathroom', and then you actually make it happen.

After quickly clarifying that he meant 'manager' as literally a person who manages things, rather than him suggesting he was my boss, I had to concede that he was right on the money. Although it obviously varies day to day, as a general rule, I push us forward with the big-picture ideas and projects, he keeps us steady and makes sure we both stay alive to reap the benefits. And we share the job of naming every cat we see on the street and giving it an in-depth backstory and rich emotional arc. It's actually a pretty good system.

But as well as our dynamic works for us at the moment, we're both very aware of the potential it has to sour if we're not careful.

Over-functioning/under-functioning

Dr Ari Tuckman, a well-known psychologist and sex therapist who literally wrote the book on intimate ADHD relationships – *ADHD after Dark*[4] – put it this way: 'ADHD doesn't invent new problems. It just exacerbates the universal ones.'

Tuckman's written a lot on how ADHD/non-ADHD couples can push each other into what he describes as the 'over-functioning/under-functioning dynamic'.[5] And I'd be lying if I said I didn't see shades of that reflected in my own relationship. So, partially for the purposes of research and partially because I had an intense personal curiosity, I reached out to him.

'When one partner has ADHD, and, really, when it's not being well attended, then it's easy for the other partner to fall into the role of doing more,' Tuckman tells me, his voice slightly distorted by his car's bluetooth mic as he drives along a busy highway in Pennsylvania. Part of this, he says, is down to the way people with ADHD experience time and urgency differently from others.

'They don't activate until the deadline gets a lot closer to the "now", whereas the non-ADHD partner usually will sort of activate first,' he says.

This could be about big things, like how far in advance holidays need to be planned or bills need to be paid, or it could be as simple as the non-ADHD partner feeling the bin needs to be emptied when it's 90 per cent full, while the ADHD partner might wait till it's overflowing.

But because it's the non-ADHDer who almost always starts feeling that urgency and anxiety first, they'll often just do it so it's done. And especially when they have a forgetful partner, this may well be the most reliable course of action.

'The problem is when the non-ADHD partner is doing that much more than fifty-fifty, they're always sort of beating the partner with ADHD to the punch, so to speak,' Tuckman says. 'So the non-ADHD partner feels like "I'm the only one who always does everything." Meanwhile, the partner with ADHD might feel like "I never had a chance to do it."'

This building tension is also complicated by many ADHDers' sensitivity around being 'parented' or told off for doing something wrong. 'You know, kids who are often off task, just, generally speaking, tend to get much more input from parents, teachers, sports coaches, whoever the adults in the room are. And they tend to be very aware of that … If you have a million experiences of this, and then your partner starts getting on your case about something, it's easy to feel like, "Oh, here we go again. Why am I destined to be the one who's always taking shit?"'

Eventually, this may lead to the ADHD partner becoming defensive or angry, and perhaps even to them lying to hide the times when they think they've failed their partner. But when this inevitably unravels the trust in the relationship, it is damaged, and the non-

ADHD partner feels even more hurt. It's the kind of thing that can very easily become a vicious cycle.

It can also seriously impact couples' sex lives – because as much as many people enjoy being bossy or bossed around in the bedroom, these roles are considerably less sexy when they start in the kitchen over a very real argument about the dishes. And, as Tuckman says, the loss of a happy sex life can have a knock-on effect, as it's just one more fun bonding activity that gets put on the backburner while a couple works through their anxiety and resentment.

There are no prizes for guessing who's the 'over-functioner' and who's the 'under-functioner' in my home. It's never bordered on being a threat to my relationship with Anthony, but once again, I reckon I might have my diagnosis to thank for this. Having a name and an explanation for what was going on helped ensure we didn't progress to the point of bitter feelings and debilitating resentment. This was just my personal theory, though, so I thought I'd check in to see if Anthony was on the same page.

I mean, you do leave wet towels on the ground a lot. [He said this laughing.]

I think at first, before you were diagnosed, maybe I was a bit standoffish about things like that, interpreting it as carelessness, I guess. But once you were diagnosed, I suddenly had a deeper explanation. I realised there were things that were genuinely out of your control, and also that there were things I could be doing to help you out, like communicating more, and knowing that sometimes a 9 am burrito just makes everything better.

Plus, you do occasionally have days that you'll just dedicate entirely to housework, and I know you'll get absolutely everything done and probably some major DIY carpentry, too. You just have a certain knack about you. You get things done, and you do them well.

And, also, I love you very much. [Eww.] So, sure, every now and then I have to step over a pile of assorted textiles in the house. But that's a very small price to pay for hanging out with you every day.

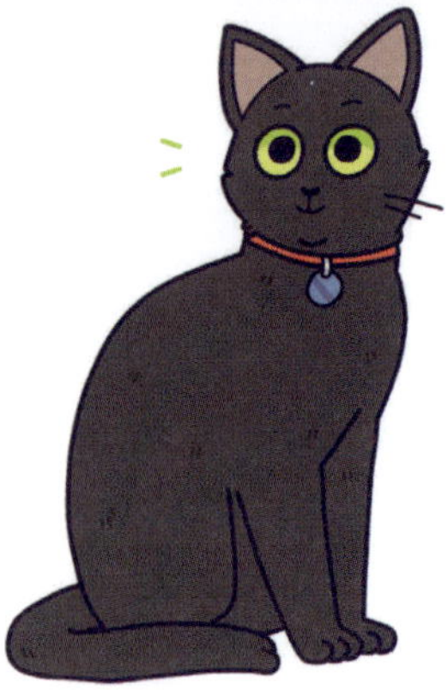

Again, the over-functioning/under-functioning dynamic is not strictly an ADHD issue – it can occur in any relationship – but it's not hard to see why an ADHDer/non-ADHDer relationship might be particularly prone to falling into it.

I'm not going to pretend I have the answers to these problems – Anthony and I are pretty much just kids who accidentally bumped into each other, share similar interests, fell in love and adopted a cat. We're still figuring this out ourselves. But one thing I can say is that the more we talk about my ADHD, the better it works.

Simple tasks, hard conversations

In the early days, before my diagnosis, I didn't realise that Anthony wouldn't always straight up ask for the things he needed. If the room was messy and it was stressing him out, he wouldn't feel that he could just request I clean it. Instead, he would make general comments hinting at the state of the room.

I come from a family that's very comfortable with asking each other to do things, so I never picked up what he was putting down. But what I did catch on to was that something was wrong, which made me feel paranoid and insecure. When I eventually dragged it out of him, I was overcome with guilt. I'd let him down. I'd been selfish. I'd been lazy, I'd been everything I'd convinced myself I was when I was growing up. But instead of actually dealing with those rather large feelings, I went for the easy option, getting defensive and angry and telling him it wasn't fair for him to be stressed and not tell me (even though he thought he had).

When I was diagnosed, I was finally able to articulate to him that while cleaning a room was a fairly easy task for him, for me it cost a lot emotionally, and even simply putting my clothes away when I took them off was often far more than I could handle at the end of the day. In turn, he got the relief of understanding that my inability to meet this need of his wasn't linked to any lack of caring or concern for him. It was about brain chemistry, not respect. So we agreed that from then on, I'd try my best to keep the floor clean and he'd tell me when it was getting too much for him.

But then we ran into another issue. When he would say, 'Hey, could you clean up the clothes?', no matter how casually he tried to deliver it, I'd immediately sink back into that guilt and shame, and start spiralling.

'Don't you get how busy work has been at the moment?' I'd snap.

I had a history that explained why I was reacting that way, but it didn't make it fair, and, as a consequence, Anthony started feeling as though he couldn't ask. When he did, his voice would be tense and worried, which came across as abrupt and harsh, and it made the problem worse.

But earlier this year, when I watched a video of Tuckman's where he described ADHDers as having a tendency to resent feeling as if they're being told what to do, I ran to Anthony and yelled, 'I've figured it out!' And by talking through how I felt, being able to articulate the baggage that's attached to housework for me, we were able to finally see eye to eye.

Nowadays, instead of asking the moment the mess overwhelms him, Anthony will let me know when it's getting a bit much, indicating that it will probably need to be dealt with soon. Without that call for immediate action, I don't feel that jolt of pressure and guilt that I've already failed. I still feel in control, Anthony still feels heard and the room gets cleaned.

Happy with the results we've had so far, but wanting to confirm with the expert, I asked Tuckman what couples need to be doing to avoid forcing each other into the over-functioning/under-functioning dynamic.

'So the obvious first answer is for the person with ADHD to better manage it . . . Start using strategies and systems that are generally helpful for people with ADHD,' Tuckman says. 'But also equally important is for the non-ADHD partner just to speak sooner, but speak nicer. Don't wait till you're fed up. Don't play the martyr and don't set up your own disappointment . . . It's also helpful for them to learn about ADHD, not as a favour to their partner, but rather as a favour to themselves.'

Assorted tips from along the way

Over the past two years, Anthony and I have developed some strategies to help me with my ADHD.

Sometimes – particularly at the end of a long and taxing day – I can get to the point where I'm utterly paralysed if I need to make even the simplest decision, overwhelmed with anxiety about making the right choice.

Should we get takeaway or eat the leftovers? My mind starts racing: I want the takeaway but we should save money, but what if I'm missing out, and what if the meals in the fridge go off, but also we should treat ourselves occasionally, and oh my god what if I choose something and he doesn't like it and then he'll be nice and not say anything?

In those moments I often just tell him to decide. Previously, sensing but not quite understanding the distress in my voice, he'd go, 'No, no, whatever you want,' or, 'No, you've had a tough day, you choose.' In different circumstances, this would be very kind, but in those moments it was the worst thing I could hear.

After I was diagnosed, and saw a few videos talking about ADHD overload, overstimulation and decision **paralysis**, I had the words (even if they weren't official, clinical terms) to explain what was happening. We spoke about it and came up with a code word for when I just desperately needed him to make a choice for me – when, wrong or right, it just needed to get done.

I think the code word was something unoriginal like 'pineapple', but, truth be told, after I used it a couple of times, Anthony got good at picking up on the signs of overload, and now more often than not he can just tell when a unilateral decision needs to be made.

Similarly, sometimes when we're out, especially when there's music pumping and everyone's talking and lots of things happening everywhere all at once, the constant distractions can wear me out after an hour or two. Previously, if I said I wanted to go home, Anthony would want to come with me, worried I wasn't okay or that I'd be upset with him for staying out without me – which of course would make me feel guilty for cutting his night short. And so I'd go hide in the bathroom on my phone instead of calling an Uber.

I actually highly recommend us ADHDers take social media bathroom breaks during parties, but these ones were so long the people we were with must have assumed something truly demonic was happening to my gastrointestinal system.

But through talking about my ADHD, I managed to explain that sometimes I need to feel like I can just scoot without ruining his good time. And once we came to this understanding, it became a lot easier for me to stick around, knowing that I wasn't obliged to be there.

He's also come to understand that one of the kindest things you can do for someone who's spent their whole life beating themselves up for not being productive enough, is noticing when they're approaching breaking point and demanding they give themselves a rest. Usually I wouldn't condone someone ordering their partner to do something, but in this case, it's more about giving an ADHDer permission to relax – a luxury so many of us don't feel we're worthy of.

And I've learnt that there are plenty of things I can do to help him, too. I can set myself reminders, bust out the chore charms, add 'empty the dishwasher' to my **habit-stacking** stack. I can channel my restlessness into cooking and meal prepping, or, if that's too overwhelming, shopping online for things we need around the house. I can leave a note on the bathroom mirror reminding myself to turn on the fan when I take a shower. And I can keep articulating and reassuring him when I fail that it's not because I don't care or I don't respect him. (The idea that forgetful=thoughtless is pretty deeply ingrained in our culture, so it can be comforting to remind our neurotypical loved ones every so often that it's not the case – god bless their poor little dopamine-filled minds.)

But probably the most important change Anthony and I have made is that we now make a concerted effort to actively tell the other that we appreciate what they do for us. He understands how much my efforts to keep everything in order mean, and I notice and appreciate all the ways he tries to lighten my mental load.

We're still tinkering, fine-tuning and working through the trial and error, but the more open we are about the stress that ADHD can cause in a relationship, the more we can enjoy all the fun parts it brings to the table. All my random hobbies that we can dive into together, spontaneous DIY projects that can transform a mundane weekend into an adventurous one, and talking for hours about the TV show we both watched, and all the theories about season two that I stayed up till 1 am reading about.

I pull him out of his shell, he keeps my feet on the ground. We complement each other in a wonderful way, and, with a bit of luck and a whole lot of forwarding each other helpful TikToks, we'll grow as a couple and, more importantly, blossom into the best possible parents we can be for our horrifically unappreciative cat, Astro.

What about a double-decker ADHD sandwich?

You might have noticed that so far, I've only really spoken about ADHD/non-ADHD relationships – romantic or otherwise. But there are plenty of people in my life with ADHD, too.

In fact, until a year or two ago, I had no idea that a huge number of my friendships fell into the 'double ADHD' variety. It seems that time and time again, people I've been drawn to, and particularly the women in my life that I've truly, deeply connected with, have been unknowing ADHDers too. And while this is mostly a net positive, it also throws up a few unique challenges.

My friends with ADHD tend to intrinsically 'get' me in a way that the general public doesn't, and that only my very closest neurotypical loved ones can replicate. There's a certain energy to them, and an immediate kinship that it turns out existed whether we knew we both had the condition or not. There's no shame in interrupting each other or going off on long tangents. We can rant about our medications and random struggles without having to explain ourselves. With some of my friends, we can go months without speaking to each other and then jump back into the conversation like no time has passed.

That being said, there's a reason we sometimes don't speak for months. With both people struggling every day with the extra weight living with ADHD brings, there's not always going to be someone who has the capacity to step up and ensure the relationship is getting the attention it needs. Often, I find that once school or work or whatever it is that mandates our consistent interactions ends, we tend to float away from each other. And, while it's true that some ADHD friends will totally understand why so much time has passed without the two of us speaking, other times our powerful emotions and heightened sensitivity to feeling unwanted can also get in the way, and one or both of us can end up deeply hurt that this person who 'got' us so well is no longer in our lives.

The friendships I've allowed to slip through the cracks are a source of huge sadness, and something I'm working really hard to correct. Because, when you can make the effort and keep the communication going, chances are these relationships might be among the most fulfilling and joyous you'll ever experience.

When it comes to cohabitation, I'm a little less qualified to give advice, as I've only lived with non-ADHDers. But, keen to hear more about what an entirely neurodivergent household was like, I rang my recently married, profoundly ADHD-ish (in a wonderful way) friends Divy and Kiz.

Just as Anthony and I had to work around my sensitivity to being told to clean and my guilt around feeling that I've somehow failed him, Divy and Kiz are both dealing with their own versions of this ADHD baggage – expressed in two very different ways.

'I was always called lazy, and that got to me,' Divy says. 'And not planning things out properly got me into some bad spots as well. So now I'm really anxious about things.'

'And I have this thing where I find it really hard to clean when Div is around,' Kiz adds. 'Which, yeah, that probably does go back to trauma related to ADHD.'

Obviously there are challenges when both people in a relationship have ADHD. (A slightly disorganised organisational schedule is one.) But Divy and Kiz have also found so much joy in their dynamic as well. For example, having someone to share your new hobbies and hyper-fixations with who is just as engrossed as you.

'I mean, the reason that we have all of these boxes around the house – like a box specifically to put the dishwashing tablets in, stuff like that – is because we were both watching this series about home organisation together, and we went out and bought, like, $300 worth of glass containers,' Divy explains.

'Yeah,' Kiz says. 'It's a bit all or nothing with us . . . but that's really nice about our relationship. We don't have the whole "Your brain doesn't work like mine" thing.'

'And,' Div adds, 'one thing I will say is that even though we do spend a lot of money on hobbies, Kiz and I have a lot of fun together.'

You, me and ADHD

Obviously, every relationship is going to be different, but ADHD wreaks the most havoc when it's hidden. There's still a significant amount of stigma in the world around having a neurological condition, but if you're in a position where it's safe to do so, talk to the people you love about it.

Tell them what's hard, what's upsetting and what they can do to help. Send them videos and articles that will help them understand – hell, show them this chapter if you think it will help. Because, while ADHDers of course have to make compromises for the people we love, there are plenty of things the people we love can be doing for us, too. But you're only going to start making that progress if you actually talk to them about what's going on.

To be perfectly honest, there's one massive element of the 'how to be a good partner and friend and child and sibling as a person with ADHD' puzzle that I've neglected to mention so far. While this is by no means an absolute requirement, a lot of people – including me – find it's way easier to implement and maintain all of these positive changes I've been asking you to make in the past few chapters, when you can take a bit of the pressure off your struggling **dopaminergic** pathways . . . and by that, I do mean chemically.

So, let's do it. Let's bite the bullet and dive into the needlessly controversial world of ADHD medication.

DIARY ENTRY

Where's my light switch?

A couple of days after my diagnosis, about half an hour before work, I sit with a glass of water on my lips and my first-ever dose of ADHD medication gripped between my teeth.

My psychiatrist told me to take one 5-milligram short-acting dexamfetamine tablet in the morning, another at lunch and then slowly build myself up to three at a time over the course of the next few weeks. Technically, I was meant to start yesterday but somehow the little white plastic bottle full of pills felt too intimidating.

It's hard to articulate exactly where my nervousness is coming from, but I think it boils down to three main worries:

1. That this medication will make me utterly lose my mind and I'll plunge into insanity, never to recover. One tablet and my life will be over, just like the stories in all those dodgy 'say no to drugs' seminars and LSD urban legends. There's absolutely no evidence to suggest this has ever been the case with prescribed stimulant medication, by the way, but safe to say the 'amphetamine' suffix in the name has got to me just a little.
2. Probably much more rationally, I'm afraid that the pill isn't going to do anything. I know stimulants don't work for everyone with ADHD, but in the back of my brain I'm convinced these tablets are my one and only shot at being a 'successful human'. And if they don't fix me, I'm essentially screwed.
3. That they'll work too well. That I'll take this tablet and suddenly I won't really be 'me' any more. What if it takes away the creativity and silliness and the part of me that decides on a whim to spend my weekends learning to skateboard, build a giant replica of the Manchester United football stadium out of Lego, or hand-sew creepy dolls of politicians just

to make my colleagues laugh? I know dexamfetamine wears off after a couple of hours, but what if by temporarily 'curing' my ADHD, I suddenly discover that without it I'm a totally different, unrecognisable person or, god forbid, a boring one? Or, even more terrifyingly, what if everything is so unbelievably easy and I'm so focused and driven and motivated that I'll be forced to realise my life up to this point has been a waste?

Oh yuck, the pill is starting to dissolve, and the unbearably bitter sludge has hit my tastebuds. Almost by instinct, I glug down the water, taking the tablet with it, and think to myself, 'Well, that's that then.' At first I don't feel anything. I start work, fire off some emails and log in to the morning conference, all while my leg is energetically bouncing up and down as normal.

But as I'm hanging up the phone from my first interview of the day, I realise something feels different. The room is too quiet. The pens aren't lightly clacking around in my Prince Charles and Princess Diana Royal Wedding memorial cup like they usually are . . . because the desk isn't moving. Because the floor isn't moving, because my leg isn't jiggling.

'Oh my god,' I think. 'It's a sign from the universe!' And I assume that the first moment of the rest of my life has just begun.

But then . . . nothing.

I notice my foot tapping again around midday as the dose wears off, but otherwise there isn't much evidence that I've taken the medication at all. Not even a hyped party buzz. Everything was just . . . normal?

At that moment I felt bloody well ripped off, but looking back, I think I had the wrong idea about what ADHD meds were there to do. I'd heard so many ADHDers describe taking medication as like 'switching a light on' or 'day and night'. It was always spoken about in terms of an immediate, drastic change.

I think I somehow expected it to turn me into a superpowered productivity machine. That I would never need to take a break, and the whole world outside my computer screen would fade away and I'd start typing at the speed of light. But no.

The first couple of days I took the meds, I'd work normally, I'd take them again at lunchtime, then work normally some more. They were just normal days. But looking back, it occurs to me that 'Oh my god, I had three whole days where I felt normal the entire time?'

Without the medication, ADHD symptoms hit me in waves. There are times when it's absolutely impossible to focus and nothing in the world can make me work, and there are times when I genuinely become that superpowered work machine and blitz through a day's work in two hours. Then there's the middle ground, where I float somewhere in the vicinity of 'normal'. I'm sure my 'normal' is still much more unfocused than the average person's, but at least these periods don't utterly drain me of energy like the two more extreme ends of my attention spectrum.

I was imagining that ADHD medication would make me hyperfocused all the time. This is how I'd always experienced 'productivity' before, so I thought that's what 'not having attention difficulties' looked like.

But as wonderful and productive as hyperfocus can be, ultimately it's just another version of being unable to regulate one's attention – only it's the inability to switch it off rather than switch it on. Some people call it a 'superpower', but it can also be super draining, and I always conveniently forget the full mind-and-body crashes I often experience for hours afterwards.

For me, ADHD meds make those 'normal' periods longer and more stable. When I began my medication, I was probably still getting about the same amount of work done in a day – but I failed to notice that this was seven or eight hours of relatively consistent chugging away rather than three hours of hating myself for being unable to start, three hours of distractedly attempting to focus, and two hours of panicked mind-boggling productivity.

The medication meant I was ending the day without feeling as if I'd used up every last skerrick of energy. I didn't need to lie on the couch and scroll TikTok for four hours while panicking about what my boss meant when they used a full stop at the end of that last email. The idea of replying to my friend who was messaging for the third time to confirm our dinner plans no longer felt utterly overwhelming. Even the concept of cooking dinner now felt borderline within reach. Well, most days at least.

For me, ADHD medication isn't a light switch, it's a discount. When I'm medicated and doing well, I'm no longer living pay cheque to pay cheque on my reserves of attention and focus. There's something left in the bank, which means I can actually enjoy my day-to-day life rather than just get through it.

I'm sure things in the attention market still cost more for me than for the average person, and I still have days that are expensive and gruelling, where all that awaits me after work is utter burnout. But they are now much fewer and further between.

This is why it now sounds so ridiculous to me when people talk about ADHD medications 'brainwashing' or 'sucking the life out of' people. I can only speak from my own experience, but that would be like telling me that getting a pay raise was going to make my life worse.

Do you know how bloody amazing it feels to do laundry at 7 pm and not want to curl up and die? Now I do! And I highly recommend it.

14

Should I take these pills?

Okay, I've delayed long enough. It's finally time to crack open the can of neurodivergent worms that is ADHD medication.

Before I'd even considered the possibility that I might have ADHD, all I knew about stimulants was that they were addictive and dangerous. As far as I could tell, ADHD drugs were either prescribed to 'bad' kids, who were being turned into little robots, or were sold on the black market to workaholic law students who were one pill away from total mental breakdown. I grew up on headlines about the 'medicated generation' of kids and the 'drug crisis no one is talking about', despite everyone talking about it . . . a lot.

This (spoiler alert) totally incorrect understanding of ADHD medication is super common. Pretty much every member of my family expressed at least some level of concern when I told them I was going to start taking stimulants to help manage my ADHD. 'Just be careful,' they'd tell me. 'You don't want too many chemicals in your head.' 'You have such a lovely brain; you need to protect it.'

But for me, taking this medication *is* protecting my lovely little brain. The meds absolutely aren't perfect, there are risks associated with them, and they don't work for everyone. However, I can't help thinking about the scores of people whose lives could be changed by these medications, who are avoiding even talking to a doctor about ADHD because no one has ever explained to them that the story they've been fed about medication is basically nonsense.

The stigma surrounding stimulants is so strong that it affects parents' willingness to allow their kids to access these treatments, despite the mountain of studies showing their effectiveness, and many countries' top medical bodies recommending them as the first line of pharmacological defence.[1,2] Instead, parents may opt for less effective treatments, or may be unwilling to get their kids diagnosed with ADHD at all.[3]

Medications aren't designed to be, and never should be, the only treatment someone receives for ADHD – it's just one piece of the puzzle.

I've experienced this firsthand. Even though I wasn't a kid when I was diagnosed, my family still urged me to ask my psychiatrist if a non-stimulant medication was available. Simply because they loved me and they were afraid.

But what's all this fuss actually about?

'In simple terms, the big problem has always been that "dexamfetamine" sounds like "methamphetamine",' says Dr Roger Paterson, an Australian psychiatrist who's been treating people with ADHD for more than thirty years. 'They're described as these dangerous amphetamines that are highly addictive and induce psychosis, yadda yadda yadda. No, no, that's *meth*amphetamine. *Dex*amfetamine is medicinal, it's been tested for many years and found to be safe and not addictive.

'I wish the stimulant medications *were* a bit addictive, so my patients would remember to take them. They don't wake up craving them, and they do not get significant withdrawal **symptoms** if they stop them.'

Basically, these medications have a massive PR problem. Even a year into taking them myself, I still harboured some concerns. So, for your benefit (and mine), why don't we run through some of the most common questions, concerns and nuggets of – what I now know to be – misinformation?

But before we jump all the way in, let me make a few things abundantly clear:

- **These medications aren't designed to be, and never should be, the only treatment someone receives for ADHD – it's just one piece of the puzzle. For a lot of people it's a pretty darn important piece, but a piece nonetheless.**
- **Not every ADHD medication is a stimulant. I'll discuss non-stimulant options in a second; however, stimulants are the most common type of ADHD medication (and the most popular subject of moral panic), so that will be where the majority of my attention lies.**
- **Not everyone with ADHD chooses to go on medication. There are a myriad of reasons for this (some more legitimate than others). But as long as you're basing your decisions on facts rather than stigma, there's no single 'correct' way to treat your ADHD.**

Ultimately, this is an important and highly personal decision that only you and your healthcare team can make. The content of this chapter isn't medical advice, merely the available scientific data and reflections from my own research and experience.

They're not a 'cure'

ADHD medication doesn't cure ADHD, it doesn't even totally eliminate your symptoms while it's active in your system. But for most ADHDers, there's a high probability that it will at least help. Because of the varied genetics for ADHD, the degree to which medication reduces **impairment** really depends on the person. It might be day and night, it might be subtle, and in some cases it might do nothing at all. The first medication you try might work wonders, or it might take you and your physician months of trial and error.

In terms of what the medication will actually do, generally speaking they help improve attention and a person's ability to control impulses.[4] It's a little less clear if they improve **working memory** (the ability to hold and manipulate multiple bits of information in the forefront of your mind) – the studies are about fifty-fifty on this one.[5] The increased attention capacity might help your memory in other ways, but you'll probably still need to incorporate reminders and ADHD-friendly memory systems into your life.

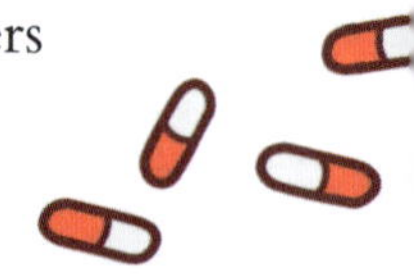

Professor David Coghill from the University of Melbourne, the world-renowned ADHD researcher and psychiatrist we met back in Chapter 1, says that medication is a means to an end. It's a way to make it easier for you to help yourself, but it's not going to magically transform your brain overnight.

> Medication is a way to make it easier for you to help yourself, but it's not going to magically transform your brain overnight.

'I mean, I am a doctor. I often prescribe medication to treat ADHD. But I also recognise that my medications are only part of the answer,' he told me. 'Different people have other needs, and so medication isn't a cure-all for those problems. We often say "Pills don't make skills" . . . there's still a lot of work to do.'

The different kinds of ADHD medication

Stimulants

Stimulants work by increasing the levels of **dopamine** and **noradrenaline** in the brain – basically giving our Ethels a good meal and a nice cup of coffee, allowing her to work more efficiently and keep all our mental paperwork in order. Despite being called 'stimulants', at the correct prescribed dosage they generally have the effect of making people feel more centred, focused and even calm. They tend to be the first port of call when medicating someone for ADHD because they're pretty bloody effective for most people.

There are a whole range of stimulants on the market, but the most famous active ingredients are:

1. **methylphenidate**, the main player in Ritalin and Artige (short-acting), or Ritalin LA and Concerta (long-acting). This family of medications is generally thought to be the best option for children and adolescents, and is the most widely used ADHD medication across the world.
2. **amphetamines**, both the short-acting dexamfetamine (which you may know from its starring role in the US brand Adderall) and its long-acting cousin lisdexamfetamine (which made its debut in the medication Vyvanse). Current studies suggest amphetamine medications may be a slightly better option for ADHD adults than methylphenidate,[6] but it depends on the individual.

Short-acting stimulants stay in your system for three to six-ish hours and are usually taken twice or three times a day. Long-acting options are taken once in the morning and usually last eight to twelve hours, depending on the type. These extended-release medications can be super helpful if, like me, you have a bad habit of forgetting to take your second dose at lunchtime because the first lot has worn off. Unfortunately, you do need to remember to take them early enough in the day, because throwing one back after lunch will (in my strictly personal, non-empirically studied experience) make you feel like you're a small Victorian-era ghost haunting your house for the rest of the afternoon. And by that I mean my tummy feels a little hollow and I experience a low buzz of anxiety that makes everything feel slightly off.

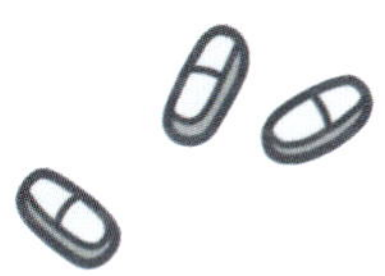

After eighteen months of adjusting and tinkering, my psychiatrist and I have landed on 70 milligrams of Vyvanse, occasionally topped up with a short-acting 5-milligram dexamfetamine tablet when I need to be ready and raring first thing in the morning, because the long-acting stuff takes bloody ages to kick in for me.

Now, I want you to really pay attention to what I say here, because I think it gets lost way too often in discussions about 'the spooky danger of ADHD drugs'. Stimulants – at least in the short term – are among the most effective psychological medications known to humankind.

It's hard to put an exact figure on how effective any psychological medicine is because there's no universally accepted definition of effective, but generally speaking, methylphenidate and amphetamines will both reduce symptoms of ADHD in about 70 per cent of ADHDers. By the time you've trialled a medication from each family, the success rate goes up to about 90 per cent.[7,8] For context, antidepressants are only 40–60 per cent effective for clinical depression.[9]

There's a reason stimulants are the first line of treatment for ADHD patients: given those odds, and the very real dangers that untreated ADHD can pose to one's life (more on this in the next chapter), it would be bordering on medical negligence to not consider them.

The big catch comes from the propensity for stimulant medications to be 'diverted' (a fancy way of saying 'people with a prescription illegally selling them to non-ADHDers to be used as a party or study drug'). For this reason they're heavily regulated in most countries and outright banned in others.

If you're travelling overseas it's imperative that you check, check and triple-check the country's laws on ADHD medications, particularly stimulants. Some countries want nothing to do with them, while others are okay with them as long as you have your prescriptions with you. Some have strict bans on short-acting medication, but they might allow you to bring a small amount of long-acting tablets for your own personal use with a doctor's note. If you don't follow the rules, you could be slapped with a big fine and have your medication confiscated. So we really don't have the luxury of just chucking a bottle of pills in our suitcase and hoping for the best.

Non-stimulants

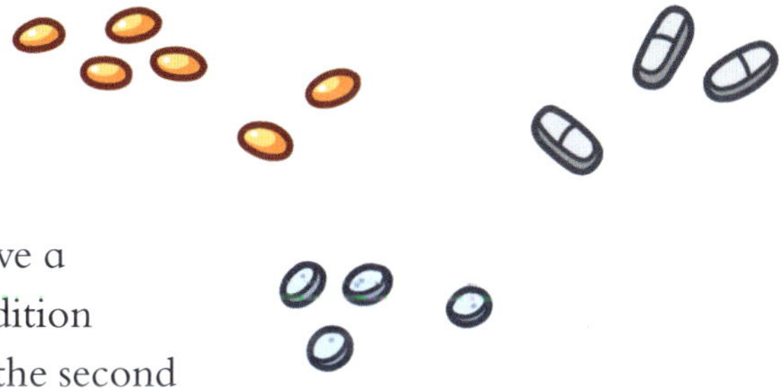

If stimulants aren't for you – maybe they just don't work, the **side effects** are too frustrating, or perhaps you have a heart condition or other medical condition that they might interfere with – then the second port of call is non-stimulant ADHD medications.

These are generally less stigmatised, less associated with misuse and less highly regulated. So why don't we switch to these and avoid all the fuss? Well, for most ADHDers, they also tend to be less effective (particularly when compared with amphetamine medications),[10] and come with their own range of side effects, too.

These types of medications target noradrenaline more than dopamine specifically (they're basically a really big cup of coffee for Ethel). Unlike stimulants – which usually start working pretty much from day one – these may take three or four weeks of daily usage for the effects to start kicking in. But once they do, they can last up to twenty-four hours, which is a neat bonus.

The exact type of non-stimulant drugs approved for use varies from country to country, but the most common varieties are atomoxetine (sold under the brand name Strattera) and guanfacine (aka Intuniv).

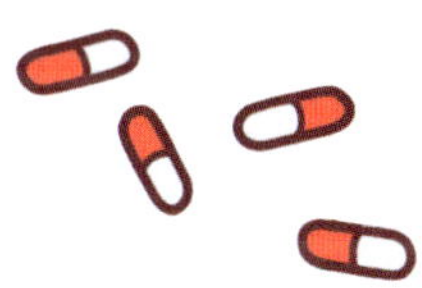

Off-label options

If non-stimulants still don't float your boat, then you may be offered an 'off-label' option.

Off-label prescribing happens when a medication has been approved for a specific use by a pharmaceutical governing body (in Australia, the Therapeutic Goods Administration), but there's also a decent amount of evidence suggesting it's both safe and potentially effective at treating another condition. In this situation, your physician is still allowed to use their discretion to prescribe this medication to you if they reckon it could help.

This may sound a bit dodgy at first, but off-label prescribing is both legal and exceedingly common. A lot of the time it's just an annoying quirk of capitalism – getting a medication officially approved for a new use is expensive and time-consuming, and if the additional condition isn't all that common, or the copyright on that drug has already lapsed (meaning consumers can buy cheaper 'generic' versions from other manufacturers), there isn't much economic motivation for a company to go through all the clinical trials and testing that are required.[11]

For example, the medication prazosin is officially approved to treat high blood pressure, but is often prescribed to help treat nightmares related to PTSD.[12]

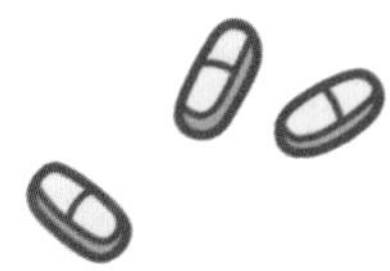

When it comes to ADHD, the most common off-label medications are antidepressants – specifically those that target dopamine and noradrenaline, such as bupropion (sold under the name Wellbutrin). Positive results have been reported by some patients, doctors and small-scale clinical trials,[13,14] but there hasn't been enough specific research to draw any definitive conclusions yet.

But it's super common for antidepressant/anti-anxiety medications to be part of an ADHDer's pharmacological routine alongside ADHD-specific medication anyway – given anxiety and depression are very often a part of an ADHDer's life.

Will I become dependent or go through withdrawals?

One of the most common fears my loved ones had when I started on ADHD meds was that I might become dependent on them. And if, for whatever reason, I was going to go off them, it could cause me to have a mental breakdown or psychotic episode. It's pretty clear where this worry comes from. The psychotropic medications that the average person knows the most about are antidepressants, which require you to take them consistently, at the same time every day, and slowly wean off them under strict medical supervision, otherwise you can experience horrible and potentially dangerous side effects.

ADHD stimulant medications don't work like this[15] – although it's still exceedingly important that you speak to your doctor before changing the way you take any medication. When used in the correct way, at the prescribed dose, stimulants rarely if ever produce withdrawal symptoms beyond perhaps a few days of feeling a bit more tired than usual.

Several experts explained to me that stimulants function in a way that's actually pretty similar to the everyday painkillers in our bathroom cabinets. You take them when you need them, they enter your body, they do their job, and then they leave. Which means you have a lot more flexibility in how you can use them.

For example, I rarely take my medications on the weekends. Partially because when there's no pressing need to focus, it's nice to just veg out and let my thoughts wander – and partially because given my high dosage level, my psychiatrist recommended taking breaks to stop my brain from building up a resistance to the medication, which – although reversible – reduces its effectiveness. (Don't worry, I'll properly explain the whole resistance thing shortly.)

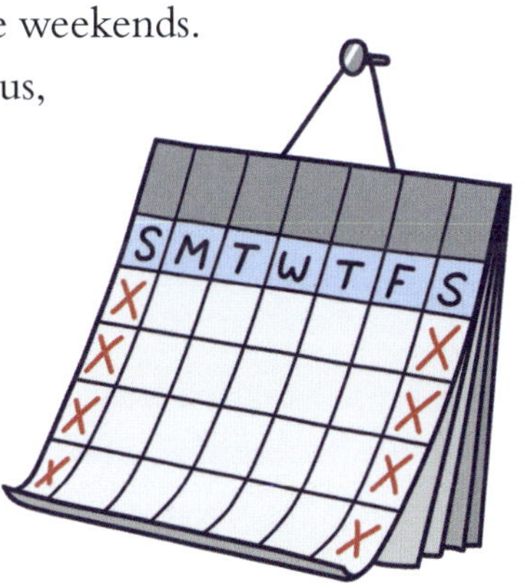

That being said, it can still be quite psychologically jarring to suddenly find yourself without medication, especially if it's caused by something unexpected – for example, realising you've left it on your bedside table while the plane you're sitting on is headed to Sydney for a week-long work trip . . . hypothetically. (Luckily for me, after a panicked and not all that productive day, I actually found the bottle of meds I'd packed last time and then forgotten about in the side pocket of my suitcase. Gosh, ADHD comes in handy sometimes! Although, that accidental stash could have been a real problem on an international flight.)

Non-stimulant ADHD medications are a bit of a different story, though. Some are fine to go cold turkey, but most act more like your classic psychotropic drugs, requiring a precise, medically supervised tapering-off period to avoid any unpleasant outcomes, so it's important to speak with your doctor about that.

What are the side effects?

Like any medication, ADHD meds come with side effects. These vary from person to person, but the most common problems with stimulants are sleep irregularities[16] and loss of appetite/weight loss.[17] Now, these are nothing to be sneezed at, especially if – like me – you have a complicated relationship with both sleep and weight to begin with.

Personally, one of the weirdest things for me about starting ADHD medication was learning how to figure out what hunger feels like without the 'hungry' part. It would get to 2 pm and I'd suddenly get really tired, my focus would slip and everyone around me would become really annoying. Turns out, that's what happens when your body runs out of fuel. So now, even if my non-existent appetite means I can't think of anything worse than eating at that moment, I try really hard to at least get some cashews or a banana into my stomach at lunchtime. (On days where that's too difficult I'll go for a glazed donut or some instant noodles or something else I really enjoy.) Also, once the medications wear off in the evening, my appetite comes back in full force, and if I haven't eaten enough during the day I will find myself absolutely ravenous, sometimes eating far too much, too quickly and tiring myself out all over again.

On the sleep side of things, at least for me, taking my medications as soon as I get up tends to ensure they've well and truly worn off by bedtime, but I certainly had some extra insomniac nights in the early days before I got the hang of things.

When used in the correct way, at the prescribed dose, stimulants rarely if ever produce withdrawal symptoms beyond perhaps a few days of feeling a bit more tired than usual.

They're also associated with a slight increase in heart and blood pressure. The majority of the time these aren't dangerous, but you should still 100 per cent tell your doctor if you notice anything like this, because in rare cases stimulants have been linked to more serious heart issues.[18] This is also why some doctors may want to run tests, such as an electrocardiogram, before you start on them, and why you should absolutely make sure to disclose any and all pre-existing conditions.

There's been some discussion of the potential for stimulants to increase the risk of psychosis. While this is a genuine danger if stimulants are being abused, the data on adults taking them as prescribed is much more reassuring.[19] The risk, if any, is very small, and symptoms usually show up early in treatment so can be quickly addressed.

Interestingly, not only did a large study using Swedish hospital records find no link between methylphenidate use and psychosis, but it showed that those with a history of psychosis were 36 per cent less likely to go to hospital because of a psychotic episode a year after starting the stimulant than they were in the period immediately before being prescribed it.[20]

Some people also feel quite anxious and jittery while on stimulants. (I used to get this way more often, but I realised it was usually coming on when I was welcoming my Vyvanse tablet into a stomach full of nothing but coffee and lychee-ice-flavoured nicotine vapour, so that's probably on me, not the meds.)

Another thing to watch for is a short period of increased fatigue and/or a bit of a bad mood as the stimulants wear off towards the end of the day.[21] I got these during my first year of taking meds, but not knowing that this was a 'thing', I referred to it as 'getting the Armageddons' because the world would occasionally start feeling rather spooky around 5.30 pm. Luckily, the Armageddons don't seem to be a problem for me any more, perhaps because my body has adjusted, or perhaps because it actually wasn't the meds but a nefarious spirit periodically visiting me who has since moved on to the next realm.

For some, these issues will be so minor and unproblematic that stimulants will have fewer adverse effects than drinking an extra cup of coffee for focus. But for others, the side effects may mean that the benefits of stimulants just don't outweigh the costs.

The good news is, the vast majority of side effects will pretty much stop immediately after you cease taking the medication. This is another reason why your doctor might be keen for you to at least try stimulants to start with (even though a lot of people are hesitant).

The side effects of non-stimulant medications vary from medication to medication but tend to be more in the realm of fatigue, nausea, dizziness and, of course, because we can't seem to escape it, loss of appetite. The most common non-stimulant, atomoxetine (Strattera), has also been known to increase blood pressure and heart rates in rare cases, so, again, if you have a history of heart issues you should definitely bring them up with your doctor before you start.[22]

My 'weird one'

I'd never had any problems with my heart rate in eighteen months of taking stimulants until – and I know how unbelievable ironic this sounds – I was writing this section about the side effects.

I was working from home, had woken up a little late, skipped breakfast and made myself a cup of coffee that I used to wash down my Vyvanse – forgetting my antidepressants altogether. As much as I've been advocating for people with ADHD to take time off, eat well, sleep well and not **burn out**, I hadn't been following my own advice.

As I gulped down the last dregs of my double-strength long black, I started to feel very weird – like I'd just been for a run but I wasn't out of breath. It felt like panic, even though I wasn't panicking. My heart was beating like crazy, and this kept on for hours, sitting at 120 beats per minute, which the internet told me isn't normal.

My heart rate probably would have gone back down if it wasn't for the fear that gripped me. I'd just spent the past four days reading all about the rare, but still possible, cardiovascular events my medication could cause, and here I was, experiencing them.

I googled 'symptoms of a heart attack in women', because I'm nothing if not dramatic, and read that one sign was shortness of breath, and suddenly I noticed that, yeah, my breath was actually a little short. Eventually, I messaged my boss to say I was sick and had to log off, called my dad in a panic telling him to come check on me, and just as he arrived . . . oh no! Now my left arm felt a tiny bit numb, coincidentally one of the heart attack symptoms I'd spent the last three hours reading about.

Tears rolling down my face, I said, 'Dad, I'm so sorry, you have to take me to Emergency.'

I knew academically that there was a 99 per cent chance I, an otherwise healthy 25-year-old, was having a panic attack, but then again I'd just read a whole lot of articles about women who dismissed heart attack symptoms and suffered the consequences.

When Dad parked across the road from the hospital, I said, 'I'm sorry, I'm just being dumb, take me home.' He looked at me and said, 'Bub, if we go in and we're wrong, the worst-case scenario is that we waste a few hours. If we go home and we're wrong, the worst-case scenario is death. Maybe let's just go in.'

So we do. And, as it turns out, a hospital emergency room is a great place to get writing done. In fact, that's where I managed to write a large portion of this chapter. After many hours, I was seen. They took some blood for testing, ran an electrocardiogram, and I got hooked up to an IV bag filled with ambiguous fluids that I was told would help bring my heart rate down. Turns out those fluids were just fancy water, because, guess what, I was incredibly dehydrated. During all those hours of panic, it never occurred to me to drink any liquids.

Eventually, the ER doctor sat next to my bed in the emergency ward, my perfectly normal blood test results in his hand, and said, 'Look, mate, I think you probably just overdid it a bit with dehydration and coffee and stimulants and a bunch of stress and anxiety all in one go.'

'Oh,' I said. 'So is there anything I need to worry about?'

'I mean, it's good you came in, but no, not really. Be more careful about taking your anti-anxiety meds consistently, maybe get your doctor to reduce your stimulant dose if this keeps happening, and probably best to avoid coffee on days you take your Vyvanse for a while. That's kind of it.'

'Oh,' I say again. 'So I just had a weird one?'

'Yeah, mate, you just had a weird one.'

And then I went home.

This definitely shook my perhaps somewhat arrogant view that everyone talking about how serious stimulant medications were was simply fearmongering. They're serious medications, and taking them is a significant decision you should be prepared to take seriously. Because ultimately, I stopped taking mine seriously, and I stopped looking after my body while I was on them. I was using my medications as a way to just 'keep going' no matter what – relying on caffeine, amphetamines and adrenaline to fuel myself rather than, you know . . . rest, food and water.

Nothing bad or dangerous came of my 'weird one', but still, it was a learning moment.

I was nervous about my medications for a few days, but I eased myself back into it, made sure to drink more water, and I haven't had any problems since.

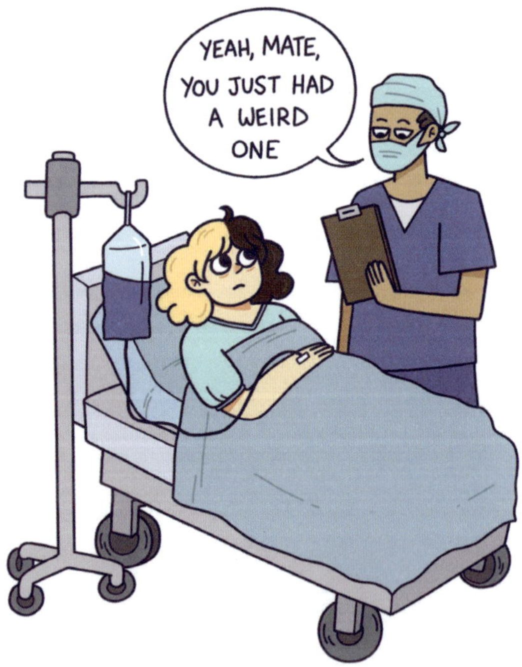

By the way, If you want to make sure you're drinking more water throughout the day, I recommend keeping water bottles on your bedside, desk and couch, so you never have to get up to get your bottle from another room. Oh, and get one with a straw – that way the barrier of having to unscrew and re-screw a lid isn't going to discourage you from having a cheeky sip between tasks.

Will I lose my sparkle?

One of the big worries about ADHD medications is that they're somehow stifling or suppressing the next generation of wonderful creative minds, putting them in a straitjacket so they can be churned through the education system or sit quietly in their small grey nine-to-five cubicles.

It stems from the idea that ADHD medication is somehow a tranquilliser or psychological numbing agent . . . but that's just not the case. With stimulants, the clue is in the name – they are stimulating your brain, powering up those neural pathways that run off dopamine, which allows us to focus our brains better. Even non-stimulant ADHD medications tend to simply increase the amount of noradrenaline in the brain, boosting our ability to stay alert rather than tranquillising it down.

But still, I've always thought of my ability to have those free-flowing twirly-whirly creative thoughts as one of my strengths (technically speaking, this is called 'diffuse attention' and is thought to be common among creative people), so I was a bit concerned that a super-focused, hyper-alert brain would ruin that. But that didn't end up happening.

The issue with my twirly and whirly creative thoughts is that often they arrive in my brain and then slip away before I can get a good grip on them. Plus, even when I can, it's difficult to turn them into concrete, actionable ideas, when I'm unable to summon the focus and motivation required for the next steps. Stimulants help me with that. Rather than lessening my creativity, they assist in channelling it into something useful.

The scientific studies we do have on the effect of stimulants on creativity have been small, with mixed or inconclusive results,[23,24] but generally any observed changes – positive or negative – have been pretty minor. And even if stimulants do slightly change the way my mind works, that's only the case while the medication is actively in my system. By the time evening rolls round, everything has gone back to the way it was. So, I could always just skip the meds if there was a day I wanted to be extra twirly and whirly.

Before I started, I was also concerned about the medication affecting my ability to **hyperfocus**. As far as I can tell, this hasn't been formally studied anywhere, but while ADHD meds have certainly evened out the peaks and troughs of my attention levels throughout the day, they haven't taken away my ability to hyperfocus altogether. When it comes to crunch time and the stress, adrenaline and panic set in, I'm still able to sit for hours, totally absorbed in the work I'm doing, and get done what needs to be done. It's just that now that I lose way less time to frustration and aimless distractibility, I'm not as reliant on these hyperfocused bursts in the first place. Which is a relief, because it's an emotionally exhausting survival tactic that I shouldn't have to lean on just to make it through day-to-day life.

My tendency to spend a week hyper-fixated on a new hobby, science fiction franchise or musical theatre cast recording has not been affected by the Vyvanse either. This isn't ideal for my bank account, or for whoever is sharing a long car trip with me, but it has eased my worries about medication somehow taking away the enjoyable parts of the condition.

Is it really just 'microdosing meth'?

I have to admit something. Despite knowing that the perceived connection between methamphetamine and stimulant medications is at the core of much of the stigma attached to ADHD, I'm still very guilty of jokingly telling people that I'm 'microdosing meth' or 'taking my morning speed', mostly because I find it extremely funny to see how confused they become for a solid five seconds before the penny finally drops.

But the more I investigate the debate that surrounds stimulants, the more I realise I need to cut this out. Because a huge chunk of the general public actually does believe that these medications are chemically identical to street meth, and it's a pretty natural human reaction to feel scared about 'giving crack to children'.

As I've mentioned before, however, these medications are not the same as methamphetamine, cocaine, MDMA or any other upper you might buy from your brother's friend's mysterious cousin.

Methylphenidate (Ritalin) is a totally different molecule. The prefix 'meth' just means it's got a group of one carbon atom and three hydrogen atoms in it somewhere – which is an extraordinarily common component in organic chemical. And while amphetamines (such as Adderall, Vyvanse etc.) are obviously in the same molecular family as methamphetamine, those extra couple of atoms make a huge, huge difference.

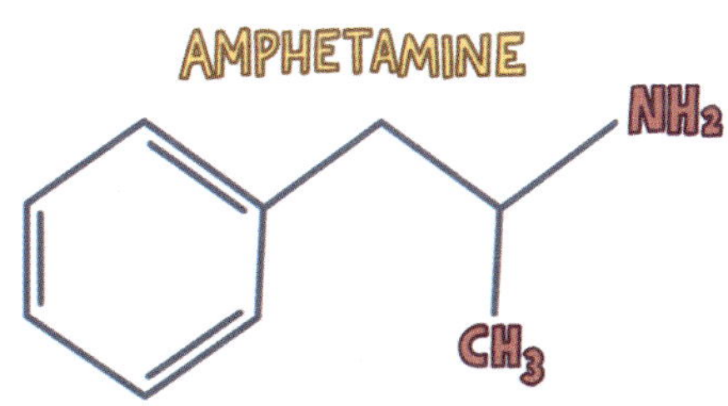

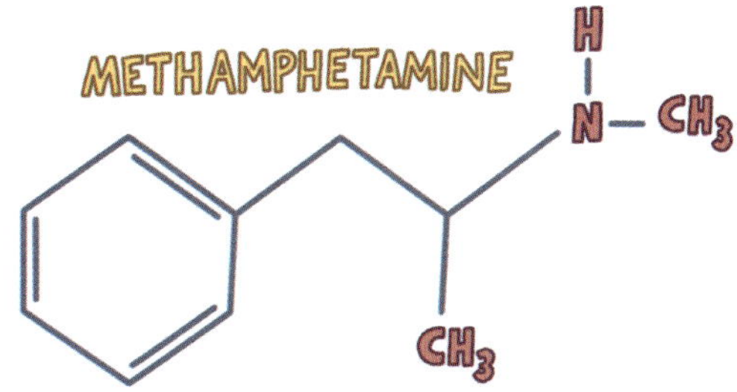

I won't bore you with the chemistry, but basically, meth's structure means a much higher percentage of the chemical gets into the brain, making it far more potent, and potentially addictive.[25] Plus there's the fact that street meth is often also laced with toxic contaminants that can wreak havoc on the body, whereas the worst thing hiding in your prescription amphetamines is a bit of starch.

Just for reference, while there are three atoms separating dexamfetamine and methamphetamine, there's only one atom separating table salt (NaCl) and bleach (NaClO). Chemistry matters!

Technically, legal, factory-produced methamphetamine (Desoxyn) is very occasionally prescribed to treat ADHD in a number of countries, but not Australia. However, the dosage is a tiny fraction of your average illicit hit.

Do ADHD meds turn people into drug addicts?

Governments tend to be pretty uptight about stimulants because of the perception that they're really easy to get addicted to. This is only kinda-sorta true. Let me explain.

Amphetamines and methylphenidate do have the potential to be abused, and can lead to other **substance-abuse** issues . . . but this is exceedingly rare if you take them orally (as opposed to being crushed up and inhaled, or injected into the vein) and at the dose prescribed by your doctor.[26] Plus, the long-acting forms are even harder to abuse.

Abuse problems tend to crop up when the medication's being taken in way higher doses than recommended, often by those who weren't prescribed it in the first place. Stimulants also have a reputation as illicit party drugs, used to achieve a high – or as study-enhancing drugs, due to the likely incorrect belief that they'll also increase the cognitive abilities of those without ADHD.[27] And while the vast majority of the time this misuse doesn't cause any lasting health effects, there have been fatal overdoses, especially when stimulants were snorted or injected.[28]

For ADHDers with a history of addiction, there are long-acting/delayed-release stimulant options, which sort of drip-feed the medication throughout the day, making it more difficult to feel any sort of 'high'. Newer medications, such as my girl lisdexamfetamine, even have molecules attached that require blood enzymes to slowly break off the lysine amino-acid before the amphetamine can be absorbed, meaning you can't even get around the delayed-release issue by inhaling or injecting it.

This isn't to say that no ADHD person has ever overused, abused or become addicted to stimulants – I mean, we're a group of people who are at increased risk of substance abuse in the first place. But all the data we have so far suggests that correct ADHD stimulant medication use is way more likely to *protect* us from addiction than to cause it.

A large-scale Swedish study following nearly 40,000 people with ADHD showed that those who were on stimulants in 2006 were about 31 per cent less likely to have a substance-abuse disorder in 2009. In fact, the longer they used prescribed stimulants, the less likely they were to struggle with addiction in general.[29] And in case that isn't a big enough subject pool for you, a 2017 study with nearly 3 million Swedes showed the same thing.[30]

However, the propensity for these medications to be diverted and abused does make life way more difficult for those of us who need them. In Australia, stimulants – short and long acting – are classified as Section 8 drugs, alongside stuff such as fentanyl, oxycodone and methadone. This means only psychiatrists can initially prescribe these medications to adults (with paediatricians also able to for children), which can make the process of getting the medication in the first place exceedingly expensive – usually hundreds of dollars even with government support, and it's not uncommon for this to run into the thousands. This excludes scores of people from ever having access to an extremely effective treatment option. Given how recently the adult form of the disorder has come into the zeitgeist, and the limited numbers of psychiatrists who will even see people for adult ADHD, wait lists in many countries have ballooned to more than a year. And despite all of this regulation and red tape, short-acting stimulant medications are still pretty darn easy to buy on the street.

I don't pretend to have the answer, but it does raise the question . . . Are our governments' skittishness and fears about the potential risks of ADHD medication actually helping prevent drug abuse, or ultimately are they just putting a group of high-risk people further at risk?

Long-term effectiveness and long-term risks

When people want to argue against the use of stimulants, they'll often mention that 'no studies have been done on the long-term effectiveness of stimulant medications or the health risks they pose'. Which sounds weird, right, given these drugs have been around since the 1950s?

Well, this is another one of those half-truths . . . or, more specifically, quarter-truths.

First, there are plenty of people looking at the long-term health outcomes of people who have used stimulant medications. Yet, in seven decades of widespread use at the prescribed dose, no significant long-term health issues have been recorded.

Pretty much the only slightly eyebrow-raising impact is that children who take the medication for several years may be a couple of centimetres shorter than their peers. But this usually corrects itself over time, meaning the kid's eventual height is unaffected, and there don't appear to be any additional medical concerns associated with this temporary front-row-of-the-school-photo status.[31]

In fact, the next chapter will make it abundantly clear that there are heaps of really positive long-term health benefits to stimulant use for ADHD people – I mean, look at the lower addiction rates we just saw.

Now onto the effectiveness question. Despite the claims of some in the anti-stimulant crowd, no reliable studies have shown that stimulants will make your baseline ADHD symptoms get worse when you stop taking them.[32] There has been some discussion in the academic work about whether long-term methylphenidate use eventually causes your brain to have a higher density of dopamine transporters[33] (the little vacuum cleaners that suck the dopamine back up into the **neuron** once it's done being useful). But there's no evidence that this actually reduces normal dopamine levels when the drug isn't in your system, or irreversibly makes the medication become less effective over time – it's just theoretical speculation. This was something I was worried about the first time I had to go without my medications during a work week (due to an ill-timed public holiday and a mix-up with my prescriptions). But ultimately I realised that my symptoms weren't actually worse than they used to be, I'd just become accustomed to work being less difficult.

When it comes to studying actual effectiveness over the course of many years or even decades, things get a bit more complicated because, well, there are a bunch of things that make studying this nearly impossible.

For the vast majority of the seventy years we've been using stimulants to treat ADHD, it was assumed that children would naturally grow out of the condition, so there wasn't much push to undertake the extremely expensive and arduous task of studying stimulants' effectiveness for longer than two years. There are also some serious ethical issues in asking a group of people not to take medication for their condition for decades at a time in order to create a 'control group', so robust clinical long-term trials are out the window.

The other problem is that currently most people tend not to use stimulants long-term, for several reasons, including but not limited to the fact that:

- **In many countries, they are difficult, expensive or even illegal to access.**
- **They do have those annoying side effects, such as loss of appetite, which may eventually outweigh the benefits for some people.**
- **The severity of ADHD symptoms is likely to fluctuate throughout a person's life, meaning the stimulants might not be necessary for a period of time, and the process of getting back on them can be really expensive.**
- **Over the years, some people are able to adapt their life and implement strategies that make it so medication is no longer required.**

This means the data on long-term effectiveness is often skewed, because the longest users tend to be those who had the most severe and impairing symptoms to begin with, and therefore the most motivation to keep going. So it's not really fair to say, 'Hey, this long-term medication-taker is functioning at the same level as this other person who decided to stop using medication ten years ago, therefore stimulants don't work long-term!'

Now, there is some evidence that stimulants may lose their effectiveness for some people over time. Again, this is really difficult to study and the data is all over the place when it comes to what percentage of ADHDers will experience it and how long it takes for tolerance to build. Like, really all over the place – one study said it was 2.7 per cent of people over ten years,[34] another said 66 per cent over three years.[35] But overall, there's a chance that after a couple of years, the effectiveness of stimulants may wane either a little or a lot.[36]

What the anti-stimulant crowd conveniently forgets to mention is that tolerance such as this can be counteracted by taking a 'medication holiday'; that is, going off your medication, even if it's just for a week or two, to 'reset' the amount of dopamine your brain feels is normal. (Which is also why your physician might recommend having at least one med-free day a week to prevent tolerance building up in the first place). If a medication holiday isn't possible, a doctor can switch the type of stimulant being used. And, if all else fails, there's always non-stimulant medications as a back-up.

Somewhat freaked out by the idea of my meds one day losing their effectiveness, I asked Professor Coghill if it was possible for someone to build up resistance to such a degree that the drug would never work again, to which he replied, 'Well, that's just not how tolerance works.'

But there are other reasons ADHD medications might not be something we can guarantee will be a part of our lives in two or twenty or fifty years' time – such as weight loss, anxiety getting worse, heart problems developing or moving to a country where they are much harder to access or are even banned. So we should be prepared for that eventuality, just in case.

The way I look at it is, hey, I've got a good thing going for now. Who knows how long it will last, so I'm going to use this time when I have all this juicy, juicy executive functioning capacity to spare to try to establish a routine, adopt habits and shape my environment to make my life as ADHD-friendly as possible. So that even if I do get unlucky one day, I'll still be a heck of a lot better off than I was before I was diagnosed.

As far as we can tell, using ADHD medications as prescribed comes with minimal long-term risks, significant short-term gains and at least a reasonable chance at long-term benefits. I get it – the field of medical research has certainly let people down in the past. (It's let me down plenty even just in the world of ADHD.) So I understand people's hesitancy in signing up for something when we're not 100 per cent sure about its long-term effects.

But what so often gets lost in this discussion about the 'risks' of ADHD medications is that we're not weighing them up against a blank, totally safe slate. We're weighing up their minor risks against something that's magnitudes more dangerous, can have way worse side effects and, we know for a fact, poses a genuine risk to lives. And that's leaving ADHD untreated.

So, let's take a look at what those dangers are.

Crying on the step machine

Just a warning: the following story contains references to disordered eating and body shaming.

When I was thirteen, I read a statistic in a magazine in the school library that said 'eight out of ten teenage girls reported being dissatisfied with their bodies and appearance'. That night, as I was changing into my pyjamas, I stood for a long time in just my bra and undies staring at my body in the mirror and thinking, 'Wow. I'm part of the two out of ten.'

When I was fourteen, my mum's extremely fashionable friend and my surrogate aunt, Lynette, brought over three big bags of her old clothes for Perrin and me to try on. It was a fantastic evening – spent darting between the living room and bedroom trying on jacket after top after skirt after jacket. Then we hit the jackpot: a shin-length black evening dress made from stretchy, form-fitting material, with little buckles over the straps. It was the most grown-up piece of clothing we'd ever seen.

Lynette handed it to Perrin, who rushed out of the room to try it first. When she walked back in my mum slapped her hands to her knees and said, 'Oh. My. God. That is just fabulous.' And it was. My sixteen-year-old sister looked utterly amazing, if slightly uncomfortable with the low neckline.

But I knew I'd have no such qualms. 'Quick, take it off and let me try,' I said.

Ever since I'd caught up to Perrin in the boob department a year or two earlier (the proudest achievement of my life to that point), I'd just assumed we now had essentially the same body. We shared clothes, we shared shoes. I never thought twice about it.

So when I went into the room, squeezed the suffocating dress over my shoulders, pulled the hem down over my knees and looked in the mirror,

I was taken aback. Rather than the single smooth curve from waist to bum that tapered down to the knees like my sister, my silhouette flared out from my midriff to the bottom of my stomach, dipped in at my hips and curved back out again around my thighs.

I'd never seen a body that looked like mine before, and I began to worry there was something medically wrong with me. I pulled out my 32GB iPod touch and googled 'more than one bump over hip and thighs'. Instantly a page full of results came up, each some variation on '16 easy exercises to make those hip dips history.'

'Oh,' I thought, '. . . oh.'

I took the dress off and quietly popped it on top of the pile to go into Perrin's wardrobe. That was the moment I joined the 80 per cent, and ever since, my relationship with my body and the food I put in it has been . . . complicated.

This seems like a pretty obvious ADHD trait now, but growing up, I always used food as a way to kill boredom – as stimulation during deeply unstimulating afternoons. But in the years AD (after dress), these boredom-induced snack sessions were plagued with a touch of guilt.

This all stayed in the realm of 'utterly emotionally devastating but relatively normal teen-girl insecurity' during high school, but as I gained weight in university, my body started taking up more and more space in my mind.

This came to a head in my early twenties. I was a baby reporter, bouncing from newsroom to newsroom, still trying to figure out what it takes to be a 'real' journalist, when someone in a position of power said that if I wanted to keep moving up, I should probably lose a few kilograms. They added that I looked much better in a dress than a skirt, tracing out the shape of my body in the air with their hands to indicate how skirts tended to emphasise my stomach rolls. At the time I knew this was unfair, and now looking back, I know that it was also blatantly untrue. But at that moment I was young, and already terrified I'd somehow be found out as the fraud I mistakenly believed I was. So I promised myself I'd go to the gym every day from then on – keenly aware of how the corners of this person's mouth would twitch up into the tiniest of smiles when they'd see my workout bag under my desk.

But at the gym I'd be consumed by nagging, insidious thoughts telling me I wasn't running fast enough, wasn't squatting deeply enough, wasn't feeling nauseated enough. It also didn't help that, despite my emotional pain and desperation, I found the gym excruciatingly, unbelievably boring.

Furious at myself for not working out harder, I started skipping meals, too. And so day after day I'd end up standing there, hungry, exhausted and crying on the step machine, consumed with self-loathing and infuriated at the pure tedium of exercise.

Eating disorders are very common among those with ADHD, especially young women. Low self-esteem, coupled with a predisposition towards hyper-fixation, perfectionism and the obsessive need to make up for perceived deficits in other areas of one's life in order to gain societal acceptance . . . it's not hard to see why.

Convinced by our society's pervasive diet culture that my habits were perfectly healthy, and that I was, in fact, just 'intermittent fasting', I never thought to bring this up with a medical professional. Therefore, it's hard to say if, in retrospect, what I was dealing with would have met the criteria of a diagnosable eating disorder. However, I think it's safe to say it was at least disordered eating.

I moved on from that job and, over time, got past the acute period of self-hatred. I started going to the gym less often, and no longer felt an overwhelming sense of panic whenever I found myself snacking. But my practice of occasionally 'forgetting' to eat throughout the workday remained.

I need to make it absolutely clear that this is not behaviour to emulate.

Nor is it even a 'secret' way to lose weight. All skipping meals ever did was make me miserable, cloud my head with fatigue and royally mess up my metabolism – fuelling even more dysmorphia as my body continued to change. But regardless, after a year or so I forgot it was even weird.

When I was diagnosed with ADHD, this habit suddenly became a much more pressing problem, because the stimulants I was prescribed are, of course, also appetite suppressants. In fact, Vyvanse's other pharmaceutical use is to help people with binge-eating disorder.

As far as I can remember, no one asked me about my relationship with food before I was put on this medication (not that I'm confident I would have been honest about it even if they had), but suddenly I, a person with a history of regularly going prolonged stretches of time without eating, was taking a pill that meant I didn't get hungry during the day.

And I leaned in.

Knowing what I know now, there's no doubt in my mind that my ADHD, and the damage to my self-esteem it caused, contributed significantly to my eating issues.

But while my diagnosis clearly made things worse at first, strangely it sort of saved me as well. A week or two into starting my meds, I was at work and having a really hard time focusing, not helped by my failure to eat breakfast. Because of this, I was behind deadline and ended up staying back a couple of hours, semi-inadvertently extending my fasting period much longer than I had before.

When I was done, I jumped on my bike and started pedalling as fast as I could, hoping to get home before Anthony, who was working the early morning shift, had to go to bed. But the combination of no food, fatigue and high-intensity exercise proved too much, and as I shot down the Albert Park Lake bike path, things started to spin, I felt nauseated, and I started to swerve. Luckily, I managed to jump off my bike and sit down on the grass, stopping the fuzzy blackness that was creeping across the edges of my vision from fully engulfing me.

I'd nearly fainted.

And in that moment, the weight of what I was doing came crashing in on me. I wish I could say it was the realisation that I was worth more than the way I was treating myself, but actually it was a little voice in my head shouting, 'For the love of god, Matilda, your reputation at the *Guardian* absolutely cannot withstand you crashing your bike into this goddamn lake for a second goddamn time.' The fear of having to explain another broken computer to the IT department proved more powerful than self-love.

From then on, I made it a rule to eat before I took my meds. I didn't always follow it at first, but slowly I got better. I now set alarms to eat lunch. I make sure I buy low-effort snack options when I'm shopping, like crackers and dip, mini cucumbers, muesli bars and yogurt cups. I've started making a game out of finding the best lunch place near my office, and thinking of the walk to the restaurants as a relaxing respite I can look forward to during long mornings. And while it's still sometimes a struggle to remember, or find the motivation, to eat, I'm getting better.

My medication has forced me to start thinking about food as a necessary, practical part of my ADHD treatment rather than an illicit indulgence I had to earn. And proactively treating my ADHD (through medication, therapy and a myriad of behavioural techniques) has reduced my anxiety and boosted my self-esteem in general.

My food-related stress and hang-ups do rear their head on a semi-regular basis (it's still a frequent topic with my therapist), but overall, the good times outweigh the bad. And despite being the largest I've ever been, my body takes up less space in my mind than it has at any time since I was fourteen, standing in front of the mirror with that stretchy black dress on.

15

What's the worst that could happen?

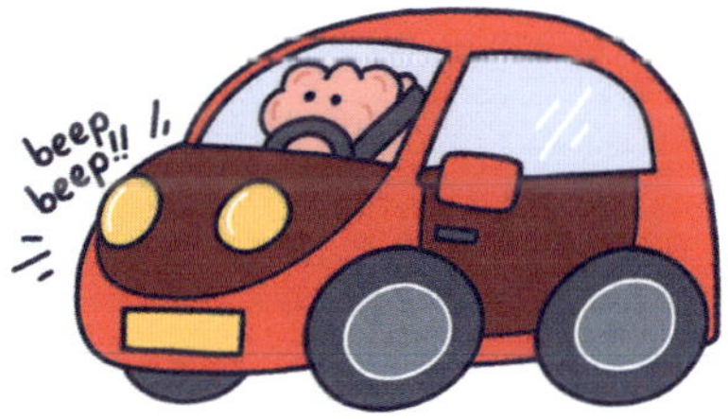

One of the most dangerous consequences of the cultural perception of ADHD as a hyperactive white boy who can't sit still at his desk is that most people only ever think about the 'harm' caused by ADHD in the context of a classroom. Like, sure, it's frustrating that it hampers that kid's learning and disrupts the students around him, but hey, that's about it.

But ADHD doesn't only exist in the relative safety of primary school. For many people, this condition, and the **inattention** and **impulsiveness** it brings, will be with them for their entire lives. It's with them during their school-leaving exams. It's with them in their job interviews. It's with them for every professional and financial decision they ever make. It's with them when someone offers them a cigarette for the first time, and when a glass of wine or two after work tips from a treat into a habit. It's there when they're driving, using power tools or hanging up holiday lights. It's there for every potential life-or-death moment, big or small.

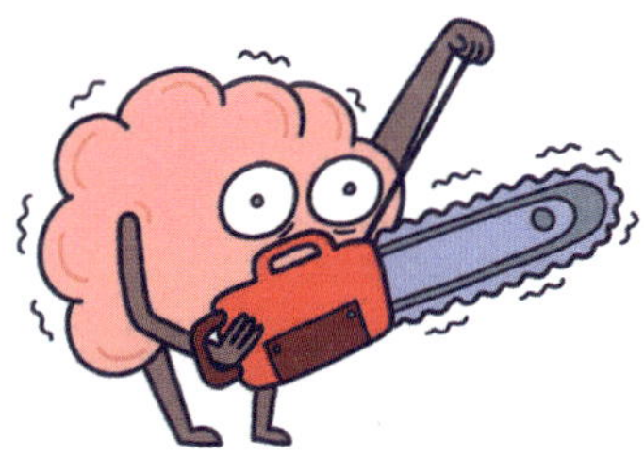

We need to drastically overhaul the way people think about ADHD treatments. We're not just talking about getting kids to sit still in class. We're talking about ensuring a really significant proportion of the earth's population aren't needlessly subjected to a more difficult, traumatic and ultimately shorter life than they deserve.

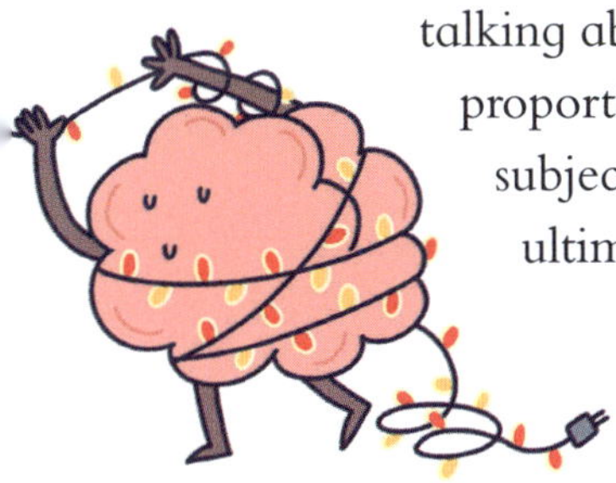

It's hard to calculate the average number of years ADHD might take off someone's life, since it impacts mortality in so many varied ways, but Professor Russell Barkley and Dr Mariellen Fischer made headlines in the late 2010s when they gathered health data from a longitudinal ADHD study and input it into an actuarial life-expectancy calculator – the super-complicated algorithm life insurance companies use to estimate how long before you cark it, and therefore how much you should be paying in premiums each year. They found that for those with **ADHD-C** (combined) that persisted into adulthood, estimated life expectancy was reduced by 12.7 years.[1]

To be clear, the study used hypothetical mortality rates, only looked at people with one kind of ADHD **presentation** and had a small subject pool (131 people), the overwhelming majority of whom were male. So, while this finding shouldn't be taken as an absolute scientific fact, it's still a stark indication of the potential consequences of not taking this condition seriously.

As we will soon see, we're more likely to be injured or accidentally killed. We're more likely to experience severe mental illness and addiction. We're more likely to grapple with entrenched poverty, unemployment and teen pregnancy. We're more likely to drop out of school and get caught up in the criminal justice system. And devastatingly, we're significantly more likely to die by suicide.

But these are not unchangeable problems with no solution. There's a huge amount of evidence showing that access to proper treatment – including, but not limited to, medications – helps keep ADHDers safe, and improves society as a whole.

Now that we find ourselves in this new, social-media-driven era of widespread ADHD awareness, especially among adults, it's about time we started taking this condition – and the stigma, cultural ignorance and economic inequity that prevents so many from accessing the treatment they need – more seriously.

Adult ADHD, adult dangers

When I first read that ADHD reduces life expectancy, I was shocked and perplexed – because I was only thinking about mortality in terms of how a disease might slowly damage one's body until it can no longer sustain life. But no, ADHD instead whittles away at our life expectancy simply by making it harder for us to protect ourselves against everything else that could potentially kill us.

We've already touched on many of the risky **side effects** of ADHD – unhealthier diets, less physical exercise, increased substance use and smoking rates, increased risk of eating disorders, and all manner of other unpleasant things. But we also have to consider how easily our 'quirky', accident-prone tendencies can become dangerous, especially in the adult world.

ADHD doesn't only exist in the relative safety of primary school. For many people, this condition, and the inattention and impulsiveness it brings, will be with them for their entire lives.

The number one cause of car accidents varies from country to country, but distractibility, making impulsive decisions and fatigue are right up there – all problems that ADHD can massively amplify. And this isn't just conjecture, we have the stats to back it up. A 2014 **meta-analysis** estimated that drivers diagnosed with ADHD were 29 per cent more likely to be involved in a vehicle accident[2] and, according to Swedish population records, this jumps up to 50 per cent when you focus in on serious accidents.

We also know medication can help with this. That Swedish study showed that male drivers with ADHD were nearly 60 per cent less likely to crash while actively taking medication, meaning more than half of these accidents could potentially have been avoided.[3] An examination of US emergency room admissions showed that ADHD men were 38 per cent less likely to be involved in a car crash during the months they were medicated, and ADHD women were 42 per cent less likely, meaning proper medication could potentially have wiped out a fifth of these accidents, too.[4]

And these are just the people who were formally diagnosed with ADHD. We have no earthly way of knowing how many millions of preventable accidents, injuries, permanent **disabilities** and deaths involve – or are caused by – **undiagnosed** and untreated ADHD drivers across the world.

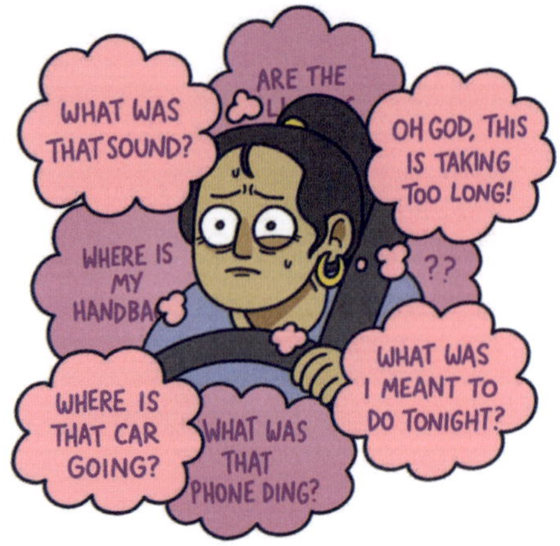

WHAT WAS THAT SOUND?
ARE THE
OH GOD, THIS IS TAKING TOO LONG!
WHERE IS MY HANDBA
??
WHAT WAS I MEANT TO DO TONIGHT?
WHERE IS THAT CAR GOING?
WHAT WAS THAT PHONE DING?

One factor that complicates transport accident statistics is that many data sets show that ADHD people tend to spend more time driving than non-ADHDers – although no papers I've found offered a theory as to why. While this doesn't change the fact that we're at higher risk of road accidents, it does tend to skew the data to make it look like we're more accident-prone than we perhaps are. Not many studies address this, but the meta-analysis I mentioned above estimated that ADHDers were still around 23 per cent more likely to be involved in a crash, even accounting for the extra time they spend behind the wheel.[5]

And it's not just vehicles we need to be worried about. Both children[6] and adults[7] with ADHD are more likely to suffer unintentional injuries, and may be 30 per cent more likely to die from incidents like these as well.[8]

In fact, people with ADHD are more likely to die prematurely in general. According to a truly massive Danish study of 1.9 million individuals, all of them aged thirty-two or younger, those with ADHD had twice the mortality rate of those without, mostly due to unnatural causes (accidents, overdoses, crime, etc.). And this rose to 5.6 times the rate if you throw in a **substance-abuse** disorder.[9]

This sounds extremely scary, but on an individual level the overall rates of premature death in countries like Denmark are in the tenths of a per cent of the population – so even when that's doubled (or quintupled), the chances of dying early are still absolutely tiny. It's more what these statistics say about the dangers of ADHD on a society-wide scale.

Interestingly, the Danish study also found that the risk of premature death among those diagnosed with ADHD as adults was 2.7 times higher than for those identified back in school. The authors of the paper speculated that this was perhaps because 'persistent' ADHD was a more 'severe' form of the disorder, but I can't help but wonder if it might also reflect the significant impact that early identification and intervention can have.

Accidental injuries contribute a lot to these premature death rates, but they don't account for all of it. People with ADHD are potentially twice as likely to be murdered as their **neurotypical** peers,[10] and more than twice as likely to attempt suicide and six times as likely to die by it.[11] Obviously, increased **impulsivity** might play a role here, but these statistics also highlight the psychological damage and degradation of **self-esteem** that ADHD can cause.

Once again, there are treatment options. While I didn't find any large studies on behavioural therapies or other interventions to prevent these accidents or injuries, the effects of medication are easier to quantify. Among young people, the use of stimulant medications led to a 10 per cent reduction in unintended injuries[12] and a 70 per cent reduction in traumatic brain injuries.[13] Three months on methylphenidate (aka Ritalin) led to a 60 per cent reduction in risk of burn injuries among ADHD youth in one review,[14] six months on methylphenidate equalled a 20 per cent reduction in bone fractures,[15] and the same drug caused a 9 per cent reduction in emergency room admissions for ADHD kids in another study.[16] ADHD adults were 40 per cent less likely to have depression after three years of taking methylphenidate,[17] while suicide attempts were reduced by as much as 60 per cent after three months of use and 70 per cent after six months.[18]

Awareness, **diagnosis**, treatment and medication save ADHDers' lives every day. But once you know that, and then look around and see how low treatment rates are in most places in the world, it becomes that much more chilling.

Climbing the life ladder

As well as these physical dangers of accident, injuries and death, ADHD poses additional risks to an individual's life and wellbeing.

Although conservative politicians may like to pretend otherwise, poverty is a cycle, one that's extraordinarily difficult to break out of. And ADHD has the capacity to lock people in even tighter. Despite sometimes being dismissed as a 'rich person's disorder' in popular media, ADHD is actually more prevalent in low-income communities.[19] This is for a number of reasons.

Firstly, low-income communities are more likely to be exposed to high levels of lead in the environment,[20,21] which you may remember is one of the environmental factors that can increase the likelihood of ADHD. But there's also a more sociological explanation.

We spoke about it briefly in Chapter 7, but one of the **DSM-5 diagnostic criteria** for ADHD is 'clear evidence that the **symptoms** interfere with, or reduce the quality of, [a person's] social, academic, or occupational functioning'.[22] There are likely many kids who experience pretty much all the classic ADHD symptoms but have enough stability, parental support and additional resources from their (well-funded) schools that this doesn't end up significantly getting in the way of their quality of life. Thus, they remain at what's known as a 'subclinical' level. Yet if that same kid grew up with the stressors of poverty – parents forced to work multiple jobs, struggles with housing and food instability, higher rates of foster and out-of-home care, higher rates of crime and over-policing in the community splitting families up – those symptoms might end up being significantly more impairing, reducing their quality of life and thus making them meet the full criteria for clinical ADHD.

Education is one of the key pathways to economic advancement in our society – or at least that's what we're promised. But ADHD kids are potentially three times as likely to drop out of high school (even after you adjust for the presence of other mental health conditions),[23] and the overcrowded and under-resourced schools where many low-income kids are educated may make it even less likely that their support needs will be met.

According to one meta-analysis, ADHDers are six and a half times less likely to attend tertiary education than non-ADHDers,[24] and the external pressures poverty places on low-income teenagers, combined with the prohibitively high cost of college in countries such as the US, don't make things any easier.

Awareness, diagnosis, treatment and medication save ADHDers' lives every day.

And ADHDers who have gone through 'female' puberty face an extra hurdle, with studies from a whole range of countries showing that they are more likely to fall pregnant in their teen years.[25] Obviously many people find great joy and fulfilment in having a child at any age, but we also have to accept that unless you have a truly legendary support system around you, having a child this early in life will likely constitute a massive economic burden.

When ADHDers do eventually make it into the workforce, they face issues there, too. Data from the US shows that ADHDers are 12 per cent less likely to have a job, and earn, on average, 34 per cent less than their non-ADHD siblings.[26] They're also nearly four times as likely to be fired and twice as likely to experience unemployment as their non-ADHD peers.[27]

These educational and financial disadvantages are only amplified for non-white ADHDers, who contend with institutionalised racism and the knock-on effects of generations of discrimination. And as we discussed previously, this is compounded yet again by the fact that racial bias makes it less likely for children of colour to be diagnosed and receive treatment in the first place.

Finally, throw in the stats about how the condition increases a person's risk of addiction, problem gambling and reckless spending, as well as making them more likely to quit their job without a plan of what to do next,[28] and it's clear that ADHDers face so many additional factors that can push them off an economic ladder that's already excruciatingly difficult to climb. Plus, because of the condition's highly heritable nature, this cycle of hardship and inequality is then entrenched deeper and deeper into our society with each generation.

Most of these studies are based on medical records, meaning we can only look at the barriers faced by people who have been formally diagnosed with ADHD. All these problems may well be magnitudes larger than we currently know, given how many undiagnosed cases are out there. This limited data also means that, unfortunately, I can't give you that same list of all the benefits that diagnosis and treatment will bring as I did when it came to accidents and injuries. But we do know that medication increases ADHD women's odds of long-term employment by 18 per cent and men's by 4 per cent,[29] boosts ADHD kids' grades, increases the odds of them completing upper secondary school by two-thirds,[30] and when used long-term also lowers the risk of teen pregnancy by 39 per cent.[31]

I'm no politician, but for me that's a strong enough indication that our governments and healthcare and education systems need to be trying harder to find those we've missed and ensure they're getting the support they need. Not only to help the individual, but in the hope of reducing entrenched poverty and improving society as a whole. The underdiagnosis and undertreatment of ADHD isn't just a medical issue: it's a human rights one.

The prison problem

One massive piece of the 'burden of not taking ADHD seriously' puzzle we haven't yet discussed is the way our social systems send so many of us to prison.

When I first read the statistics on what percentage of the average prison population meets the diagnostic criteria for ADHD, I rubbed my eyes, re-read it six or seven times, and then closed my laptop and went to bed, figuring I must be missing something and was simply too tired to keep working. But there it was the next morning, those same numbers in black and white.

Around 2.8 per cent of the general adult population has ADHD, but in prisons it's closer to 25.5 per cent.[32] That means not only are ADHDers more than 800 per cent overrepresented in prisons, but we potentially make up a quarter of all prisoners. This holds true for both men and women, and in juvenile prisons ADHD rates sit between 17 and 25 per cent as well.[33]

These statistics are from studies where researchers get clinicians to go in and assess large groups of incarcerated people for ADHD, with diagnosis then made through stringent diagnostic interviews so as to rule out other conditions, including PTSD or acquired brain injuries, which can present with similar symptoms. I mention this because it's important to realise that a huge proportion of those with ADHD in prisons likely have no idea they have the condition and will never receive any treatment for it.

Socioeconomic status, systemic disadvantage and a tendency towards substance abuse play a huge role in these inflated numbers, likely amplified by the difficulties many ADHDers face with impulsivity, inhibition control, **novelty seeking** and weighing up the potential rewards and consequences of actions. These symptoms may also seriously impair one's ability to successfully navigate the court system. And, to make matters worse, a large Icelandic study suggests that, among adolescents interrogated by police, those with ADHD were twice as likely to make a false confession.[34]

Once again, non-white ADHDers are placed at an even higher risk given the vast overrepresentation of certain racial groups in prison systems, such as African Americans in the US and First Nations people in Australia.

In my research for this chapter, I spoke to a number of social service workers, all of whom stressed to me that reintegration into society after being released from prison is already extraordinarily difficult – from finding stable housing to getting employment, and even just the extremely complex logistical requirements of fulfilling one's parole obligations. It's the kind of thing where having a brain that isn't that great at organisation and consistency puts you at a profound disadvantage. So it follows that diagnosis and adequate treatment for ADHD could be revolutionary in getting people's lives back on track.

Now, to be clear, the vast majority of people with ADHD have never been arrested or convicted of a crime, nor can we assume that every person with ADHD in prison is there directly because of the condition. But given the sheer magnitude of these numbers, the idea of screening all incarcerated adults for ADHD has been gaining traction in a number of countries. In fact, the UK technically adopted this approach way back in 2009,[35] although the UK ADHD Foundation has questioned how adequately it's been implemented.[36]

In my conversations with social workers and others who interact regularly with the criminal justice system, however, most were fairly tepid about exactly how much this sort of universal screening might achieve. Even in some of the wealthiest countries on earth, prison systems are still massively underfunded. And, as several case workers pointed out, as the system currently stands, mental health interventions tend to be reserved for those in the midst of crisis.

Despite prisons purportedly being places of rehabilitation, there's often little to no focus on proactively helping people with underlying mental health problems, even for conditions as common as anxiety and depression. So, while an ADHD diagnosis in and of itself can be utterly life-changing, and, in an ideal (and just) world, treatment for the condition should be accessible in correctional centres, this is just one of hundreds, if not thousands of issues with the system that need to be addressed. So perhaps the more immediate focus should be on trying to ensure people with undiagnosed ADHD don't needlessly end up in the criminal justice system to begin with.

Once again, this is an area where we know medication works. Multiple large studies have found that criminality among ADHD adults is reduced drastically during periods when they are medicated – by between 30 and 40 per cent.[37,38] That is *a lot* of crimes that could be prevented, and a lot of lives that wouldn't be derailed by incarceration.

But, hey, even if a government doesn't particularly care about preventing crime, breaking the cycle of poverty or, you know, lessening human suffering in general, they probably should still care about ADHD, because it turns out this condition costs our economies a staggering amount of money, too.

Untreated ADHD costs society

Let's start on my home turf of Australia, because there happens to be some really thorough accounting on the topic from down under. A Deloitte Access Economics report, commissioned by the Australian ADHD Professionals Association, estimated that the condition costs our economy up to AU$12.83 billion (approximately US$8.7 billion) a year.[39] Here's why: AU$1.23 billion of the ADHD bill is due to direct costs – things like increased emergency room visits and the extra burden placed on the education system. But the largest chunk, a whopping AU$10.19 billion, was in loss of productivity. ADHDers tend to take more days off due to illness (physical or mental), and when we're at work lose productive hours due to the symptoms of our condition. That's an economic cost that builds up . . . fast.

This Australian report also listed AU$7.59 billion (about US$5.14 billion) in 'wellbeing costs'. This is basically a calculation of the total number of healthy years of life lost to a disability, which is then assigned a dollar figure based on the estimated value a society places on an anonymous life (in Australia, apparently, just under AU$200,000). I've chosen not to include this in my total, partially because the whole concept of placing a monetary value on human lives kind of freaks me out, but also because we're not concerning ourselves here with trivial things like 'happiness' or 'the betterment of society for society's sake'. We're strictly talking cold, hard cash.

A **systematic review** of studies looking at the yearly economic burden of ADHD in the US placed it somewhere between US$196 billion and US$365 billion in 2023 money (around AU$289–539 billion).[40]

Underdiagnosis is expensive on a countrywide scale. But the issue is, there are some very serious access issues when it comes to acquiring an ADHD diagnosis in the first place. There's no doubt in my mind that plenty of you reading this will have a hefty suspicion that you have ADHD but simply can't afford the hundreds, if not thousands, of dollars that a proper clinical diagnosis would cost.

Even in Australia, where we love to boast about our universal healthcare system, the vast majority of the extremely limited pool of psychiatrists who are willing to treat adult ADHD patients operate only within the private system, with private-system fees.

ADHD naysayers panic about 'medicating normal human behaviours' and 'turning to drugs to force people to become cogs in the machine', but in plenty of countries the drugs are the only form of ADHD treatment that is subsidised by the government. No one, and I repeat, *no one*, is saying that medications should be the only form of ADHD treatment, but what other options do people have? In Australia, we're lucky that we get ten therapy sessions a year that are at least partially paid for by the government, but it's unlikely this will be anywhere near enough for the kind of life-altering work people need to do in the years after diagnosis.

It's clear from the data we've seen that the hardships ADHD causes are a massive issue in today's society. It's a burden on our systems, and more importantly, it's a burden on those of us who carry it throughout our lives. But it doesn't *have* to be. Because, as corny as it sounds, there are some amazing, nourishing, beautiful things about having brains like ours. By failing to properly invest in ADHD awareness, diagnosis and support, however, we as a society are setting ourselves up for failure – locking many of the extremely valuable things that ADHD adults could be contributing behind walls of inequality and vicious cycles of disadvantage.

Over the course of this year, I've become extremely keen on the idea of redefining ADHD as something more than just 'a disorder'. To embrace it as an identity and a way of existing in the world. This is at the core of the **neurodiversity movement**.

But before we turn our focus to ADHD acceptance and self-love, it's worth acknowledging that this simply isn't a reality for most ADHD people across the world – especially those who didn't win the genetic lottery of economic privilege, whiteness and low support needs. And unless the movement towards ADHD acceptance, and neurodivergent empowerment more generally, is also pushing for systemic, concrete changes to our healthcare and justice systems, the advances we're making will only be to the benefit of the privileged few.

DIARY ENTRY

Foot glue

By now you should know how much I truly hate the 'Oh look, a butterfly' memeification of ADHD. But I have to admit, this morning I did accidentally superglue my foot into my shoe.

I need to go into the office, so naturally I'm running late. The last possible train that will allow me to get in before the morning conference is arriving in fourteen minutes and the station is a twelve-minute walk away. All that's left to do is put on the gold boots I've assembled my outfit around. But, whoops – part of the inside lining has come loose and is making my foot feel weird.

Aware of my rapidly declining seconds, I grab the superglue from the shoebox full of random screws, picture-hanging strips and 700 of the allen keys that come with flat-pack furniture. Forgetting superglue's signature watery consistency, I squirt far too much onto the loose shoe material, shove my hand in and press it to the top. As I pull my fingers away, some of the fake suede lining comes with them. No time to think too much about that – I only have fifteen seconds left. I shove my foot inside and try to pretend I don't feel the still-wet glue seeping through the fabric of my stockings onto my skin.

I chuck on the other boot, and as I stand up, I feel a distinct, uncomfortable tug on the flesh at the top of my foot. Shit.

But I genuinely can't bear the idea of being late yet again, so I decide not to think about that either and instead hope that foot sweat happens to also function as an adhesive solvent. Behind schedule, I'm forced to jog the last 500 metres to the station, wincing very slightly each time my right foot shifts back and forth in my shoe, tugging at my glued skin. I just slip through the closing train doors, saved only by the fact that the Melbourne rail network is even worse at time management than I am.

On the train I decide that this whole situation is actually very funny and I'll tweet about it. As a result, when I walk through the office door, one of my co-workers immediately questions me about my foot-glue situation. I then show off by unzipping the back of my boot and knocking the heel against the ground to demonstrate the degree to which my foot simply won't budge. My wacky antics are an absolute hit, so, intoxicated by the laughter and attention of others, I motion to my boss as I see her leaving a meeting room. 'Come see this!' I say, whacking my shoe one last time against the carpet. But much to my horror, it turns out sweat actually is pretty good at diminishing the structural integrity of glue. This last bump finally breaks the stocking free from the boot's lining and my shoe goes flying off across the room, colliding with the window.

Let me be clear. My boss hasn't seen my tweet. From her point of view, she has simply come out of a meeting to see me arrive late, beckon her over, kick off my boot and show her my foot for no reason at all.

This was one little moment. A fun quirk of living a life full of time crunches, impulsive decisions and unforeseen consequences. At first, I thought it was too small and insignificant to include in this account of my year, but it was as I burst out laughing, trying to explain the situation to my frankly startled manager, that I realised I wasn't laughing as a defence any more. I wasn't trying to get in first to prove that I can make fun of myself and so therefore can't be made fun of. This wasn't going to haunt me in the days to come. This was just funny.

Sometimes ADHD is funny. I'm allowed to enjoy the joke, too.

16

So, should I love my brain or not?

It's nearly the end of the year now, and yet, through all these months of academic articles, interviews, diagnostic manuals and oh-so-many contrasting opinions, I've felt as if there's been a little knot in my brain that I can't quite untie. I didn't even realise exactly what the issue was until recently.

Now that we've entered this new era in awareness of adult ADHD, it feels as if there's an ever-growing tension between the concept of ADHD the medical disorder and ADHD the identity. Rather than being a dark omen of all the difficulties we may face in the future, for many of us who find out we have ADHD as an adult, it's amazing news. It's the answer to the questions we never knew we had. It's the thing we need to be able to finally start healing and forgiving ourselves.

Rather than being a dark omen of all the difficulties we may face in the future, for many of us who find out we have ADHD as an adult, it's amazing news.

ADHDers now have their own online communities and spaces, and while we're talking about the struggles that come along with the condition, we're also discussing all the bits that are neutral and even positive. We've started viewing ourselves as ADHD people, not just people with ADHD, and we're learning to think about our brain differences as intrinsic parts of who we are.

I'm delving into the world of philosophy more than science here, but to me, ADHD feels like it's so much more than the **impairments** it causes me.

The good and the grey

This idea is something that really struck me while I was talking to comedian and presenter Em Rusciano. We spoke just a week or two after she'd given a major speech in front of Australia's top politicians and journalists about receiving an ADHD **diagnosis** in her forties.[1] As she was delivering it, five different people texted me to tell me to turn on the TV, but there was no need – I was already watching, and, to be perfectly honest, softly crying as she discussed the courage required for ADHDers, and women in particular, to be our unfiltered selves.

Rusciano spoke a lot about the struggles and challenges that come with the condition, but what made me really, desperately want to speak to her was the way she talked about it contributing to her successes, too.

'Nuance is never really part of the conversation when it comes to people like us,' she tells me. 'Like, there's some great things, and also, fuck, it takes me ten times longer to do everything than a **neurotypical** person.'

And the 'great things' Rusciano talks about are the same things many other ADHD adults have described to me. They're the same things I feel a deep sense of pride about in myself. 'I just had this relentless drive to understand things. I'm always in motion, my brain is always seeking to really latch on to something, and I can feel the **hyper-fixation** settling into my bones,' she says.

'I didn't know that that's what it was until a year and a half ago, but all of a sudden it's like being in love with a new person. You get obsessed, it's all you think about, you don't sleep, you forget to shower. It's all you talk about. Sometimes I'm just hanging on to wee because I don't want to leave my computer because I'm in love with what I'm doing.

'Everything great I've ever made has been a result of a hyper-fixation trance.'

And while **impulsivity** is associated with so many of the dangers and horrors of ADHD, very occasionally it pays to jump in headfirst before giving yourself time to reason your way out. Rusciano started in the entertainment industry almost by accident, deciding on a whim at twenty-four to audition for *Australian Idol* – despite never having sung in public before – and then making it all the way to the finals.

'I'm a total risk-taker,' she says, before pausing. 'Mind you, I'm a very anxious person. But I definitely have been like, "Yeah, I've never sung before, but I'll try out." "Yeah, I'll go do a commercial radio job, even though I don't ever listen to the radio." "Yeah, sure, I'll try a TV show." "I'll do stand up." All my career has been me stepping into arenas that I have no business being in, but just believing a little bit more that I can than I can't. And it's so exciting, because the stakes are so high, you know, and my brain, being a **dopamine** demon, seeks it out.'

I've spoken a lot about the horrific impact ADHD can have on **self-esteem**, but I can't help but wonder if in saying this, I'm only telling half the story. Because, for many of us, the blows we've faced have led to a profound resilience and the ability to persist despite our fears. It's not really fair that we've had to develop this shield. In a better world, we wouldn't have to. Still, it can be a powerful tool.

'It's not confidence, it's courage,' Rusciano says. 'I have courage and resilience because I've been told since I was so young that I was wrong. I know how to keep getting back up again after knock-downs. So I think that I've fostered a resilience and a courage in me that was like, "Yeah, fuck, why not?"

'However, although I'm really good at hard stuff, I'm not good at the easy stuff, you know. And that can be really hard . . .

I'm in turmoil a lot about all the easy stuff I haven't done. I feel guilty all the time . . . I probably would have been less tortured mentally without it,' she says.

It can be difficult to talk about this duality when it comes to ADHD. Many (often neurotypical people) are quick to jump in to call it a 'superpower'. Their intentions are good, but when you've been struggling your whole life, being told you have a 'superpower' can sound perilously similar to 'So why are you complaining?' On the flipside, when you only ever hear about the struggles, it's dangerously easy to get bogged down in despair and feel like your brain is irreparably broken.

'When people talk about ADHD it's always feast or famine, all good or all bad, you know,' Rusciano says. 'Grey is not interesting to people, but for people like us, our brains live in the grey.'

I agree with her in a lot of ways. I've been nervous to talk about this – aware of how many of my opportunities have been a function of luck and privilege – but I really do think my ADHD helped give me the career I have today, too.

I'm so passionate about journalism because it means I get to dive in to a new topic every day, totally engrossing myself in the details, nuances and history. I have to problem-solve and think outside the box, and I experience a rush as all the little pieces click into place. And then I get to flex my creative muscles writing a story or making a video and sharing it with everyone else.

There's a lot of contention about the connection between ADHD and creativity. But the data we have so far does show at least some relationship between our chaotic minds – more scientifically known as our 'diffuse attention' style – and one of the core components of creativity: divergent thinking, aka the ability to take one idea and sprout dozens more out of it.[2]

I wonder if part of the reason I'm good at making short news-explainer TikTok videos, the thing I've become known for in the Aussie journalism world, is that I've spent so much of my life having to think about structuring all my chaotic ideas into simple sentences that make sense for the rest of the world. I've been teaching myself about succinct communication from day one.

Yes, my ADHD makes so many aspects of my job harder. There are plenty of things I'd change if I were given the choice. It absolutely is a disorder. But at the same time – precisely because of my ADHD – I've also found a passion that fits my brain like a glove, and that I'm actually pretty darn good at.

So I can't bring myself to say this is *only* a disorder, at least for me.

'I have courage and resilience because I've been told since I was so young that I was wrong. I know how to keep getting back up again after knock-downs.'

Disorder by design

Sometimes I wonder if the fact that ADHD is only ever defined by the harm and impairments it causes is more a function of how the term was invented than a reflection of some universal truth.

It's the mid-1800s, universal primary education is becoming widespread. Suddenly, the grown-ups notice a pattern among the kids who are acting up. Their behaviour is causing problems. Problems have to be fixed. And to fix something, you have to name it and define it. Thus, this deviation from the norm was named and defined by the problems it caused. In fact, in 1902, when Sir George Frederic Still first formally laid out the **symptoms** of the condition that would one day become 'ADHD', he referred to it only as 'the morbid defect of moral control'.[3]

The name and definition have changed a bit over the years, but the core idea that it's 'primarily a problem' has remained. There was no need to add creativity, a spark for life and the broad imaginative thinking that may well also come with ADHD to the definition, because good things don't need solutions. And there was also no need to really study those elements in the intervening years either because, well, doctors and scientists want to help people. They want to make people's lives better. You do that by fixing problems, not documenting assets.

And there was never really cause to question the framework through which we defined this condition, because, for a hundred years or so, it was a label we really only ever gave children. These kids don't even know who they are yet, so of course they can't stand up and say, 'Hey, honestly, the way I critically conceptualise my ADHD is much more broad-reaching than your medicalised definition, and it would probably be more constructively discussed as a distinct identity or even perhaps "neurotype" for want of a better word. Because, while I accept that I experience some extremely real defects and impairments due to the way my brain works, probably only, like, 30 per cent of them are inherent or biological and the rest are merely symptoms of living within a system built by and for people whose cognition functions differently from mine . . . and also can I go to the bathroom? I really have to pee.'

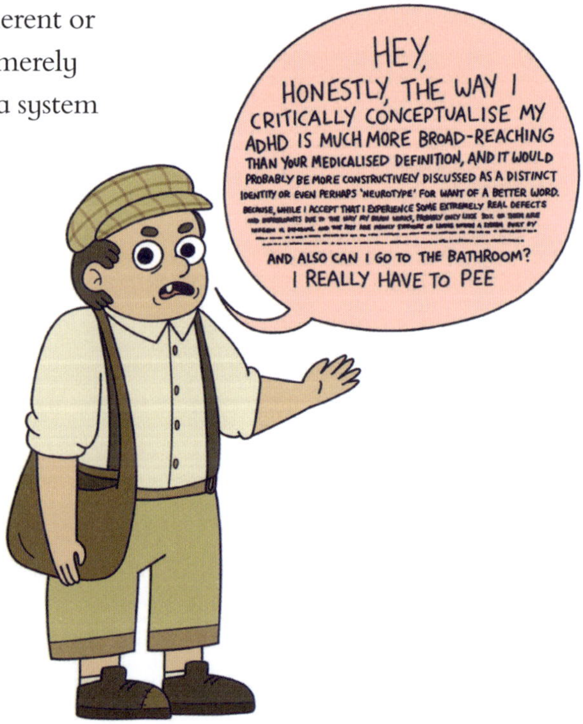

It's only now, in the past couple of decades (well, past couple of years really), as the psychiatric community has started to come to terms with

ADHD as a lifelong condition, that we have the capacity to truly form a community and start questioning if 'disorder' is the best word for it at all. Not the 'wrong' word, exactly, just far, far too narrow.

Outgrowing the medical model

Remember how I mentioned earlier that it's possible that, for most people, ADHD isn't so much something you 'recover from' as it is a diagnosable threshold that you might move above and below throughout your life? Well, that's been making me question the entire system through which we understand the condition.

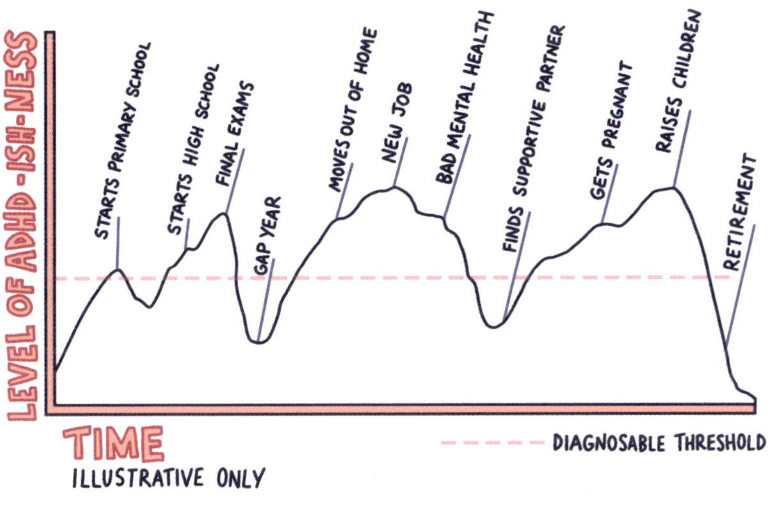

Obviously, when things like medications and educational funding are involved, we do need to have a cut-off point. And, for something that's exclusively a medical disorder, I totally agree with the line that has currently been drawn, marking the point where symptoms have a clear negative impact on one's functioning and quality of life.

But does that mean I could have a **neurodevelopmental** disorder one day and not the next? What if I got so good at coping and adapting that my symptoms no longer impaired me? Medically speaking, I wouldn't have ADHD any more. That just doesn't make sense to me. It doesn't feel right that this entire aspect of my being is only ever defined by the suffering it causes.

The scientific world has also been grappling with the issue of defining ADHD as something that can come and go, and recent papers often discuss the importance and significance of 'subclinical ADHD', where people don't meet the full criteria but share a lot of ADHD traits. The **DSM-5** also mentions 'ADHD in partial **remission**', where the impairment is still there but the person now displays fewer than the five required symptoms. It doesn't seem like the researchers have really agreed on how to handle these terms yet, but they're still intrinsically linked to 'the problem' – so they don't really solve my issue.

For argument's sake, let's say that instead of someone living in our society with ADHD, we're talking about someone travelling to the US but only speaking French. They would have trouble communicating, it would be hard for them to get an education, it would be difficult to get work, they might struggle to make friends and keep relationships, and the social isolation could even lead to things like depression and anxiety. For all intents and purposes, that person is disabled in that situation. But the fact that they speak French isn't inherently a **disability**. In fact, there are heaps of situations where speaking French might be super useful. If they wanted to 'cure' their disability, they wouldn't have to unlearn French, they'd just need to pick up enough English to get by. And once they did, no one would ever think to suggest that they're not French any more just because they know enough of the King's tongue to have a steady work life and robust social circle. They would just be a French person who is now significantly less impaired in that specific environment.

Now, this isn't a perfect metaphor, because, unlike the traveller, there are some aspects of ADHD that are always going to be a problem no matter what society looks like – for example, making impulsive decisions that increase our risk of fatal injuries. But I'm not convinced that the majority of my impairments are inherently biological.

A new normal

So, what if, as a culture, we started thinking about ADHD more as the 'flavour' of mind some people are born with, rather than just 'a problem'?

It doesn't feel right that this entire aspect of my being is only ever defined by the suffering it causes me.

This is what the **neurodiversity movement** is about. Asking what society would look like if our educational institutions, workplaces and social systems were more flexible – adapting to accommodate those whose brains work differently rather than building a wall around what's 'normal' and asking those who fall outside to find a way to climb over in order to fit in.

There's a lot to be said for this framework, and I agree with so much of it . . . but I'd be lying if I said it didn't make me a little nervous as well, because of the potential for the conversation to race from one extreme to another, and leave people in the dust as it does.

As much as I don't think terms like 'severe', 'mild' or 'high-' and 'low-functioning' are particularly useful or accurate when it comes to ADHD, I still clearly have a version of the disorder that allowed me to live a relatively normal life before ever receiving a lick of treatment. I don't want to blithely dismiss the struggles that I've faced, but in my case, the disorder was more about making things much harder instead of utterly impossible. And the truth is, a lot of us newly diagnosed adult ADHDers who are now joining this conversation tend to be towards the low end of the support-needs spectrum.

I'm worried that if we're all shouting 'ADHD isn't a disorder', we'll drown out the rest of our community's calls for better access to treatment, workplace and educational accommodations, and governmental support. And unfortunately, ADHD medications are still so controversial and stigmatised that there are plenty of people out there who will hear 'ADHD is just a different version of normal' and twist that into 'and therefore we shouldn't diagnose or medicate for it'. We can't afford to let that happen.

But surely there's a way we can talk about all the things we love about having the minds we do without dismissing how excruciatingly hard it can be? There must be a way I can come to terms with the harm my condition has done to my life while still loving my mind for the wonderful things it's brought, too.

Ocean brain

This year I've spent a lot of time trying to explain the differences in the way my brain works to the neurotypical people in my life, and I've come up with a pretty decent metaphor to help them get the gist.

It's the difference between having a land brain and an ocean brain.

For neurotypicals, getting things done is like walking on land. You're taught how to do it basically from birth, and most of the time you can head in a fairly straight line. Sure, there are hills and obstacles to avoid, but you can usually see them coming, and ultimately your speed really just depends on how much energy you have. It's not always easy to start running, but it's usually still within your control.

But – at least for me – getting stuff done is much closer to trying to sail a little boat through a big old ocean. If you've never been taught to sail, you're really at the mercy of the winds and the waves. Sometimes they speed you along, propelling you forwards at breakneck speed. Sometimes the water is so choppy and rough, it's hard to move anywhere as you're buffeted in every direction. You might not even realise your boat has a sail, so you've sat there rowing for years and years, exhausted, getting pummelled every time the storms get too rough. But once you learn how to navigate, you can start controlling where you're going, and maybe even how quickly you get there. You can use the winds and the waves to your advantage, easing your way out of the storms and finding the currents that will whisk you where you need to go. Sometimes the journey will still be slow and rough, but with the right training, and the right crew of people to help, you might even find that you can get there faster than those travelling on foot.

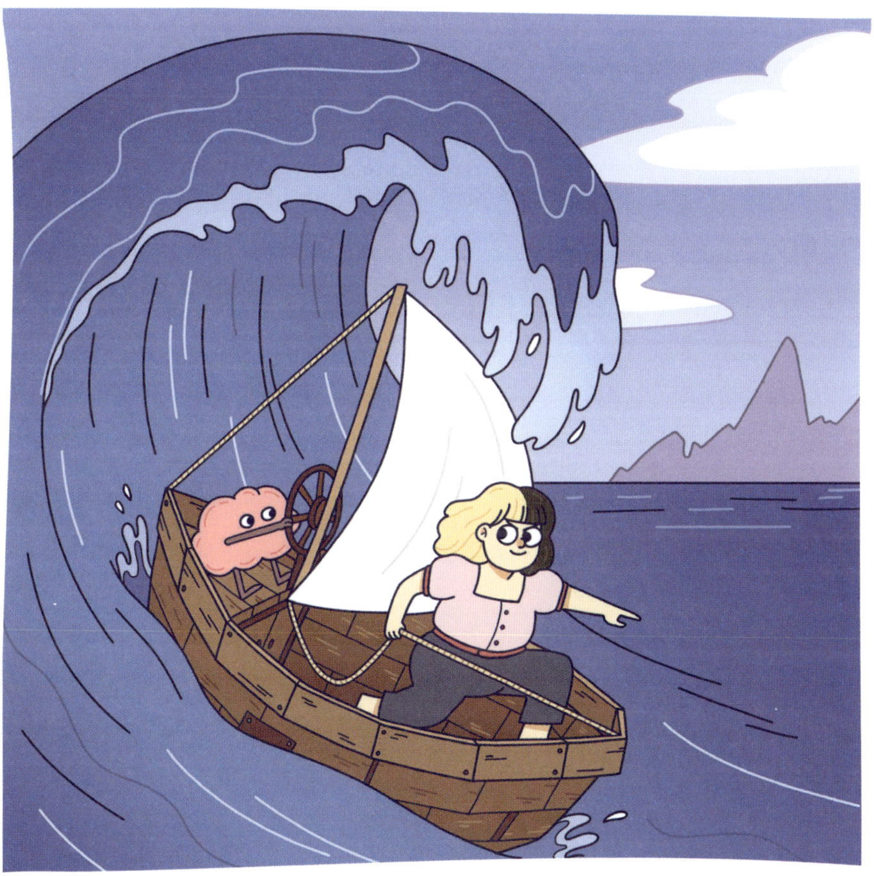

Stay with me, but I wonder if part of the cultural 'ADHD' conundrum we're facing comes from how much pressure we're putting on an initialism that was only ever meant to be a diagnostic term. 'ADHD' was never intended to represent an identity, a way to travel through the world, an all-encompassing description of the flavour of brain one has. It was meant to decide who would benefit from legal access to prescription medications and specific support services.

And I also wonder if this tension could be released if we just had another word for everything else that comes with an ADHD mind. Something cultural rather than diagnostic.

Because, at least from what I've seen of the world, plenty of people have 'ocean brains', whether they meet all the criteria for a formal ADHD diagnosis or not. And it feels like education systems could really benefit if we talked to children about what kind of terrain they are working with, and adjusted the way we taught them to match. Hell, it would help grown-ups in the workplace to have some kind of non-stigmatised, non-medicalised language to describe our patterns of productivity.

The problem is, while 'ocean brain' would be excellent for teaching kids, it's a bit new-age hippy-dippy for my grown-up ears. Also, just personally, I'd like something that ends with '-ic' so we can have a cool way of describing ourselves, like **autism** has with 'autistic'.

But luckily, there's actually already a word in English we could adopt that fits the bill perfectly: 'pelagic', meaning 'relating to the open sea'.

Imagine – we could have a whole bunch of people with all different varieties and levels of symptoms identifying as pelagic, coming together as a community around the shared life experience that having this kind of brain brings. Then, alongside this, we could continue to use the legal/medical term for those of us experiencing the disorder that is commonly associated with pelagism: ADHD.

(Which, by the way, means those of us with the disorder could then say, 'Oh, yeah, I'm seasick at the moment.' And I think that's pretty darn cute.)

Drs Edward Hallowell and John Ratey put forward a somewhat similar idea in their book *ADHD 2.0* – suggesting the term 'VAST', which stands for Variable Attention Stimuli Trait. However, they described this as ADHD-like symptoms that are brought on by the demands of our technologically dense world.[4] This isn't really what I'm going for, and I'm also not convinced we should just replace one (only partially accurate) initialism with a (only slightly more accurate) acronym.

I don't know if this will fit for everyone, but having a cultural word for my type of brain would really help me come to terms with the interwoven web of my identity and my disorder. In a world where we have these two separate words, then yes, I want to cure my ADHD, no doubt in my mind about that. But that doesn't mean I don't want to be pelagic.

Surely that's what we – as the generation of newly discovered ADHD adults – should be using our voices to call for, right?

1. **Understanding and acknowledgement of the hardships this condition brings.**
2. **Systemic change to address the injustices we face and guarantee equal access to diagnosis and treatment.**
3. **A cultural shift to ensure it's only the impairments, not our identities, that society is attempting to correct.**

I love the ocean that is my brain. I know a lot of other people who love their ocean brains, too. We just want help learning to sail, and maybe some seasickness tablets to ease the way.

Conclusion: Nice to meet you

It's December now. Anthony and I have put up the Christmas tree, turned on the air conditioner, and started planning where we'll be at midnight on December 31st.

Thinking back to the start of this year, it's only now that I realise how scared I was. I was living in the wake of a life-changing revelation with absolutely no clue what it meant for me, my identity, my relationships or my future.

I was happy to have been diagnosed a year earlier, but I was happy because I thought diagnosis meant I'd been handed a map that would show me which direction to row in to reach 'normal' – a mystical land that had always eluded me. I figured, with the right pills and enough determination, I would get there. But there I was, twelve months after I first got the news, and although the medication was helping . . . I was still lost. And because of this, part of me still felt like I was failing.

'Okay,' I thought. 'If the map I've been handed isn't working, then *this* year – with all the research and pondering about my own brain that will go into writing this book – I'll be able to create my own, better map instead.'

But that's not what happened either. Because the more I learnt about my brain, the more I realised that I should actually listen to it. Here I was on a little boat, paddling for my life, trying to force my way through the waves, when really I needed to learn to move with them. And that's what I started doing:

- I complemented my medication with better life skills, healthier breakfasts, more exercise, and occasionally even a full night's sleep.
- I began using my chore charms again, bought some fidget toys, rearranged my fridge and started paying attention to the way my period affected my brain.
- I put proper time and energy into forgiving myself for all the ways

I thought I'd failed, I talked to my loved ones about how they can help me, and I can help them, and I stopped fighting against every single wave no matter how small.

- I learnt to take rests when I needed them, hone my focus when it was abundant and use my unique way of looking at the world to my advantage.
- I learnt why I had been missed as a child and started to grasp the scale of just how many more of us there are out there.
- I learnt how much more needs to be done to ensure that ADHDers can thrive, and I began to comprehend the responsibility those of us with a platform and voice have to advocate for ADHDers who were forced down a different path by chance, circumstance and discrimination.

And, somewhere along the way, I realised I wasn't scouring the horizon for land any more.

I'm still not perfect when it comes to living with the brain I have. Doctor's appointments still get forgotten, chores still go undone, I still get overwhelmed and burnt out and frustrated. But nowadays I'm much better at thinking, 'Well, that was annoying' rather than 'Do better, be better, don't be a failure.' Because it no longer feels like every mistake is pushing me further and further away from my destination.

There might come a time when I no longer meet the full diagnostic criteria for ADHD, but I realise now that I'm never going to be neurotypical. I'm always going to be pelagic. And I'm going to get much further by letting down the sails and accepting and loving my brain for what it is, rather than by constantly struggling against the tide and trying to force it to be something it's not.

So, now that the introductions are over, I guess my brain and I should probably get on with living the rest of our lives together. There's a big, wide world of distractions out there waiting for a team like us to take notice and turn them into something wonderful.

And, okay, yes, I'm ending with a little corniness, but whatever. Let me have this one. I'm proud of myself.

It's been one hell of a year.

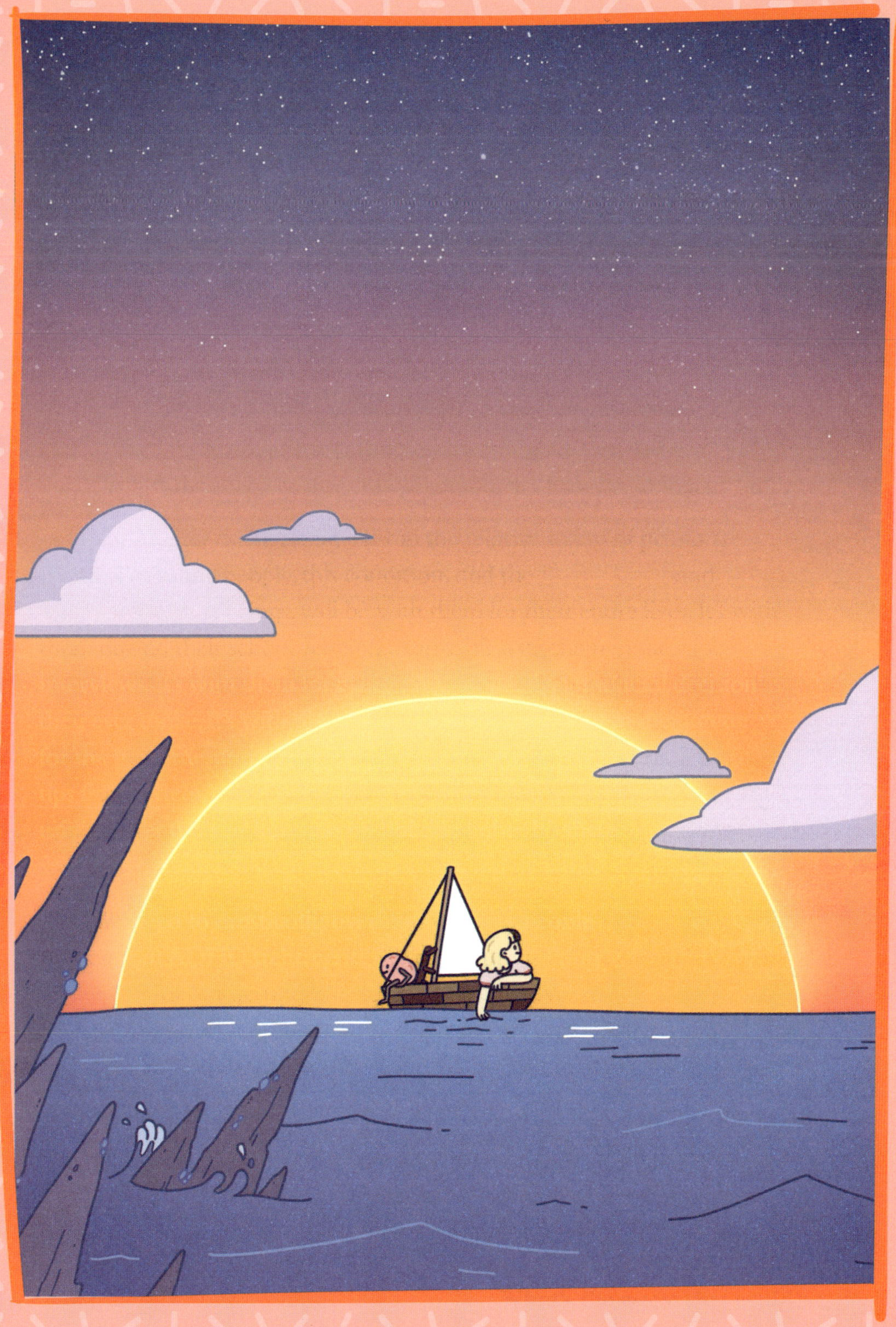

Appendix

Diagnostic criteria for ADHD from the *DSM-5-TR*

This is an excerpt from the most recent edition of the *Diagnostic and Statistical Manual of Mental Disorders* which was created by the American Psychiatric Association and is the most widely used clinical definition of ADHD. The manual serves as a guide for medical professionals, describing the traits, symptoms and criteria that are generally required for a diagnosis of ADHD. However, it's important to stress that this is not a diagnostic test in and of itself, and only specific, highly trained medical professionals can make a diagnosis of ADHD. This is a complex condition that shares traits with many other physiological and somatic disorders (which means relating to the body rather than the mind), and simply fulfilling the criteria listed here does not automatically mean that an individual has ADHD.

Attention-Deficit/Hyperactivity Disorder

Diagnostic criteria

A. A persistent pattern of inattention and/or hyperactivity-impulsivity that interferes with functioning or development, as characterized by (1) and/or (2):

1. **Inattention:** Six (or more) of the following symptoms have persisted for at least 6 months to a degree that is inconsistent with developmental level and that negatively impacts directly on social and academic/occupational activities:
   Note: The symptoms are not solely a manifestation of oppositional behavior, defiance, hostility, or failure to understand tasks or instructions. For older adolescents and adults (age 17 and older), at least five symptoms are required.

a. Often fails to give close attention to details or makes careless mistakes in schoolwork, at work, or during other activities (e.g., overlooks or misses details, work is inaccurate).

b. Often has difficulty sustaining attention in tasks or play activities (e.g., has difficulty remaining focused during lectures, conversations, or lengthy reading).

c. Often does not seem to listen when spoken to directly (e.g., mind seems elsewhere, even in the absence of any obvious distraction).

d. Often does not follow through on instructions and fails to finish schoolwork, chores, or duties in the workplace (e.g., starts tasks but quickly loses focus and is easily sidetracked).

e. Often has difficulty organizing tasks and activities (e.g., difficulty managing sequential tasks; difficulty keeping materials and belongings in order; messy, disorganized work; has poor time management; fails to meet deadlines).

f. Often avoids, dislikes, or is reluctant to engage in tasks that require sustained mental effort (e.g., schoolwork or homework; for older adolescents and adults, preparing reports, completing forms, reviewing lengthy papers).

g. Often loses things necessary for tasks or activities (e.g., school materials, pencils, books, tools, wallets, keys, paperwork, eyeglasses, mobile telephones).

h. Is often easily distracted by extraneous stimuli (for older adolescents and adults, may include unrelated thoughts).

i. Is often forgetful in daily activities (e.g., doing chores, running errands; for older adolescents and adults, returning calls, paying bills, keeping appointments).

2. **Hyperactivity and impulsivity:** Six (or more) of the following symptoms have persisted for at least 6 months to a degree that is inconsistent with developmental level and that negatively impacts directly on social and academic/occupational activities:

Note: The symptoms are not solely a manifestation of oppositional behavior, defiance, hostility, or a failure to understand tasks or instructions. For older adolescents and adults (age 17 and older), at least five symptoms are required.

a. Often fidgets with or taps hands or feet or squirms in seat.

b. Often leaves seat in situations when remaining seated is expected (e.g., leaves his or her place in the classroom, in the office or other workplace, or in other situations that require remaining in place).

c. Often runs about or climbs in situations where it is inappropriate. (**Note:** In adolescents or adults, may be limited to feeling restless.)

d. Often unable to play or engage in leisure activities quietly.

e. Is often 'on the go,' acting as if 'driven by a motor' (e.g., is unable to be or uncomfortable being still for extended time, as in restaurants, meetings; may be experienced by others as being restless or difficult to keep up with).

f. Often talks excessively.

g. Often blurts out an answer before a question has been completed (e.g., completes people's sentences; cannot wait for turn in conversation).

h. Often has difficulty waiting his or her turn (e.g., while waiting in line).

i. Often interrupts or intrudes on others (e.g., butts into conversations, games, or activities; may start using other people's things without asking or receiving permission; for adolescents and adults, may intrude into or take over what others are doing).

B. Several inattentive or hyperactive-impulsive symptoms were present prior to age 12 years.

C. Several inattentive or hyperactive-impulsive symptoms are present in two or more settings (e.g., at home, school, or work; with friends or relatives; in other activities).

D. There is clear evidence that the symptoms interfere with, or reduce the quality of, social, academic, or occupational functioning.

E. The symptoms do not occur exclusively during the course of schizophrenia or another psychotic disorder and are not better explained by another mental disorder (e.g., mood disorder, anxiety disorder, dissociative disorder, personality disorder, substance intoxication or withdrawal).

Specify whether:

F90.2 Combined presentation: If both Criterion A1 (inattention) and Criterion A2 (hyperactivity-impulsivity) are met for the past 6 months.

F90.0 Predominantly inattentive presentation: If Criterion A1 (inattention) is met but Criterion A2 (hyperactivity-impulsivity) is not met for the past 6 months.

F90.1 Predominantly hyperactive/impulsive presentation: If Criterion A2 (hyperactivity-impulsivity) is met and Criterion A1 (inattention) is not met for the past 6 months.

Specify if:

In partial remission: When full criteria were previously met, fewer than the full criteria have been met for the past 6 months, and the symptoms still result in impairment in social, academic, or occupational functioning.

Specify current severity:

Mild: Few, if any, symptoms in excess of those required to make the diagnosis are present, and symptoms result in no more than minor impairments in social or occupational functioning.

Moderate: Symptoms or functional impairment between 'mild' and 'severe' are present.

Severe: Many symptoms in excess of those required to make the diagnosis, or several symptoms that are particularly severe, are present, or the symptoms result in marked impairment in social or occupational functioning.

Glossary

ADHD-C the combined **presentation** of ADHD (Aka 'the hurricane'. See p. 38)

ADHD-H the primarily **hyperactive presentation** of ADHD (Aka 'the class clown'. See p. 35)

ADHD-I the primarily **inattentive presentation** of ADHD (Aka 'the space cadet'. See p. 37)

ADHD paralysis a community-driven, non-scientific term used to describe an ADHDer feeling unable to make themselves do something, despite wanting to, or of being so overwhelmed by information and environmental factors that they freeze. Also sometimes called 'task paralysis'

autism another form of neurodivergence; a neurological and developmental disorder that is commonly **comorbid** with ADHD. Also called autism spectrum disorder (ASD). 'AuDHD' is sometimes used to describe having both ASD and ADHD

bias in science and research, bias is a systematic flaw in a study or information collection that can lead to skewed results. Often the result of human error, either conscious or unconscious

body doubling a tool some ADHDers use to help them start and complete projects. Sometimes referred to as an accountability partner, a body double is a friend or partner who is present and/or works simultaneously, either in the same room or connected through technology

burnout a state of mental, physical and emotional exhaustion brought on by extended periods of stress or dysregulation

circadian rhythm physical, mental and behavioural changes in the human body that follow a 24-hour cycle, including sleeping and waking

cognitive behavioural therapy (CBT) a form of psychological treatment that focuses on correcting unhelpful thoughts, patterns or behaviour

comorbidity a condition or disease that exists alongside another. The existence of these two conditions can be unrelated, but sometimes there is a **correlation** between them

consensus in the scientific world, this refers to the generally held position or opinion of the majority of scientists in a particular field of study

correlation used in science and academia to describe a situation where there's enough evidence to show that two things are related in some way or frequently co-occur, but not that one necessarily causes the other

delay discounting the decline in the perceived value of an outcome or reward based on how far into the future it will be received. All humans experience this, but ADHDers in particular struggle with it

diagnosis the formal process of process of identifying a disease, condition or injury from its signs and **symptoms**

diagnostic criteria (or diagnostic requirements) a set of signs, **symptoms** and tests used to determine the **diagnosis** of a condition and guide the care of the person with the condition

disability people with disability have long-term physical, mental, intellectual or sensory differences that, when interacting with inaccessible communities and environments, prevent their full and equal participation

dopamine a **neurotransmitter** that can affect a person's mood, attention, motivation and movement. Also regulates the brain's mesolimbic reward system (Aka Ethel's biscuits. See p. 50)

dopaminergic involving or related to **dopamine** as a **neurotransmitter**

DSM-5 the *Diagnostic and Statistical Manual of Mental Disorders*, fifth edition. Published by the American Psychiatric Association, this is a tool for classification and **diagnosis** of mental disorders used by mental health professionals in many parts of the world

emotional dysregulation difficulty in managing emotions or keeping them in check, characterised by more rapid and dramatic emotional shifts, with frequent highs and lows

executive dysfunction the inability to self-regulate one's **executive functions**

executive function all the higher-order self-regulation skills our brains use to organise themselves and make it easy for us to get complicated things done – controlling inhibitions, sustaining attention, problem-solving, switching between tasks or ways of thinking, etc.

habit stacking a concept that involves purposely creating associations between something you already instinctively do and something you're more likely to forget to do

hereditary meaning genetically transmitted or transmittable from parent to offspring

hyperactivity refers to excessive movement such as fidgeting, excessive energy and not sitting still, and being talkative

hyper-fixation a colloquial term for a deep and intense concentration on an interest or activity for an extended period of time

hyperfocus a colloquial term for becoming fully immersed in something that interests you

impairment any significant difference in a person's body structure or function, or mental functioning

impulse control the ability to think through the consequences of behaviour or decisions before acting

impulsivity/impulsiveness refers to decisions or actions taken without thinking through the consequences

inattention/inattentiveness refers to challenges with staying on task, focusing and organisation

masking when a person hides or suppresses symptoms, behaviours or difficulties they are experiencing in order to fit in or gain social acceptance

melatonin the chemical that makes you sleep in response to darkness; also used by some ADHDers as a pharmaceutical sleep aid or supplement

mesolimbic pathway a **dopaminergic** pathway in the brain which connects all the areas that make up the brain's reward system

meta-analysis the combination of data from several independent primary studies that address the same question to produce a single estimate of the answer

neuron the fundamental units of the brain and nervous system, responsible for receiving sensory input from the external world and sending commands from our brain to our body

neurodevelopmental relating to or involving the development of the nervous system. Neurodevelopmental disorders are a group of conditions where the function of the nervous system is impacted during critical periods of brain development

neurodivergence a way of talking about groups of people within society whose brains have developed or function differently from the majority

neurodiversity movement a human rights movement aimed at supporting **neurodivergent** people, with a focus on destigmatisation, acceptance and treatment equity rather than solely medicalising the brains of those who aren't **neurotypical**

neurotransmitters molecules used by the nervous system to transmit messages between neurons (or from neurons to muscles)

neurotype a sociological rather than clinical term referring to the different ways the brain can work. **Neurotypical** and **neurodivergent** are both neurotypes

neurotypical a way of describing people with neurological development or functioning that is considered the norm; i.e. who are not **neurodivergent**

noradrenaline a **neurotransmitter** and hormone. In the brain, it plays a role in focus and alertness (Aka norepinephrine, aka Ethel's cups of coffee. See p. 50)

novelty-seeking a personality trait common among ADHDers that involves seeking out the excitement of novel stimuli

object permanence a community-driven, non-scientific term used to describe difficulty with remembering something exists when it is out of sight

prefrontal cortex a part of the brain at the front of the frontal lobe which plays a crucial role in regulating attention, behaviour, emotion and inhibition

presentation a way of describing the three 'flavours' of ADHD – **ADHD-H**, **ADHD-I** and **ADHD-C**

prevalence in medicine, a measure of the total number of people in a specific group who have a certain disease, condition or risk factor at a specific time

rejection-sensitive dysphoria a community-driven, non-scientific term for the feeling many ADHDers describe of intense emotional pain because of a failure or feeling rejected

remission when the signs and symptoms of a condition disappear or fall below the threshold of **diagnostic criteria**

restlessness sometimes used to mean **hyperactivity**, but can also be an intense inner yearning to take action and frustration when you feel you can't

self-efficacy an individual's belief in their ability to take steps and execute the behaviours required to succeed at a task

self-esteem an individual's subjective sense of their personal worth or value

self-medicating conscious or unconscious use of alcohol or other drugs to manage symptoms of a health issue, rather than prescribed medications

side effect any unintended effect of a medicine or treatment

substance abuse the harmful or hazardous use of psychoactive substances, including alcohol and illicit drugs

symptom a physical or mental state experienced by a person who has a condition, disease or disorder

systematic review an authoritative summary of the existing scientific literature on a subject, which synthesises the results of multiple related primary studies by using strategies that reduce **biases** and random errors

time blindness a colloquial term for the inability to accurately measure time and to conceive of the future, such as in **delay discounting**

undiagnosed describes living with the symptoms of a condition prior to a formal medical **diagnosis** or without knowing that the disorder is the cause

working memory the cognitive system that relates to our limited capacity to hold information temporarily. It is important for reasoning and for the guidance of decision-making and behaviour

Resources

This book has covered a number of the serious issues that can come along with living with ADHD. If any of these topics have brought up difficult emotions for you, please consider reaching out and getting some extra support from one of the organisations listed below. You do not have to go through these struggles alone. These services operate in Australia, but many countries have resources like this, so if you are reading this somewhere else in the world, you should be able to find services relevant to you with a quick internet search.

ReachOut
Anonymous and confidential mental health and wellbeing support for young people
au.reachout.com

Lifeline
Crisis support and suicide prevention services
lifeline.org.au
13 11 14

Beyond Blue
Mental health support services for anxiety, depression and suicide
beyondblue.org.au
1300 224 636

headspace

Mental health support for young people

headspace.org.au

1800 650 890

The Butterfly Foundation

Support for eating disorders and body image issues

butterfly.org.au

1800 33 4673

13YARN

For Aboriginal and Torres Strait Islander people who are going through a tough time and feel like having a yarn

13yarn.org.au

13 92 76

1800RESPECT

Confidential information, counselling and support for domestic, family and sexual violence

1800respect.org.au

1800 737 732

Relationships Australia

Relationship support services for individuals, families and communities

relationships.org.au

1300 364 277

MensLine

Relationship advice and mental health support for men

mensline.org.au

1300 78 99 78

Notes

Introduction

1 Faraone, S.V., et al. (2021). 'The World Federation of ADHD International Consensus Statement: 208 evidence-based conclusions about the disorder'. *Neuroscience & Biobehavioral Reviews, 128*, 789–818. doi.org/10.1016/j.neubiorev.2021.01.022

1. Why is everyone suddenly talking about ADHD?

1 Sciutto, M. J., & Eisenberg, M. (2007). 'Evaluating the evidence for and against the overdiagnosis of ADHD'. *Journal of Attention Disorders, 11*(2), 106–13. doi.org/10.1177/1087054707300094

2 Willcutt, E. G. (2012). 'The prevalence of *DSM-IV* attention-deficit/hyperactivity disorder: A meta-analytic review'. *Neurotherapeutics, 9*(3), 490–9. doi.org/10.1007/s13311-012-0135-8

3 Thomas, R., et al. (2015). 'Prevalence of attention-deficit/hyperactivity disorder: A systematic review and meta-analysis'. *Pediatrics, 135*(4), e994–1001. doi.org/10.1542/peds.2014-3482

4 Willcutt, 'The prevalence of *DSM-IV* attention-deficit/hyperactivity disorder'

5 Fayyad, J., et al. (2017). 'The descriptive epidemiology of *DSM-IV* adult ADHD in the World Health Organization world mental health surveys'. *ADHD Attention Deficit and Hyperactivity Disorders, 9*, 47–65. doi.org/10.1007/s12402-016-0208-3

6 Australian Bureau of Statistics. (2021). *Population: Census*. ABS. abs.gov.au/statistics/people/population/population-census/2021#key-statistics. Accessed 7 June 2023

7 Department of Health. (2021). Public Release Document, June 2021 DUSC Meeting. pbs.gov.au/industry/listing/participants/public-release-docs/2021-06/guanfacine-prd-2021-06-FINAL.PDF. Accessed 7 June 2023

8 Raman, S. R., et al. (2018). 'Trends in attention-deficit hyperactivity disorder medication use: A retrospective observational study using population-based databases'. *Lancet Psychiatry, 5*(10), 824–35. doi.org/10.1016/S2215-0366(18)30293-1

9 Lee, S. M., et al. (2021). 'Nationwide rate of adult ADHD diagnosis and pharmacotherapy from 2015 to 2018'. *International Journal of Environmental Research and Public Health, 18*(21), 11322. doi.org/10.3390/ijerph182111322

10 Hinshaw, S. P. & Scheffler, R. M. (2014). Chapter 5, 'What a difference a state makes: How educational policy determines diagnosis and treatment' in *The ADHD Explosion: Myths, medication, money, and today's push for performance*. Oxford University Press, New York. 67–82

11 Centers for Disease Control and Prevention. (2022). 'State-based prevalence of ADHD diagnosis and treatment 2016–2019'. CDC. cdc.gov/ncbddd/adhd/data/diagnosis-treatment-data.html. Accessed 23 May 2023

12 Polanczyk, G.V., et al. (2014). 'ADHD prevalence estimates across three decades: An updated systematic review and meta-regression analysis'. *International Journal of Epidemiology, 43*(2), 434–42. doi.org/10.1093/ije/dyt261

13 van Lieshout, M., et al. (2016). 'A 6-year follow-up of a large European cohort of children with attention-deficit/hyperactivity disorder-combined subtype: Outcomes in late adolescence and young adulthood'. *European Child & Adolescent Psychiatry, 25*, 1007–17. doi.org/10.1007/s00787-016-0820-y

14 Cheung, C. H., et al. (2016). 'Cognitive and neurophysiological markers of ADHD persistence and remission'. *British Journal of Psychiatry*, *208*(6), 548–55. doi:10.1192/bjp.bp.114.145185

15 Sibley, M. H., et al. (2022). 'Variable patterns of remission from ADHD in the multimodal treatment study of ADHD'. *American Journal of Psychiatry*, *179*(2), 142–51. doi.org/10.1176/appi.ajp.2021.21010032

16 Sibley, 'Variable patterns of remission from ADHD in the multimodal treatment study of ADHD'

2. What's wrong with me?

1 Momany, A. M., et al. (2018). 'A meta-analysis of the association between birth weight and attention deficit hyperactivity disorder'. *Journal of Abnormal Child Psychology*, *46*, 1409–26. doi.org/10.1007/s10802-017-0371-9

2 Lindström, K., et al. (2011). 'Preterm birth and attention-deficit/hyperactivity disorder in schoolchildren'. *Pediatrics*, *127*(5), 858–65. doi.org/10.1542/peds.2010-1279

3 Nilsen, F. M., & Tulve, N. S. (2020). 'A systematic review and meta-analysis examining the interrelationships between chemical and non-chemical stressors and inherent characteristics in children with ADHD'. *Environmental Research*, *180*, 108884. doi.org/10.1016/j.envres.2019.108884

4 Faraone, S.V., et al. (2021). 'The World Federation of ADHD International Consensus Statement: 208 evidence-based conclusions about the disorder'. *Neuroscience & Biobehavioral Reviews*, *128*, 789–818 (795). doi.org/10.1016/j.neubiorev.2021.01.022

5 Starck, M., et al. (2016). 'Occurrence of ADHD in parents of ADHD children in a clinical sample'. *Neuropsychiatric Disease and Treatment*, *12*, 581–8. doi.org/10.2147/NDT.S100238

6 Smalley, S. L., et al. (2000). 'Familial clustering of symptoms and disruptive behaviors in multiplex families with attention-deficit/hyperactivity disorder'. *Journal of the American Academy of Child & Adolescent Psychiatry*, *39*(9), 1135–43. doi.org/10.1097/00004583-200009000-00013

7 Uchida, M., et al. (2021). 'Assessing the magnitude of risk for ADHD in offspring of parents with ADHD: A systematic literature review and meta-analysis'. *Journal of Attention Disorders*, *25*(13), 1943–8. doi.org/10.1177/1087054720950815

8 Miller, M., et al. (2019). 'Sibling recurrence risk and cross-aggregation of attention-deficit/hyperactivity disorder and autism spectrum disorder'. *JAMA Pediatrics*, *173*(2), 147–52. doi:10.1001/jamapediatrics.2018.4076

9 Kooij, S. J., et al. (2010). 'European consensus statement on diagnosis and treatment of adult ADHD: The European Network Adult ADHD'. *BMC Psychiatry*, *10*, 67. doi.org/10.1186/1471-244X-10-67

10 Willcutt, E. G. (2012). 'The prevalence of *DSM-IV* attention-deficit/hyperactivity disorder: A meta-analytic review'. *Neurotherapeutics*, *9*(3), 490–9. doi.org/10.1007/s13311-012-0135-8

11 Gibbins, C., et al. (2010). 'ADHD-hyperactive/impulsive subtype in adults'. *Mental Illness*, *2*(1), 41–5. doi.org/10.4081/mi.2010.e9

12 Willcutt, E. G., et al. (2012). 'Validity of *DSM-IV* attention deficit/hyperactivity disorder symptom dimensions and subtypes'. *Journal of Abnormal Psychology*, *121*(4), 991–1010. doi.org/10.1037/a0027347

13 Willcutt, 'The prevalence of *DSM-IV* attention-deficit/hyperactivity disorder'

14 Willcutt, 'Validity of *DSM-IV* attention deficit/hyperactivity disorder symptom dimensions and subtypes'

15 Willcutt, 'The prevalence of DSM-IV attention-deficit/hyperactivity disorder'

3. What's going on inside my brain?

1 Hoogman, M., et al. (2017). 'Subcortical brain volume differences in participants with attention deficit hyperactivity disorder in children and adults: A cross-sectional mega-analysis'. *Lancet Psychiatry, 4*(4), 310–19. doi.org/10.1016/S2215-0366(17)30049-4

2 Scheres, A., et al. (2007). 'Ventral striatal hyporesponsiveness during reward anticipation in attention-deficit/hyperactivity disorder'. *Biological Psychiatry, 61*(5), 720–4. doi.org/10.1016/j.biopsych.2006.04.042

3 ibid., 722

4. What does ADHD mean for a grown-up?

1 Faraone, S.V., et al. (2021). 'The World Federation of ADHD International Consensus Statement: 208 evidence-based conclusions about the disorder'. *Neuroscience & Biobehavioral Reviews, 128*, 789–818 (793). doi.org/10.1016/j.neubiorev.2021.01.022

2 American Psychiatric Association. (1980). Attention Deficit Disorder with Hyperactivity. In *Diagnostic and Statistical Manual of Mental Disorders* (3rd edition), 41–5; American Psychiatric Association. (1968). Hyperkinetic reaction of childhood (or adolescence). In *Diagnostic and Statistical Manual of Mental Disorders* (2nd edition), 50

3 Kooij, S. J., et al. (2010). 'European consensus statement on diagnosis and treatment of adult ADHD: The European Network Adult ADHD'. *BMC Psychiatry, 10*, 67. doi.org/10.1186/1471-244X-10-67

4 Faraone, 'The World Federation of ADHD International Consensus Statement', 801

5 Ennitis, M., et al. (2021). 'Substance-specific variability of ADHD symptoms in riga psychiatry and addiction medicine centre treatment-seeking substance use disorder outpatient population'. *European Psychiatry, 64*(S1), S89–90. doi:10.1192/j.eurpsy.2021.264

6 Kooij, 'European consensus statement on diagnosis and treatment of adult ADHD'

7 Beheshti, A., et al. (2020). 'Emotion dysregulation in adults with attention deficit hyperactivity disorder: A meta-analysis'. *BMC Psychiatry, 20*(120), 1–11 (9). doi.org/10.1186/s12888-020-2442-7

8 Kooij, 'European consensus statement on diagnosis and treatment of adult ADHD', 6

9 Beheshti, 'Emotion dysregulation in adults with attention deficit hyperactivity disorder', 6

10 Retz, W., et al. (2012). 'Emotional dysregulation in adult ADHD: What is the empirical evidence?'. *Expert Review of Neurotherapeutics, 12*(10), 1241–51. doi.org/10.1586/ern.12.109

11 Surman, C. B., et al. (2013). 'Understanding deficient emotional self-regulation in adults with attention deficit hyperactivity disorder: A controlled study'. *ADHD Attention Deficit and Hyperactivity Disorders, 5*, 273–81. doi.org/10.1007/s12402-012-0100-8

12 Corbisiero, S., et al. (2013). 'Is emotional dysregulation part of the psychopathology of ADHD in adults?'. *ADHD Attention Deficit and Hyperactivity Disorders, 5*, 83–92. doi.org/10.1007/s12402-012-0097-z

13 Beheshti, 'Emotion dysregulation in adults with attention deficit hyperactivity disorder'

14 Hirsch, O., et al. (2018). 'Emotional dysregulation is a primary symptom in adult attention-deficit/hyperactivity disorder (ADHD)'. *Journal of Affective Disorders, 232*, 41–7. doi.org/10.1016/j.jad.2018.02.007

15 American Psychiatric Association. (2022). Attention-deficit/hyperactivity disorder: Diagnostic criteria. In *Diagnostic and Statistical Manual of Mental Disorders* (5th ed., text rev.), 69. doi.org/10.1176/appi.books.9780890425787

16 UNC Learning Centre. 'Russell A. Barkley: 2012 Burnett Lecture: Part 2 ADHD, Self-regulation and

executive functioning theory'. YouTube, 2 November 2012. youtube.com/watch?v=QZpF2_IelWo. Accessed 26 May 2023

17 Zheng, Q., et al. (2022). 'Time perception deficits in children and adolescents with ADHD: A meta-analysis'. *Journal of Attention Disorders, 26*(2), 267–81. doi.org/10.1177/1087054720978557

18 Pollak, Y., et al. (2009). 'Testing possible mechanisms of deficient supra-second time estimation in adults with attention-deficit/hyperactivity disorder'. *Neuropsychology, 23*(5), 679 –86. doi.org/10.1037/a0016281

19 Prevatt, F., et al. (2011). 'Time estimation abilities of college students with ADHD'. *Journal of Attention Disorders, 15*(7), 531–8. doi.org/10.1177/1087054710370673

20 Patros, C. H., et al. (2016). 'Choice-impulsivity in children and adolescents with attention-deficit/hyperactivity disorder (ADHD): A meta-analytic review'. *Clinical Psychology Review, 43*, 162–74. doi.org/10.1016/j.cpr.2015.11.001

21 Jackson, J. N., & MacKillop, J. (2016). 'Attention-deficit/hyperactivity disorder and monetary delay discounting: A meta-analysis of case-control studies'. *Biological Psychiatry: Cognitive neuroscience and neuroimaging, 1*(4), 316–25. doi.org/10.1016/j.bpsc.2016.01.007

22 American Psychiatric Association. (1980). Diagnostic criteria for Attention Deficit Disorder with Hyperactivity. In *Diagnostic and Statistical Manual of Mental Disorders* (3rd edition), 44

23 Yoon, S.Y. R., et al. (2013). 'Sleep and daytime function in adults with attention-deficit/hyperactivity disorder: Subtype differences'. *Sleep Medicine, 14*(7), 648–55. doi.org/10.1016/j.sleep.2013.03.003

24 Weiss, M. D., & McBride, N. M. (2018). ' ADHD: A 24-Hour Disorder'. *Psychiatric Times, 35*(10), 16–18.psychiatrictimes.com/view/adhd-24-hour-disorder. Accessed 26 May 2023

25 Sedky, K., et al. (2014). 'Attention deficit hyperactivity disorder and sleep disordered breathing in pediatric populations: A meta-analysis'. *Sleep Medicine Reviews, 18*(4), 349–56. doi.org/10.1016/j.smrv.2013.12.003

26 Roy, M., et al. (2018). 'Association between restless legs syndrome and adult ADHD in a German community-based sample'. *Journal of Attention Disorders, 22*(3), 300–8. doi.org/10.1177/10870547145612

27 Coogan, A. N., & McGowan, N. M. (2017). 'A systematic review of circadian function, chronotype and chronotherapy in attention deficit hyperactivity disorder'. *ADHD Attention Deficit and Hyperactivity Disorders, 9*, 129–47. doi.org/10.1007/s12402-016-0214-5

28 Van der Heijden, K. B., et al. (2005). 'Idiopathic chronic sleep onset insomnia in attention-deficit/hyperactivity disorder: A circadian rhythm sleep disorder'. *Chronobiology International, 22*(3), 559–70. doi.org/10.1081/CBI-200062410

29 Van Veen, M. M., et al. (2010). 'Delayed circadian rhythm in adults with attention-deficit/hyperactivity disorder and chronic sleep-onset insomnia'. *Biological Psychiatry, 67*(11), 1091–6. doi.org/10.1016/j.biopsych.2009.12.032

30 Gruber, R., et al. (2012). 'Short sleep duration is associated with teacher-reported inattention and cognitive problems in healthy school-aged children'. *Nature and Science of Sleep, 4*, 33–40. doi.org/10.2147/NSS.S24607

31 Gamble, K. L., et al. (2013). 'Delayed sleep timing and symptoms in adults with attention-deficit/hyperactivity disorder: A controlled actigraphy study'. *Chronobiology International, 30*(4), 598–606. doi.org/10.3109/07420528.2012.754454

32 Barkley, R. A., & Brown, T. E. (2008). 'Unrecognized attention-deficit/hyperactivity disorder in

adults presenting with other psychiatric disorders'. *CNS Spectrums*, *13*(11), 977–84. doi:10.1017/S1092852900014036
33 Hvolby, A. (2015). 'Associations of sleep disturbance with ADHD: Implications for treatment'. *ADHD Attention Deficit and Hyperactivity Disorders*, 7, 1–18 (2). doi.org/10.1007/s12402-014-0151-0
34 ibid.
35 Almey, A., et al. (2015). 'Estrogen receptors in the central nervous system and their implication for dopamine-dependent cognition in females'. *Hormones and Behavior*, *74*, 125–38. doi.org/10.1016/j.yhbeh.2015.06.010
36 Littman, E., et al. (2021). 'ADHD in females across the lifespan and the role of estrogen'. *The ADHD Report*, *29*(5), 1–8. doi.org/10.1521/adhd.2021.29.5.1
37 Roberts, B., et al. (2018). 'Reproductive steroids and ADHD symptoms across the menstrual cycle'. *Psychoneuroendocrinology*, *88*, 105–14 (113). doi.org/10.1016/j.psyneuen.2017.11.015
38 Young, S., et al. (2020). 'Females with ADHD: An expert consensus statement taking a lifespan approach providing guidance for the identification and treatment of attention-deficit/hyperactivity disorder in girls and women'. *BMC Psychiatry*, *20*(1), 404. doi.org/10.1186/s12888-020-02707-9
39 Roberts, 'Reproductive steroids and ADHD symptoms across the menstrual cycle', 113
40 Hupfeld, K. E., et al. (2019). 'Living "in the zone": Hyperfocus in adult ADHD'. *ADHD Attention Deficit and Hyperactivity Disorders*, *11*, 191–208. doi.org/10.1007/s12402-018-0272-y
41 Lee, S. S., et al. (2011). 'Prospective association of childhood attention-deficit/hyperactivity disorder (ADHD) and substance use and abuse/dependence: A meta-analytic review'. *Clinical Psychology Review*, *31*(3), 328–41. doi.org/10.1016/j.cpr.2011.01.006
42 Groenman, A. P., et al. (2017). 'Childhood psychiatric disorders as risk factor for subsequent substance abuse: A meta-analysis'. *Journal of the American Academy of Child & Adolescent Psychiatry*, *56*(7), 556–69. doi.org/10.1016/j.jaac.2017.05.004
43 Chen, Q., et al. (2018). 'Common psychiatric and metabolic comorbidity of adult attention-deficit/hyperactivity disorder: A population-based cross-sectional study'. *PLoS one*, *13*(9), e0204516. doi.org/10.1371/journal.pone.0204516
44 Nazar, B. P., et al. (2016). 'The risk of eating disorders comorbid with attention-deficit/hyperactivity disorder: A systematic review and meta-analysis'. *International Journal of Eating Disorders*, *49*(12), 1045–57. doi.org/10.1002/eat.22643
45 ibid., 1054
46 American Psychiatric Association. (2022). Attention-deficit/hyperactivity disorder: Differential diagnosis. In *Diagnostic and Statistical Manual of Mental Disorders* (5th ed., text rev.), 74. doi.org/10.1176/appi.books.9780890425787
47 American Psychiatric Association. (2022). Attention-deficit/hyperactivity disorder: Comorbidity. In *Diagnostic and Statistical Manual of Mental Disorders* (5th ed., text rev.), 75. doi.org/10.1176/appi.books.9780890425787
48 Jensen, C. M., & Steinhausen, H. C. (2015). 'Comorbid mental disorders in children and adolescents with attention-deficit/hyperactivity disorder in a large nationwide study'. *ADHD Attention Deficit and Hyperactivity Disorders*, 7, 27–38. doi.org/10.1007/s12402-014-0142-1
49 Antshel, K. M., et al. (2016). 'An update on the comorbidity of ADHD and ASD: A focus on clinical management'. *Expert Review of Neurotherapeutics*, *16*(3), 279–93 (279). doi.org/10.1586/14737175.2016.1146591
50 Antshel, 'An update on the comorbidity of ADHD and ASD', 280

51 Ghirardi, L., et al. (2018). 'The familial co-aggregation of ASD and ADHD: A register-based cohort study'. *Molecular Psychiatry*, *23*, 257–62. doi.org/10.1038/mp.2017.17

52 Kern, J. K., et al. (2015). 'Are ASD and ADHD a continuum? A comparison of pathophysiological similarities between the disorders'. *Journal of Attention Disorders*, *19*(9), 805–27. doi.org/10.1177/1087054712459886

53 Instanes, J. T., et al. (2018). 'Adult ADHD and comorbid somatic disease: A systematic literature review'. *Journal of Attention Disorders*, *22*(3), 203–28. doi:10.1177/1087054716669589

54 Chen, M. H., et al. (2018). 'Sexually transmitted infection among adolescents and young adults with attention-deficit/hyperactivity disorder: A nationwide longitudinal study'. *Journal of the American Academy of Child & Adolescent Psychiatry*, *57*(1), 48–53. doi.org/10.1016/j.jaac.2017.09.438

5. Am I okay?

1 Jellinek, M. S. 'Don't let ADHD crush children's self-esteem'. *Clinical Psychiatry News*, May 2012. cdn.mdedge.com/files/s3fs-public/issues/articles/70231_main_7.pdf. Accessed 26 May 2023

2 Psychogiou, L., et al. (2007). 'Mothers' expressed emotion toward their school-aged sons: Associations with child and maternal symptoms of psychopathology'. *European Child & Adolescent Psychiatry*, *16*, 458–64. doi.org/10.1007/s00787-007-0619-y

3 Musser, E. D., et al. (2016). 'Attention-deficit/hyperactivity disorder developmental trajectories related to parental expressed emotion'. *Journal of Abnormal Psychology*, *125*(2), 182–95. doi.org/10.1037/abn0000097

4 Hoza, B. (2007). 'Peer functioning in children with ADHD'. *Journal of Pediatric Psychology*, *32*(6), 655–63. doi.org/10.1093/jpepsy/jsm024

5 Taylor, L. A., et al. (2010). 'Adding insult to injury: Bullying experiences of youth with attention deficit hyperactivity disorder'. *Children's Health Care*, *39*(1), 59–72. doi.org/10.1080/02739610903455152

6 Becker, S. P., et al. (2017). 'Rates of peer victimization in young adolescents with ADHD and associations with internalizing symptoms and self-esteem'. *European Child & Adolescent Psychiatry*, *26*, 201–14. doi.org/10.1007/s00787-016-0881-y

7 Strine, T. W., et al. (2006). 'Emotional and behavioral difficulties and impairments in everyday functioning among children with a history of attention-deficit/hyperactivity disorder'. *Preventing Chronic Disease*, *3*(2), A52

8 Ros, R., & Graziano, P. A. (2018). 'Social functioning in children with or at risk for attention deficit/hyperactivity disorder: A meta-analytic review'. *Journal of Clinical Child & Adolescent Psychology*, *47*(2), 213–35. doi.org/10.1080/15374416.2016.1266644

9 Harpin, V., et al. (2016). 'Long-term outcomes of ADHD: A systematic review of self-esteem and social function'. *Journal of Attention Disorders*, *20*(4), 295–305. doi.org/10.1177/1087054713486516

10 Shaw, M., et al. (2012). 'A systematic review and analysis of long-term outcomes in attention deficit hyperactivity disorder: Effects of treatment and non-treatment'. *BMC Medicine*, *10*, 99. doi.org/10.1186/1741-7015-10-99

11 Newark, P. E., et al. (2016). 'Self-esteem, self-efficacy, and resources in adults with ADHD'. *Journal of Attention Disorders*, *20*(3), 279–90. doi.org/10.1177/1087054712459561

12 Pawaskar, M., et al. (2020). 'Comparison of quality of life, productivity, functioning and self-esteem in adults diagnosed with ADHD and with symptomatic ADHD'. *Journal of Attention Disorders*, *24*(1), 136–44. doi.org/10.1177/1087054719841129

6. Where did all the girls go?

1 Willcutt, E. G. (2012). 'The prevalence of *DSM-IV* attention-deficit/hyperactivity disorder: A meta-analytic review'. *Neurotherapeutics*, *9*(3), 490–9 (492). doi.org/10.1007/s13311-012-0135-8

2 Quinn, P. O., & Madhoo, M. (2014). 'A review of attention-deficit/hyperactivity disorder in women and girls: Uncovering this hidden diagnosis'. *Primary Care Companion for CNS Disorders*, *16*(3). doi:10.4088/PCC.13r01596

3 Price, A., et al. (2020). 'Regional analysis of UK primary care prescribing and adult service referrals for young people with attention-deficit hyperactivity disorder'. *BJPsych Open*, *6*(1), e7. doi:10.1192/bjo.2019.94

4 Kooij, S. J., et al. (2010). 'European consensus statement on diagnosis and treatment of adult ADHD: The European Network Adult ADHD'. *BMC Psychiatry*, *10*, 67. doi.org/10.1186/1471-244X-10-67

5 De Rossi, P., et al. (2022). 'Gender-related clinical characteristics in children and adolescents with ADHD'. *Journal of Clinical Medicine, 11*(2), 385. doi.org/10.3390/jcm11020385

6 Wang, L., et al. (2017). 'Prevalence rates of youths diagnosed with and medicated for ADHD in a nationwide survey'. *Epidemiology and Psychiatric Sciences*, *26*(6), 624–34. doi:10.1017/S2045796016000500

7 Jensen, C. M., & Steinhausen, H. C. (2015). 'Time trends in incidence rates of diagnosed attention-deficit/hyperactivity disorder across 16 years in a nationwide Danish registry study'. *Journal of Clinical Psychiatry*, *76*(3), e334–41. doi:10.4088/JCP.14m09094

8 Lange, K. W., et al. (2010). 'The history of attention deficit hyperactivity disorder'. *ADHD Attention Deficit and Hyperactivity Disorders*, *2*, 241–55. doi.org/10.1007/s12402-010-0045-8

9 ibid.

10 Willcutt, 'The prevalence of *DSM-IV* attention-deficit/hyperactivity disorder'

11 American Psychiatric Association. (1980). Attention Deficit Disorder with Hyperactivity. In *Diagnostic and Statistical Manual of Mental Disorders* (3rd edition), 41–5; American Psychiatric Association. (1968). Hyperkinetic reaction of childhood (or adolescence). In *Diagnostic and Statistical Manual of Mental Disorders* (2nd edition), 50

12 Young, S., et al. (2020). 'Females with ADHD: An expert consensus statement taking a lifespan approach providing guidance for the identification and treatment of attention-deficit/hyperactivity disorder in girls and women'. *BMC Psychiatry*, *20*(1), 404. doi.org/10.1186/s12888-020-02707-9

13 ibid.

14 ibid.

15 ibid.

16 Grevet, E. H., et al. (2006). 'Lack of gender effects on subtype outcomes in adults with attention–deficit/hyperactivity disorder: Support for the validity of subtypes'. *European Archives of Psychiatry and Clinical Neuroscience*, *256*, 311–19. doi.org/10.1007/s00406-006-0639-5

17 Solberg, B. S., et al. (2018). 'Gender differences in psychiatric comorbidity: A population-based study of 40,000 adults with attention deficit hyperactivity disorder'. *Acta Psychiatrica Scandinavica*, *137*(3), 176–86. doi.org/10.1111/acps.12845

18 Grevet, 'Lack of gender effects on subtype outcomes in adults with attention–deficit/hyperactivity disorder'

19 Quinn, P., & Wigal, S. (2004). 'Perceptions of girls and ADHD: Results from a national survey'. *Medscape General Medicine*, *6*(2), 2

20 Sciutto, M. J., et al. (2004). 'Effects of child gender and symptom type on referrals for ADHD by

elementary school teachers'. *Journal of Emotional and Behavioral Disorders*, *12*(4), 247–53. doi.org/10.1177/10634266040120040.

21 Ohan, J. L., & Visser, T. A. (2009). 'Why is there a gender gap in children presenting for attention deficit/hyperactivity disorder services?'. *Journal of Clinical Child & Adolescent Psychology*, *38*(5), 650–60. doi.org/10.1080/15374410903103627

22 Coles, E. K., et al. (2012). 'Exploring the gender gap in referrals for children with ADHD and other disruptive behavior disorders'. *Journal of Attention Disorders*, *16*(2), 101–8. doi.org/10.1177/1087054710381481

23 Moldavsky, M., et al. (2013). 'Teachers' recognition of children with ADHD: Role of subtype and gender'. *Child and Adolescent Mental Health*, *18*(1), 18–23. doi.org/10.1111/j.1475-3588.2012.00653.x

24 Mowlem, F., et al. (2019). 'Do different factors influence whether girls versus boys meet ADHD diagnostic criteria? Sex differences among children with high ADHD symptoms'. *Psychiatry Research*, *272*, 765–73. doi.org/10.1016/j.psychres.2018.12.128

25 Morris, E. W., & Perry, B. L. (2017). 'Girls behaving badly? Race, gender, and subjective evaluation in the discipline of African American girls'. *Sociology of Education*, *90*(2), 127–48. doi.org/10.1177/0038040717694876

26 Hinshaw, S. P., et al. (2022). 'Annual Research Review: Attention-deficit/hyperactivity disorder in girls and women: Underrepresentation, longitudinal processes, and key directions'. *Journal of Child Psychology and Psychiatry*, *63*(4), 484–96. doi.org/10.1111/jcpp.13480

27 Willcutt, 'The prevalence of *DSM-IV* attention-deficit/hyperactivity disorder'

28 Rucklidge, J. J., & Kaplan, B. J. (1997). 'Psychological functioning of women identified in adulthood with attention-deficit/hyperactivity disorder'. *Journal of Attention Disorders*, *2*(3), 167–76. doi.org/10.1177/108705479700200303

29 ibid.

30 Biederman, J., et al. (2012). 'Predictors of persistence in girls with attention deficit hyperactivity disorder: Results from an 11-year controlled follow-up study'. *Acta Psychiatrica Scandinavica*, *125*(2), 147–56. doi.org/10.1111/j.1600-0447.2011.01797.x

31 Skoglund, C., et al. (2019). 'Association of attention-deficit/hyperactivity disorder with teenage birth among women and girls in Sweden'. *JAMA Network Open*, *2*(10), e1912463. doi:10.1001/jamanetworkopen.2019.12463

32 Quinn, P. O., & Madhoo, M. (2014). 'A review of attention-deficit/hyperactivity disorder in women and girls: Uncovering this hidden diagnosis'. *Primary Care Companion for CNS Disorders*, *16*(3). doi:10.4088/PCC.13r01596

33 Newark, P. E., et al. (2016). 'Self-esteem, self-efficacy, and resources in adults with ADHD'. *Journal of Attention Disorders*, *20*(3), 279–90. doi.org/10.1177/1087054712459561

7. How does race factor into this?

1 Ayano, G., et al. (2020). 'Epidemiology of attention-deficit/hyperactivity disorder (ADHD) in children and adolescents in Africa: A systematic review and meta-analysis'. *Annals of General Psychiatry*, *19*, 21. doi.org/10.1186/s12991-020-00271-w

2 Cenat, J. M., et al. (2021). 'Prevalence and risk factors associated with attention-deficit/hyperactivity disorder among US Black individuals: A systematic review and meta-analysis'. *JAMA Psychiatry*, *78*(1), 21–8. doi:10.1001/jamapsychiatry.2020.2788

3 Morgan, P. L., et al. (2014). 'Racial/ethnic disparities in ADHD diagnosis by kindergarten entry'. *Journal of Child Psychology and Psychiatry, 55*(8), 905–13. doi.org/10.1111/jcpp.12204
4 Coker, T. R., et al. (2016). 'Racial and ethnic disparities in ADHD diagnosis and treatment'. *Pediatrics, 138*(3), e20160407. doi.org/10.1542/peds.2016-0407
5 Morgan, 'Racial/ethnic disparities in ADHD diagnosis by kindergarten entry'
6 Coker, 'Racial and ethnic disparities in ADHD diagnosis and treatment'
7 Faraone, S.V., et al. (2021). 'The World Federation of ADHD International Consensus Statement: 208 evidence-based concluoions about the disorder'. *Neuroscience & Biobehavioral Reviews, 128*, 789–818 (800). doi.org/10.1016/j.neubiorev.2021.01.022
8 Young, S., et al. (2015). 'A meta-analysis of the prevalence of attention deficit hyperactivity disorder in incarcerated populations'. *Psychological Medicine, 45*(2), 247–58. doi:10.1017/S0033291714000762

Hobbies can hurt

1 Ruiz-Goikoetxea, M., et al. (2018). 'Risk of unintentional injuries in children and adolescents with ADHD and the impact of ADHD medications: A systematic review and meta-analysis'. *Neuroscience & Biobehavioral Reviews, 84*, 63–71. doi.org/10.1016/j.neubiorev.2017.11.007

8. How did the internet know?

1 Yeung, A., et al. (2022). 'TikTok and attention-deficit/hyperactivity disorder: A cross-sectional study of social media content quality'. *Canadian Journal of Psychiatry*, 67(12), 899–906. doi.org/10.1177/070674372210828
2 Dodson, W. W. 'Emotional Regulation'. *Attention*, October 2016, 8–11. chadd.org/wp-content/uploads/2016/10/ATTN_10_16_EmotionalRegulation.pdf. Accessed 17 May 2023
3 Beheshti, A., et al. (2020). 'Emotion dysregulation in adults with attention deficit hyperactivity disorder: A meta-analysis'. *BMC Psychiatry, 20*(120), 1–11 (6). doi.org/10.1186/s12888-020-2442-7
4 Brown, T. E. (2009). 'ADD/ADHD and impaired executive function in clinical practice'. *Current Attention Disorders Reports*, 1, 37–41. doi.org/10.1007/s12618-009-0006-3
5 Faraone, S.V., et al. (2021). 'The World Federation of ADHD International Consensus Statement: 208 evidence-based conclusions about the disorder'. *Neuroscience & Biobehavioral Reviews, 128*, 789–818. doi.org/10.1016/j.neubiorev.2021.01.022

10. How do I live with it?

1 Knouse, L. E., et al. (2017). 'Meta-analysis of cognitive–behavioral treatments for adult ADHD'. *Journal of Consulting and Clinical Psychology, 85*(7), 737–50. doi.org/10.1037/ccp0000216
2 Young, Z., et al. (2020). 'The efficacy of cognitive behavioral therapy for adults with ADHD: A systematic review and meta-analysis of randomized controlled trials'. *Journal of Attention Disorders, 24*(6), 875–88. doi.org/10.1177/1087054716664413
3 Vysniauske, R., et al. (2020). 'The effects of physical exercise on functional outcomes in the treatment of ADHD: A meta-analysis'. *Journal of Attention Disorders, 24*(5), 644–54. doi.org/10.1177/1087054715627489
4 Mehren, A., et al. (2019). 'Acute effects of aerobic exercise on executive function and attention in adult patients with ADHD'. *Frontiers in Psychiatry, 10*, 132. doi.org/10.3389/fpsyt.2019.00132

5 Vysniauske, 'The effects of physical exercise on functional outcomes in the treatment of ADHD'
6 Zang, Y. (2019). 'Impact of physical exercise on children with attention deficit hyperactivity disorders: Evidence through a meta-analysis'. *Medicine, 98*(46), e17980. doi:10.1097/MD.0000000000017980
7 Rebar, A. L., et al. (2015). 'A meta-meta-analysis of the effect of physical activity on depression and anxiety in non-clinical adult populations'. *Health Psychology Review, 9*(3), 366–78. doi.org/10.1080/17437199.2015.1022901
8 Morgan, A. J., et al. (2013). 'Exercise and mental health: An Exercise and Sports Science Australia commissioned review'. *Journal of Exercise Physiology Online, 16*(4), 64–73
9 Flannery, S., & Ruggiero, S. 'What we know about ADHD and food: Does your child's diet play a role in their symptoms?'. Child Mind Institute, 6 March 2023. childmind.org/article/what-we-know-about-adhd-and-food. Accessed 26 May 2023
10 Li, L., et al. (2020). 'Attention-deficit/hyperactivity disorder symptoms and dietary habits in adulthood: A large population-based twin study in Sweden'. *American Journal of Medical Genetics Part B: Neuropsychiatric Genetics, 183*(8), 475–85. doi.org/10.1002/ajmg.b.32825
11 Akmatov, M. K., et al. (2021). 'Psychiatric and nonpsychiatric comorbidities among children with ADHD: An exploratory analysis of nationwide claims data in Germany'. *Journal of Attention Disorders, 25*(6), 874–84. doi.org/10.1177/1087054719865779
12 Galioto, R., & Spitznagel, M. B. (2016). 'The effects of breakfast and breakfast composition on cognition in adults'. *Advances in Nutrition,* 7(3), 576S–89S. doi.org/10.3945/an.115.010231
13 Children and Adults with Attention-Deficit/Hyperactivity Disorder, 'Breakfast tips for busy minds', CHADD, chadd.org/adhd-weekly/breakfast-tips-for-busy-minds. Accessed 26 May 2023
14 Bloch, M. H., & Qawasmi, A. (2011). 'Omega-3 fatty acid supplementation for the treatment of children with attention-deficit/hyperactivity disorder symptomatology: Systematic review and meta-analysis'. *Journal of the American Academy of Child & Adolescent Psychiatry, 50*(10), 991–1000. doi.org/10.1016/j.jaac.2011.06.008
15 Lentjes, M. A. (2019). 'The balance between food and dietary supplements in the general population'. *Proceedings of the Nutrition Society, 78*(1), 97–109. doi:10.1017/S0029665118002525
16 'Drug interactions between amphetamine and vitamin C'. Drugs.com. drugs.com/drug-interactions/amphetamine-with-vitamin-c-2543-0-238-3823.html. Accessed 26 May 2023
17 Therapeutic Goods Administration. (2023.) Australian Product Information: Vyvanse® (Lisdexamfetamine dimesilate), 9. TGA. ebs.tga.gov.au/ebs/picmi/picmirepository.nsf/pdf?OpenAgent=&id=CP-2013-PI-02051-1&d=20230609172310101. Accessed 10 June 2023
18 Therapeutic Goods Administration. (2021.) Australian Product Information: Aspen Dexamfetamine (dexamfetamine sulfate) tablets, 5. TGA. ebs.tga.gov.au/ebs/picmi/picmirepository.nsf/pdf?OpenAgent=&id=CP-2017-PI-01667-1&d=20230605172310101. Accessed 10 June 2023
19 Hvolby, A. (2015). 'Associations of sleep disturbance with ADHD: Implications for treatment'. *ADHD Attention Deficit and Hyperactivity Disorders,* 7, 1–18 (2). doi.org/10.1007/s12402-014-0151-0
20 Yoon, S.Y. R., et al. (2013). 'Sleep and daytime function in adults with attention-deficit/hyperactivity disorder: Subtype differences'. *Sleep Medicine, 14*(7), 648–55. doi.org/10.1016/j.sleep.2013.03.003
21 Coogan, A. N., & McGowan, N. M. (2017). 'A systematic review of circadian function, chronotype and chronotherapy in attention deficit hyperactivity disorder'. *ADHD Attention Deficit and Hyperactivity Disorders, 9,* 129–47. doi.org/10.1007/s12402-016-0214-5
22 Van der Heijden, K. B., et al. (2007). 'Effect of melatonin on sleep, behavior, and cognition in ADHD

and chronic sleep-onset insomnia'. *Journal of the American Academy of Child & Adolescent Psychiatry*, *46*(2), 233–41. doi.org/10.1097/01.chi.0000246055.76167.0d

23 Weiss, M. D., et al. (2006). 'Sleep hygiene and melatonin treatment for children and adolescents with ADHD and initial insomnia'. *Journal of the American Academy of Child & Adolescent Psychiatry*, *45*(5), 512–19. doi.org/10.1097/01 chi.0000205706.78818.ef

24 Rybak, Y. E., et al. (2006). 'An open trial of light therapy in adult attention-deficit/hyperactivity disorder'. *Journal of Clinical Psychiatry*, *67*(10), 1527–35. doi.org/10.4088/JCP.v67n1006

25 Fargason, R. E., et al. (2017). 'Correcting delayed circadian phase with bright light therapy predicts improvement in ADHD symptoms: A pilot study'. *Journal of Psychiatric Research*, *91*, 105–10. doi.org/10.1016/j.jpsychires.2017.03.004

26 ibid.

13. How do I live with other people?

1 Beheshti, A., et al. (2020). 'Emotion dysregulation in adults with attention deficit hyperactivity disorder: A meta-analysis'. *BMC Psychiatry*, *20*(120), 1–11 (6). doi.org/10.1186/s12888-020-2442-7

2 Marsh, L. E., et al. (2015). 'ADHD symptomatology, fear of intimacy, and sexual anxiety and behavior among college students in China and the United States'. *Journal of Attention Disorders*, *19*(3), 211–21. doi.org/10.1177/108705471245348

3 Wymbs, B. T., et al. (2017). 'ADHD symptoms as risk factors for intimate partner violence perpetration and victimization'. *Journal of Interpersonal Violence*, *32*(5), 659–81. doi.org/10.1177/0886260515586371

4 Tuckman, A. (2019). *ADHD After Dark: Better sex life, better relationship.* Routledge, New York

5 Tuckman, A. (2020). *ADHD, Relationships, and Sex: Strategies to overcome the over/under-functioner dynamic.* PESI, Eau Claire. catalog.pesi.com/item/adhd-relationships-sex-strategies-overcome-overunderfunctioner-dynamic-71783. Accessed 17 May 2023

14. Should I take these pills?

1 ADHD Guideline Development Group. (2022). *Australian evidence-based clinical practice guideline for Attention Deficit Hyperactivity.* Australian ADHD Professionals Association, Melbourne. adhdguideline.aadpa.com.au/wp-content/uploads/2022/10/ADHD-Clinical-Practice-Guide-041022.pdf. Accessed 26 May 2023

2 Kooij, S. J., et al. (2010). 'European consensus statement on diagnosis and treatment of adult ADHD: The European Network Adult ADHD'. *BMC Psychiatry*, *10*, 67 (3). doi.org/10.1186/1471-244X-10-67

3 Mueller, A. K., et al. (2012). 'Stigma in attention deficit hyperactivity disorder'. *ADHD Attention Deficit and Hyperactivity Disorders, 4*, 101–14. doi.org/10.1007/s12402-012-0085-3

4 Tamminga, H. G. H., et al. (2016). 'Effects of methylphenidate on executive functioning in attention-deficit/hyperactivity disorder across the lifespan: A meta-regression analysis'. *Psychological Medicine*, *46*(9), 1791–807. doi:10.1017/S0033291716000350

5 Rubia, K., et al. (2014). 'Effects of stimulants on brain function in attention-deficit/hyperactivity disorder: A systematic review and meta-analysis'. *Biological Psychiatry*, *76*(8), 616–28. doi.org/10.1016/j.biopsych.2013.10.016

6 Cortese, S., et al. (2018). 'Comparative efficacy and tolerability of medications for attention-deficit hyperactivity disorder in children, adolescents, and adults: A systematic review and network meta-analysis'. *Lancet Psychiatry*, *5*(9), 727–38. doi.org/10.1016/S2215-0366(18)30269-4

7 Centers for Disease Control and Prevention. (2022). 'Treatment of ADHD'. CDC. cdc.gov/ncbddd/adhd/treatment.html. Accessed 23 May 2023

8 Kolar, D., et al. (2008). 'Treatment of adults with attention-deficit/hyperactivity disorder'. *Neuropsychiatric Disease and Treatment*, *4*(2), 389–403. doi.org/10.2147/ndt.s6985

9 InformedHealth.org. (2006; updated 2020). *Depression: How effective are antidepressants?* Institute for Quality and Efficiency in Health Care (IQWiG), Cologne, Germany. ncbi.nlm.nih.gov/books/NBK361016. Accessed 26 May 2023

10 Cortese, 'Comparative efficacy and tolerability of medications for attention-deficit hyperactivity disorder in children, adolescents, and adults'

11 Bell, J. S., & Richards, G. C. (2021). 'Off-label medicine use: Ethics, practice and future directions'. *Australian Journal of General Practice*, *50*(5), 329–31. doi.org/10.31128/AJGP-08-20-5591

12 Togno, J., & Eaton, S. (2015). 'Is there a role for prazosin in the treatment of post-traumatic stress disorder?'. *Australian Family Physician*, *44*(9), 647–9

13 Barrickman, L. L., et al. (1995). 'Bupropion versus methylphenidate in the treatment of attention-deficit hyperactivity disorder'. *Journal of the American Academy of Child & Adolescent Psychiatry*, *34*(5), 649–57. doi.org/10.1097/00004583-199505000-00017

14 Conners, C. K., et al. (1996). 'Bupropion hydrochloride in attention deficit disorder with hyperactivity'. *Journal of the American Academy of Child & Adolescent Psychiatry*, *35*(10), 1314–21. doi.org/10.1097/00004583-199610000-00018

15 Shapiro, D. 'Discontinuing ADHD Meds'. *Attention*, February 2018, 6–9. chadd.org/attention-article/discontinuing-adhd-meds-when-the-only-way-to-move-forward-is-to-stop. Accessed 26 May 2023

16 Kidwell, K. M., et al. (2015). 'Stimulant medications and sleep for youth with ADHD: A meta-analysis'. *Pediatrics*, *136*(6), 1144–53. doi.org/10.1542/peds.2015-1708

17 Holmskov, M., et al. (2017). 'Gastrointestinal adverse events during methylphenidate treatment of children and adolescents with attention deficit hyperactivity disorder: A systematic review with meta-analysis and Trial Sequential Analysis of randomised clinical trials'. *PLoS One*, *12*(6), e0178187. doi.org/10.1371/journal.pone.0178187

18 Dalsgaard, S., et al. (2014). 'Cardiovascular safety of stimulants in children with attention-deficit/hyperactivity disorder: A nationwide prospective cohort study'. *Journal of Child and Adolescent Psychopharmacology*, *24*(6), 302–10. doi.org/10.1089/cap.2014.0020

19 Man, K. K., et al. (2016). 'Methylphenidate and the risk of psychotic disorders and hallucinations in children and adolescents in a large health system'. *Translational Psychiatry*, *6*(11), e956. doi.org/10.1038/tp.2016.216

20 Hollis, C., et al. (2019). 'Methylphenidate and the risk of psychosis in adolescents and young adults: A population-based cohort study'. *Lancet Psychiatry*, *6*(8), 651–8. doi.org/10.1016/S2215-0366(19)30189-0

21 Kolar, 'Treatment of adults with attention-deficit/hyperactivity disorder'

22 Therapeutic Goods Administration. (2020.) Australian Product Information: Strattera (atomoxetine hydrochloride). TGA. ebs.tga.gov.au/ebs/picmi/picmirepository.nsf/pdf?OpenAgent&id=CP-2010-PI-04269-3&d=20230606172310101. Accessed 7 June 2023

23 Ten, W., et al. (2020). 'Creativity in children with ADHD: Effects of medication and comparisons with normal peers'. *Psychiatry Research*, *284*, 112680. doi.org/10.1016/j.psychres.2019.112680

24 Farah, M. J., et al. (2009). 'When we enhance cognition with Adderall, do we sacrifice creativity? A preliminary study'. *Psychopharmacology*, *202*, 541–7. doi.org/10.1007/s00213-008-1369-3

25 National Institue on Drug Abuse. 'What is methamphetamine?'. NIDA, 9 June 2022. nida.nih.gov/publications/research-reports/methamphetamine/what-methamphetamine. Accessed 26 May 2023

26 Kuczenski, R., & Segal, D. S. (2002). 'Exposure of adolescent rats to oral methylphenidate: Preferential effects on extracellular norepinephrine and absence of sensitization and cross-sensitization to methamphetamine'. *Journal of Neuroscience*, *22*(16), 7264–71. doi.org/10.1523/JNEUROSCI.22-16-07264.2002

27 McCabe, S. E., et al. (2017). 'Adolescents' prescription stimulant use and adult functional outcomes: A national prospective study. *Journal of the American Academy of Child & Adolescent Psychiatry*, *56*(3), 226–33.e4. doi.org/10.1016/j.jaac.2016.12.008

28 Faraone, S.V., et al. (2020). 'Systematic review: nonmedical use of prescription stimulants: Risk factors, outcomes, and risk reduction strategies'. *Journal of the American Academy of Child & Adolescent Psychiatry*, *59*(1), 100–12. doi.org/10.1016/j.jaac.2019.06.012

29 Chang, Z., et al. (2014). 'Stimulant ADHD medication and risk for substance abuse'. *Journal of Child Psychology and Psychiatry*, *55*(8), 878–85. doi.org/10.1111/jcpp.12164

30 Quinn, P. D., et al. (2017). 'ADHD medication and substance-related problems'. *American Journal of Psychiatry*, *174*(9), 877–85. doi.org/10.1176/appi.ajp.2017.16060686

31 Faraone, S.V., et al. (2008). 'Effect of stimulants on height and weight: A review of the literature'. *Journal of the American Academy of Child & Adolescent Psychiatry*, *47*(9), 994–1009. doi.org/10.1097/CHI.ObO13e31817eOea7

32 Fredriksen, M., et al. (2013). 'Long-term efficacy and safety of treatment with stimulants and atomoxetine in adult ADHD: A review of controlled and naturalistic studies'. *European Neuropsychopharmacology*, *23*(6), 508–27. doi.org/10.1016/j.euroneuro.2012.07.016

33 Wang, G. J., et al. (2009). 'Chronic treatment with methylphenidate increases dopamine transporter density in patients with attention deficit hyperactive disorder'. *Journal of Nuclear Medicine*, *50*(s2), 1283

34 Safer, D. J., & Allen, R. P. (1989). 'Absence of tolerance to the behavioral effects of methylphenidate in hyperactive and inattentive children'. *Journal of Pediatrics*, *115*(6), 1003–8. doi.org/10.1016/S0022-3476(89)80759-0

35 Swanson, J. M., et al. (2007). 'Secondary evaluations of MTA 36-month outcomes: Propensity score and growth mixture model analyses'. *Journal of the American Academy of Child & Adolescent Psychiatry*, *46*(8), 1003–14. doi.org/10.1097/CHI.0b013e3180686d63

36 Handelman, K., & Sumiya, F. (2022). 'Tolerance to stimulant medication for attention deficit hyperactivity disorder: Literature review and case report'. *Brain Sciences*, *12*(8), 959. doi.org/10.3390/brainsci12080959

15. What's the worst that could happen?

1 Barkley, R. A., & Fischer, M. (2019). 'Hyperactive child syndrome and estimated life expectancy at young adult follow-up: The role of ADHD persistence and other potential predictors'. *Journal of Attention Disorders*, *23*(9), 907–23. doi.org/10.1177/1087054718816164

2 Vaa, T. (2014). 'ADHD and relative risk of accidents in road traffic: A meta-analysis'. *Accident Analysis & Prevention*, *62*, 415–25. doi.org/10.1016/j.aap.2013.10.003

3 Chang, Z., et al. (2014). 'Serious transport accidents in adults with attention-deficit/hyperactivity disorder and the effect of medication: A population-based study'. *JAMA Psychiatry*, *71*(3), 319–25. doi:10.1001/jamapsychiatry.2013.4174

4 Chang, Z., et al. (2017). 'Association between medication use for attention-deficit/hyperactivity disorder and risk of motor vehicle crashes'. *JAMA Psychiatry*, *74*(6), 597–603. doi:10.1001/jamapsychiatry.2017.0659

5 Vaa, 'ADHD and relative risk of accidents in road traffic'

6 Ruiz-Goikoetxea, M., et al. (2018). 'Risk of unintentional injuries in children and adolescents with ADHD and the impact of ADHD medications: A systematic review and meta-analysis'. *Neuroscience & Biobehavioral Reviews*, *84*, 63–71. doi.org/10.1016/j.neubiorev.2017.11.007

7 Swensen, A., et al. (2004). 'Incidence and costs of accidents among attention-deficit/hyperactivity disorder patients'. *Journal of Adolescent Health*, *35*(4), 346.e1–346.e9. doi.org/10.1016/j.jadohealth.2003.12.003

8 Chen, V. C. H., et al. (2019). 'Attention-deficit/hyperactivity disorder and mortality risk in Taiwan'. *JAMA Network Open*, *2*(8), e198714, doi:10.1001/jamanetworkopen.2019.8714

9 Dalsgaard, S., et al. (2015). 'Mortality in children, adolescents, and adults with attention deficit hyperactivity disorder: A nationwide cohort study'. *Lancet*, *385*(9983), 2190–6. doi.org/10.1016/S0140-6736(14)61684-6

10 Chen, 'Attention-deficit/hyperactivity disorder and mortality risk in Taiwan'

11 Septier, M., et al. (2019). 'Association between suicidal spectrum behaviors and attention-deficit/hyperactivity disorder: A systematic review and meta-analysis'. *Neuroscience & Biobehavioral Reviews*, *103*, 109–18. doi.org/10.1016/j.neubiorev.2019.05.022

12 Ruiz-Goikoetxea, 'Risk of unintentional injuries in children and adolescents with ADHD and the impact of ADHD medications'

13 Ghirardi, L., et al. (2020). 'Use of medication for attention-deficit/hyperactivity disorder and risk of unintentional injuries in children and adolescents with co-occurring neurodevelopmental disorders'. *Journal of Child Psychology and Psychiatry*, *61*(2), 140–7. doi.org/10.1111/jcpp.13136

14 Chen, V. C. H., et al. (2020). 'Methylphenidate and the risk of burn injury among children with attention-deficit/hyperactivity disorder'. *Epidemiology and Psychiatric Sciences*, *29*, e146. doi:10.1017/S2045796020000608

15 Chen, V. C. H., et al. (2017). 'The association between methylphenidate treatment and the risk for fracture among young ADHD patients'. *PLoS ONE*, *12*(3), e0173762. doi.org/10.1371/journal.pone.0173762

16 Man, K. K., et al. (2015). 'Methylphenidate and the risk of trauma'. *Pediatrics*, *135*(1), 40–8. doi.org/10.1542/peds.2014-1738

17 Chang, Z., et al. (2016). 'Medication for attention-deficit/hyperactivity disorder and risk for depression: A nationwide longitudinal cohort study'. *Biological Psychiatry*, *80*(12), 916–22. doi.org/10.1016/j.biopsych.2016.02.018

18 Liang, S. H.Y., et al. (2018). 'Suicide risk reduction in youths with attention-deficit/hyperactivity disorder prescribed methylphenidate'. *Research in Developmental Disabilities*, *72*, 96–105. doi.org/10.1016/j.ridd.2017.10.023

19 Keilow, M., et al. (2020). 'Cumulative social disadvantage and risk of attention deficit hyperactivity disorder: Results from a nationwide cohort study'. *SSM-Population Health*, *10*, 100548. doi.org/10.1016/j.ssmph.2020.100548

20 Hauptman, M., et al. (2021). 'Individual-and community-level factors associated with detectable and elevated blood lead levels in US children: Results from a national clinical laboratory'. *JAMA Pediatrics*, *175*(12), 1252–60. doi:10.1001/jamapediatrics.2021.3518

21 Kim, E., et al. (2018). 'How does low socioeconomic status increase blood lead levels in Korean children?'. *International Journal of Environmental Research and Public Health, 15*(7), 1488. doi.org/10.3390/ijerph15071488

22 American Psychiatric Association. (2022). Attention-deficit/hyperactivity disorder: Diagnostic criteria. In *Diagnostic and Statistical Manual of Mental Disorders* (5th ed., text rev.), 69. doi.org/10.1176/appi.books.9780890425787

23 Erskine, H. E., et al. (2016). 'Long-term outcomes of attention-deficit/hyperactivity disorder and conduct disorder: A systematic review and meta-analysis'. *Journal of the American Academy of Child & Adolescent Psychiatry, 55*(10), 841–50. doi.org/10.1016/j.jaac.2016.06.016

24 ibid.

25 Østergaard, S. D., et al. (2017). 'Teenage parenthood and birth rates for individuals with and without attention-deficit/hyperactivity disorder: A nationwide cohort study'. *Journal of the American Academy of Child & Adolescent Psychiatry, 56*(7), 578–84.e3. doi.org/10.1016/j.jaac.2017.05.003

26 Fletcher, J. M. (2014). 'The effects of childhood ADHD on adult labor market outcomes'. *Health Economics, 23*(2), 159–81. doi.org/10.1002/hec.2907

27 Erskine, 'Long-term outcomes of attention-deficit/hyperactivity disorder and conduct disorder'

28 Bernardi, S., et al. (2012). 'The lifetime impact of attention deficit hyperactivity disorder: Results from the National Epidemiologic Survey on Alcohol and Related Conditions (NESARC)'. *Psychological Medicine, 42*(4), 875–87. doi:10.1017/S003329171100153X

29 Li, L., et al. (2022). 'Association between pharmacological treatment of attention-deficit/hyperactivity disorder and long-term unemployment among working-age individuals in Sweden'. *JAMA Network Open, 5*(4), e226815. doi:10.1001/jamanetworkopen.2022.6815

30 Jangmo, A., et al. (2019). 'Attention-deficit/hyperactivity disorder, school performance, and effect of medication'. *Journal of the American Academy of Child & Adolescent Psychiatry, 58*(4), 423–32. doi.org/10.1016/j.jaac.2018.11.014

31 Hua, M. H., et al. (2021). 'Early pregnancy risk among adolescents with ADHD: A nationwide longitudinal study'. *Journal of Attention Disorders, 25*(9), 1199–206. doi.org/10.1177/1087054719900232

32 Young, S., et al. (2015). 'A meta-analysis of the prevalence of attention deficit hyperactivity disorder in incarcerated populations'. *Psychological Medicine, 45*(2), 247–58. doi:10.1017/S0033291714000762

33 Beaudry, G., et al. (2021). 'An updated systematic review and meta-regression analysis: Mental disorders among adolescents in juvenile detention and correctional facilities'. *Journal of the American Academy of Child & Adolescent Psychiatry, 60*(1), 46–60. doi.org/10.1016/j.jaac.2020.01.015

34 Gudjonsson, G. H., et al. (2016). 'A national epidemiological study investigating risk factors for police interrogation and false confession among juveniles and young persons'. *Social Psychiatry and Psychiatric Epidemiology 51*, 359–67. doi.org/10.1007/s00127-015-1145-8

35 Hill, Amelia. 'All prisoners to be tested for ADHD'. *Guardian*, 27 December 2009. theguardian.com/uk/2009/dec/27/adhd-prisons-mental-health-crime. Accessed 17 May 2023

36 Campbell, Denis. 'One in four UK prisoners has attention deficit hyperactivity disorder, says report'. *Observer*, 19 June 2022. theguardian.com/society/2022/jun/18/uk-prisoners-attention-deficit-disorder-adhd-prison. Accessed 17 May 2023

37 Lichtenstein, P., et al. (2012). 'Medication for attention deficit–hyperactivity disorder and criminality'. *New England Journal of Medicine, 367*(21), 2006–14. doi:10.1056/NEJMoa1203241

38 Mohr-Jensen, C., et al. (2019). 'Attention-deficit/hyperactivity disorder in childhood and adolescence and the risk of crime in young adulthood in a Danish nationwide study'. *Journal of the American Academy of Child & Adolescent Psychiatry*, *58*(4), 443–52. doi.org/10.1016/j.jaac.2018.11.016

39 Deloitte Access Economics. (2019). *The social and economic costs of ADHD in Australia: Report prepared for the Australian ADHD Professionals Association*. AADPA. aadpa.com.au/wp-content/uploads/2019/07/Economic-Cost-of-ADHD-To-Australia.pdf. Accessed 26 May 2023

40 Doshi, J. A., et al. (2012). 'Economic impact of childhood and adult attention-deficit/hyperactivity disorder in the United States'. *Journal of the American Academy of Child & Adolescent Psychiatry*, *51*(10), 990–1002.e2. doi.org/10.1016/j.jaac.2012.07.008

16. So, should I love my brain or not?

1 ABC News (Australia). 'In full: Comedian Em Rusciano shines a light on ADHD at the National Press Club | ABC News'. YouTube, 24 August 2022, youtube.com/watch?v=4v88Wd20GiU. Accessed 7 June 2023

2 Hoogman, M., et al. (2020). 'Creativity and ADHD: A review of behavioral studies, the effect of psychostimulants and neural underpinnings'. *Neuroscience & Biobehavioral Reviews*, *119*, 66–85. doi.org/10.1016/j.neubiorev.2020.09.029

3 Lange, K. W., et al. (2010). 'The history of attention deficit hyperactivity disorder'. *ADHD Attention Deficit and Hyperactivity Disorders*, *2*, 241–55. doi.org/10.1007/s12402-010-0045-8

4 Hallowell, E. M. & Ratey, J. J. (2021). *ADHD 2.0: New science and essential strategies for thriving with distraction – from childhood through adulthood*. Ballantine Books, New York

Acknowledgements

I would like to thank Kathryn Knight, Isabelle Yates, Adam Laszczuk and the whole team from Penguin Random House Australia for your patience and support as I embarked on writing my first book. Thank you for trusting in me, taking a chance and giving me the opportunity to share my story, and to Justin Ractliffe for believing I could do it in the first place. To Caitlan Cooper-Trent from Curtis Brown Australia, thank you for swooping in and guiding me through the labyrinth of the publishing world, for encouraging me every step of the way, for reminding me why on earth I am doing this and why it's worth it, and for being my trusted sounding-board no matter how bizarre the idea. Thank you to Nicola Young for taking this rough rock, polishing it until it shone and cutting out at least half of my 'So the thing is'–es. They needed to go. Thanks also to Bronwyn Sweeney for her killer proofreading skills. And, of course, to Evie Hilliar. You are my favourite comic artist in the world, and I pinch myself every day that it's you who turned my bizarre little 2 am ideas for drawings into works of art. You brought this book to life, and your wit and flair inspire me constantly.

The world's biggest thank-you to my family and friends who wrote about their experiences for this book. Anthony, you are the love of my life and the most wonderful man I know. Thank you for telling me I could do this, helping me through every day of the writing process, forgiving me for all the events this book forced you to go to alone and for holding me tight in the moments when it felt like I'd never finish. This is just as much yours as it is mine. To my mum, Jo Bell, thank you for reading every page of this book at least five times, for working through each and every chapter to help it find its shape and for being honest enough to tell me when something needed to go – helping your baby kill her babies, if you will.

You are amazingly talented, and this book would be so much the poorer without you. And to Andrea, my soulmate, the most beautiful woman in the world and the best thing ever to come out of Norway. Thank you for always being there for me, for forgiving me when I come up short and for reminding me who I am when I forget. I'm so lucky to have you.

To my dad, Ray Boseley, your creative ability and drive inspire me every day. Thank you for helping me believe I could be an author, and reading and giving me notes on every chapter I sent your way. Now there are two writers in the family staying up till 3 am and never seeing the sunlight. I couldn't be prouder to be following in your footsteps. To my sister, Perrin, thank you for the kindness, generosity and understanding you showed me as I was writing this book, and thank you so much again for doing my Christmas shopping for me – I'll never be able to express how much that meant. To Loki Cavanga, the best brother-in-law I could ask for. Thank you for letting me share your story and for being the person I can always go to to talk about any and all things ADHD. To the person whose name isn't really Olivia, you are one of the smartest, most brilliant people I know. Thank you for the thirteen years of friendship. You have seen the best and the worst of me and decided to stick around anyway, bringing constant laughs and joy. I'm so grateful you allowed me to include your experiences in this book.

Speaking of the courage and generosity it takes to allow someone to share your story, thank you to Emily Johnson, Kiz and Divina Blanca-Jackson, Ksa Curry and Cate Osborn. You made this book what it is. You provided brilliant insights and much-needed perspective, and constantly made me pause and reflect, which is the best gift anyone can give to an author. A huge thank-you to Em Rusciano, not just for your time but for your work to help ADHD adults all over the country. Your speech brought this conversation into the limelight and gave thousands of us ADHDers hope along the way. And thank you to the countless other ADHD adults I spoke with over the course of the year – you are truly champions.

Thank you to all the brilliant and talented experts who gave up their precious free time to be interviewed by me. To Prof David Coghill, Dr Roger Paterson, Prof Stephen Faraone, Prof Stephen Hinshaw, Dr Ari Tuckman, Dr Ellen Littman,

Dr Paul Morgan, Dr Anthony Yeung, A/Prof Marc Seal, Prof Mark Bellgrove, Prof Christel Middeldorp and Dr Cory Lane, I can't thank you enough for your patience and generosity in helping this little Bachelor of Arts graduate understand the science and medicine that underpins all discussion of this condition. A special thank you to A/Prof Katherine Johnson for always being available for a chat, willing to answer any and all questions I had, and even taking an afternoon out of your busy day to let me experience firsthand some of the ADHD testing systems you use. You made this huge, scary world of ADHD seem approachable and helped me believe this was a story I could tell.

To all the social workers who spoke to me about their experiences treating people with ADHD within the prison system, your insights were invaluable. And thanks to staff at the Australian Community Support Organisation for helping me connect with and speak to so many interesting people in this field. Thank you as well to the staff at the Butterfly Foundation for your guidance and advice on some of the most serious, personal and difficult topics in this book.

To the best primary school teacher anyone could ask for, Susan Bishop. Although you weren't aware I was an ADHDer, you accepted me for who I was, found a way to work with my brain and brought out the best in me. You taught a bullied little kid to love and value themselves again, and that's a gift I will carry with me for the rest of my life. To my favourite university lecturer, and overseer of my student magazine, Corinna Hente. You saw something in me, reminded me of my love of writing and always challenged me to be better. There's no way I could ever have done this without the foundation you helped me to build. And to my football club – you are some of the funniest and most positive people I know. Thank you for your patience and guidance, for forgiving me when I occasionally zone out mid-game, and for motivating me to get out of the house and take a much-needed break even during the most intense times.

To all the writers, editors, sub editors and staff at the *Guardian* Australia, thank you for showing me what courageous, powerful journalism looks like, for giving me the space to first tell my ADHD story and for always being so kind and understanding about my conditions, not just on the good days but on the bad ones too. I'd especially like to thank Miles Martignoni, Alyx Gorman, Tamsin Rose, Calla Wahlquist and Melissa Davey for being among my first confidants. To my manager, Molly Glassey, and colleagues Lisa Grace and Bertin Huynh, you listened to me complain about book work day in and day out, told me to look after my mental health when I needed to and never once questioned the dark circles under my eyes after a long night of writing. And to my editor and (now) fellow author, Gabrielle Jackson – when I asked if I should write this book you said, 'It will be the worst year of your life, you're going to hate every second of it, but it's also the best, most rewarding thing you will ever do. You'll love it more than life and you absolutely must do it.' You were completely spot on.

And, finally, to all the social media ADHD educators whose videos helped me realise who I was. There are too many of you to count, but your research, labour and willingness to share the most personal experiences with the big scary internet changed my life forever. I can never thank you enough.

Index

PENGUIN LIFE

UK | USA | Canada | Ireland | Australia
India | New Zealand | South Africa | China

Penguin Life is part of the Penguin Random House group of companies
whose addresses can be found at global.penguinrandomhouse.com

Penguin Random House Australia

First published by Penguin Life in 2023

Cover design and internal design by Adam Laszczuk © Penguin Random House Australia Pty Ltd
Internal illustrations by Evie Hilliar © Penguin Random House Australia Pty Ltd
Index by Puddingburn Publishing Services
Typeset in 12/16 pt Bembo Infant MT by Post Pre-Press Group, Australia

Printed and bound in China by 1010 Printing International Co. Ltd

NATIONAL LIBRARY OF AUSTRALIA
A catalogue record for this book is available from the National Library of Australia

ISBN 978 0 14377 977 3

penguin.com.au

We at Penguin Random House Australia acknowledge that Aboriginal and Torres Strait Islander peoples are the Traditional Custodians and the first storytellers of the lands on which we live and work. We honour Aboriginal and Torres Strait Islander peoples' continuous connection to Country, waters, skies and communities. We celebrate Aboriginal and Torres Strait Islander stories, traditions and living cultures; and we pay our respects to Elders past and present.